HIV in US Communities of Color

Bisola O. Ojikutu • Valerie E. Stone
Editors

HIV in US Communities of Color

Second Edition

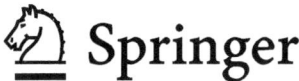 Springer

Editors
Bisola O. Ojikutu
Division of Global Health Equity
Division of Infectious Diseases
Department of Medicine
Brigham and Women's Hospital
Harvard Medical School
Boston, MA
USA

Valerie E. Stone
Division of General Internal Medicine
Division of Infectious Diseases
Department of Medicine
Brigham and Women's Hospital
Harvard Medical School
Boston, MA
USA

ISBN 978-3-030-48743-0   ISBN 978-3-030-48744-7   (eBook)
https://doi.org/10.1007/978-3-030-48744-7

This Springer imprint is published by the registered company Springer Nature Switzerland AG
The registered company address is: Gewerbestrasse 11, 6330 Cham, Switzerland

Preface

Although significant progress has been made in the prevention and treatment of HIV, racial and ethnic inequity remains a persistent and pervasive feature of the epidemic in the USA. Published in 2009, *HIV/AIDS in U.S. Communities of Color*, an in-depth guide to the HIV epidemic among Black and Latino individuals living in the USA, edited by Valerie E. Stone, Bisola O. Ojikutu, M. Keith Rawlings, and Kimberly Y. Smith, provided the first comprehensive guide to the epidemiology, clinical characteristics, and treatment of HIV/AIDS in people of color in the USA. The current text, *HIV in US Communities of Color: Second Edition* builds upon the previous work by comprehensively updating important epidemiologic and clinical content. In addition, this edition integrates expert review of critical aspects of the structural and social environment that may compromise our ability to decrease HIV risk and improve outcomes, such mass incarceration, neighborhood-level disadvantage, discrimination, and mistrust. Further, we review the impact of significant advances in HIV prevention, such as pre-exposure prophylaxis (PrEP), within Black and Latino communities.

New chapters dedicated to highly vulnerable populations, transgender individualsof color and Black immigrants from sub-Saharan Africa and the Caribbean, whohave unique needs and face a myriad of challenges related to HIV risk, prevention, care, and treatment have also been included.

This text is intended for a multidisciplinary audience. Healthcare providers, trainees, community-based leadership, advocates, and public health professionals will find that the information contained herein provides useful insight into their work. The expert faculty who have been selected as chapter authors have dedicated their careers to their respective content areas, and we sincerely appreciate their contribution to this textbook. We hope that this resource will lead to a better understanding of the needs of people of color who are at risk or living with HIV and ultimately improve care and treatment outcomes in US communities of color.

Boston, MA, USA   Bisola O. Ojikutu
Boston, MA, USA   Valerie E. Stone

Contents

Contributors

Yazan A. Al-Ajlouni, BS Columbia Spatial Epidemiology Lab, Department of Epidemiology, Mailman School of Public Health, Columbia University, New York, NY, USA

Laura M. Bogart, PhD RAND Corporation, Santa Monica, CA, USA

Denton Callander, PhD Columbia Spatial Epidemiology Lab, Department of Epidemiology, Mailman School of Public Health, Columbia University, New York, NY, USA

Nicholas Campalans, BS University of Texas Southwestern Medical Center, Dallas, TX, USA

Victoria A. Cargill, MD, MSCE HIV/STD Services and Community Risk Reduction, Baltimore City Health Department, Baltimore, MA, USA

Chinazo Cunningham, MD, MS Department of Medicine, Albert Einstein College of Medicine, Bronx, NY, USA

William E. Cunningham, MD, MPH, Deceased Division of General Internal Medicine, Department of Medicine, University of California Los Angeles (UCLA), Los Angeles, CA, USA

Jessy G. Dévieux, PhD Department of Health Promotion and Disease Prevention, Florida International University, Miami, FL, USA

Dustin T. Duncan, ScD Columbia Spatial Epidemiology Lab, Department of Epidemiology, Mailman School of Public Health, Columbia University, New York, NY, USA

Charlene A. Flash, MD, MPH Legacy Community Health Center, Houston, TX, USA

Baylor College of Medicine, Houston, TX, USA

Alex González, MD, MPH Fenway Health, Boston, MA, USA

Emily Hoff, MD University of Texas Southwestern Medical Center/Parkland Health and Hospital Systems, Dallas, TX, USA

Syundai R. Johnson, MPH Baylor College of Medicine, Houston, TX, USA

Byoungjun Kim, MUP Columbia Spatial Epidemiology Lab, Department of Epidemiology, Mailman School of Public Health, Columbia University, New York, NY, USA

Florence M. Momplaisir, MD, MSHP Department of Medicine, University of Pennsylvania Perelman School of Medicine, Philadelphia, PA, USA

Ank Nijhawan, MD, MPH Division of Infectious Diseases, University of Texas Southwestern Medical Center, Dallas, TX, USA

Chioma Nnaji, MEd, MPH Multicultural AIDS Coalition, Boston, MA, USA

Bisola O. Ojikutu, MD, MPH Divisions of Global Health Equity, Division of Infectious Diseases, Department of Medicine, Brigham and Women's Hospital, Harvard Medical School, Boston, MA, USA

Deborah Parham-Hopson, PhD, MSPH, RN MayaTech Corporation, Silver Spring, MD, USA

Tonia Poteat, PhD, MPH, PA-C Department of Social Medicine, University of North Carolina Chapel Hill, Chapel Hill, NC, USA

Asa E. Radix, MD, MPH Callen-Lorde Community Health Center, New York, NY, USA

M. Keith Rawlings, MD ViiV Healthcare, Research Triangle Park, Durham, NC, USA

Deepika Slawek, MD, MPH Department of Medicine, Albert Einstein College of Medicine, Bronx, NY, USA

Dawn K. Smith, MD, MS, MPH Division of HIV/AIDS Prevention, National Center for HIV/AIDS, STD, Viral Hepatitis, and TB Prevention, Centers for Disease Control and Prevention, Atlanta, GA, USA

Valerie E. Stone, MD, MPH Divisions of General Internal Medicine, Division of Infectious Diseases, Department of Medicine, Brigham and Women's Hospital, Harvard Medical School, Boston, MA, USA

Sae Takada, MD, PhD Division of General Internal Medicine, Department of Medicine, University of California Los Angeles (UCLA), Los Angeles, CA, USA

Leo Wilton, PhD, MPH Department of Human Development, College of Community and Public Affairs (CCPA), State University of New York at Binghamton, Binghamton, NY, USA

Chapter 1
Achieving Health Equity Among US Communities of Color at Risk for or Living with HIV

Bisola O. Ojikutu and Valerie E. Stone

Introduction

In the United States (US), disparities by race and ethnicity have been noted across the HIV care continuum. Black and Latinx individuals who are living with HIV are less likely than their White counterparts to be diagnosed, to be engaged in care, and to be virologically suppressed [1–4]. From a clinical perspective, these disparities increase the risk for suboptimal health outcomes. From the public health perspective, lack of virologic suppression increases the likelihood of HIV transmission to uninfected individuals. Although significant progress has been made in the development of biomedical HIV prevention (i.e., pre-exposure prophylaxis [PrEP]) and in the availability of antiretroviral therapy for treatment as prevention, racial and ethnic disparities in new HIV diagnoses have persisted [5]. This is due in part to suboptimal uptake of currently available biomedical prevention strategies. Compared to other races and ethnicities, Black and Latinx men and women who are at risk are less likely to be aware of and utilize PrEP [6–9]. If barriers to uptake of PrEP within communities of color are not addressed, existing racial and ethnic disparities in HIV incidence will widen.

The root causes of these pervasive health disparities are complex and include historical and contemporary structural inequity and racism. Manifestations of structural racism, such as mass incarceration and residential segregation, have resulted in the unjust distribution of resources and opportunities and left Black and Latinx individuals with lower rates of employment, higher rates of uninsurance and limited

B. O. Ojikutu (✉)
Division of Global Health Equity, Division of Infectious Diseases, Department of Medicine, Brigham and Women's Hospital, Harvard Medical School, Boston, MA, USA
e-mail: bojikutu@mgh.harvard.edu

V. E. Stone
Divisions of General Internal Medicine, Division of Infectious Diseases, Department of Medicine, Brigham and Women's Hospital, Harvard Medical School, Boston, MA, USA

© Springer Nature Switzerland AG 2021
B. O. Ojikutu, V. E. Stone (eds.), *HIV in US Communities of Color*,
https://doi.org/10.1007/978-3-030-48744-7_1

access to quality health care. These overlapping and reinforcing determinants of health place uninfected Black and Latinx individuals at higher risk of HIV acquisition and predispose those living with HIV to poorer outcomes. Implementing interventions and policies that are fundamentally grounded in the pursuit of health equity (i.e., striving for the highest possible standard of health for all people while focusing on those who are marginalized or most at risk) is necessary to mitigate disproportionate risk and poor outcomes [10]. Undoubtedly, achieving health equity within the domestic HIV epidemic will entail the development of strategies that acknowledge and successfully tackle the long-standing root causes of racial and ethnic disparities. This will demand an unprecedented, multilevel commitment to change at the individual, the community, the clinical, and the broader systems level.

In 2019, *Ending the HIV Epidemic: A Plan for America (EHE)*, a federal initiative to address HIV in the US was launched. The goal of this initiative is to reduce new HIV infections in the United States by 75% in 5 years and by 90% by 2030. The plan will fund selected geographic "hot spots" of HIV infection around the country to implement strategies that utilize advances in HIV prevention, diagnosis, treatment, and outbreak response [11]. However, it is unclear how successful many of these jurisdictions around the country will be in reaching the targeted goals. To address this question, Nosyk et al. used a dynamic HIV transmission model to identify the optimal, cost-effective combination of evidence-based interventions to reach the EHE goal of 90% reduction of incidence in 10 years in six cities that comprise one-quarter of people living with HIV in the United States [12]. Under ideal implementation conditions, the targets for ending the HIV epidemic were not reached within any of the selected cities, although several cities were close to reaching the EHE goal. The authors concluded that, in addition to HIV-specific interventions, efforts to overcome social and structural inequity would be required. This study and others demonstrate the importance of addressing the root causes of racial and ethnic disparities to ending the HIV epidemic [13, 14]. Hence, the purpose of this chapter is to highlight strategies for overcoming racial and ethnic disparities in HIV, and thereby achieve health equity with respect to HIV prevention, care and treatment outcomes.

Acknowledge and Address Structural Racism

There is growing acknowledgment that multilevel factors, including the structural and cultural environments in which risk behaviors, care, and treatment occur, drive HIV-related disparities. Extant literature has highlighted the individual level of influence, which include mental health disorders (e.g., depression), substance use, stigma, and health system mistrust [15–17]. The focus on proximal causes of health disparities is justified because these factors are critical to health and well-being, are unique to individual circumstance, and may be modifiable. However, the epidemic of HIV within communities of color is persistent because it is interconnected and co-occurring with other complex, broader conditions that have not been fully addressed. Syndemic theory, which posits that individual epidemics are "sustained in a community or population *because of harmful social conditions and injurious social connections*," best explains the persistence of HIV within Black and Latinx communities [18]. Therefore, identifying and addressing these "conditions" is of paramount importance to ending the HIV epidemic within communities of color in the US.

Structural racism is inarguably the primary "condition" driving HIV persistence within Black and Latinx communities. Defined as the macro-level system that promotes and reinforces inequities among racial and ethnic groups, structural racism is an overarching system of hierarchy, privilege, and power that excludes people of color [19]. Unlike interpersonal racism, structural racism functions as an aspect of the external environment, circumscribes options, and delimits opportunities throughout one's life course [20]. Structural racism impacts all health disorders from cardiovascular disease to mental health disorders to cancer and to HIV infection. Studies have described the pathways linking structural racism and HIV infection [13, 21]. For example, it is well established that residential segregation, a mechanism driven by structural racism and a fundamental cause of health disparities, restricts employment opportunities and exacerbates the concentration of poverty in the US. Further, residential segregation in poverty-stricken urban centers has led to circumscribed sexual and drug use networks through which HIV has spread [22, 23]. For many Black and Latinx individuals, residential segregation also limits access to well-resourced health care services and high-quality HIV prevention, care, and treatment [24, 25].

A second manifestation of structural racism is the evolution and aftermath of the crack cocaine epidemic of the mid-1980s. The rise in the sale and use of crack cocaine was potentiated by progressive socioeconomic decline within inner cities where many Black and Latinx individuals reside [26]. Crack cocaine was easily made, affordable, and a profitable source of income, particularly at a time when few other viable opportunities existed. By 1985, there were 1.6 million new users of cocaine and a fourfold increase in cocaine-related emergency department visits [27]. Instead of initiating a public health response, the US government expanded the "War on Drugs," a federal initiative begun in the 1970s that imposed mandatory prison sentencing for drug crimes and increased federal antidrug laws. One of the consequences of these excessively punitive, racist policies is the mass incarceration of Black and Latinx men, which has been associated with increased HIV transmission risk behavior and new diagnoses within communities of color [28–33]. In addition, drug use has had a devastating impact on women of color. Crack cocaine has been independently associated with the disproportionate rate of HIV diagnoses among Black/African-American women through transactional sex, high-risk male sexual partners, and polysubstance use [34–37].

To address structural racism, health care providers should be taught to combat the structural context in which race impacts health, specifically HIV risk and outcomes [38]. Instead of becoming culturally competent, HIV care providers must become structurally competent [39]. In order to become structurally competent, providers should: (1) acknowledge how structural racism operates, privileges certain groups, erects barriers to healthy outcomes, and impacts our patients' lives [40]; (2) demonstrate to patients that they have this understanding by showing respect for their thoughts, beliefs, and experiences; (3) establish programming on the clinic and health system levels that addresses manifestations of structural racism (e.g., community outreach to re-engage patients in care and development of partnerships with community-based organizations (CBOs) that provide needed services such as legal assistance); and lastly (4) recognize that *individuals* can dismantle structures through advocacy and leadership. Training efforts that include these action-oriented strategies should focus on all levels and cadres of health care professions, including seasoned HIV care providers.

Improve Patient-Provider Relationships

Effective patient-provider relationships are central to the delivery of high-quality health care and are associated with improved health outcomes, higher patient satisfaction, and reduced health disparities [41–43]. Since early in the HIV epidemic, studies noted that Black and Latinx patients living with HIV reported less satisfaction with their care and challenges with communication [44–48]. More recent studies have documented persistent challenges with patient-provider communication. For example, Zhang et al. found that poor communication was significantly associated with suboptimal HIV-related outcomes among Black men and with low psychosocial well-being among Latinx men living with HIV [49]. Black and Latinx MSM living with HIV have also identified that provider empathy and respect are essential to communication and ongoing engagement in care [50]. In addition, women living with HIV face communication challenges. In a cross-sectional study to determine attitudes, opinions, and perceived health needs among women living with HIV, most of whom where Black or Latinx, 43% indicated that they had switched providers because of communication issues. Furthermore, many study participants noted that they had not discussed critical sexual health and gender-specific concerns, such as pre-conception health, with their health care providers [51]. These data highlight the need to address gaps in provider communication among Black and Latinx men and women living with HIV.

Among at risk patients, poor patient-provider interaction has also been identified as a barrier to PrEP uptake. Black and Latinx MSM are at highest risk of HIV acquisition, and may face specific challenges in health care settings. In a qualitative study of at-risk, young Black MSM, participants described ineffective communication with their health care providers due to medical mistrust, perceived discrimination, and differences in cultural norms. Racism and homonegativity within the health care system, and among health care providers, were also identified as barriers to communication and subsequent PrEP uptake [52]. To elucidate the association between racism and provider intentions to prescribe PrEP, Calebrese et al. surveyed more than one hundred US medical students and found that heterosexism, not racism, indirectly affected prescribing intention [53].

Suboptimal PrEP use has also been documented among Black and Latinx transgender individuals who are also at high risk of HIV acquisition. Studies have documented transphobia within health care settings, which discourages engagement in biomedical prevention and retention in care [54, 55]. Cisgender women of color also face communication challenges with health care providers. Studies have demonstrated that once women are made aware of PrEP, they are often interested in using it as an HIV prevention strategy [56, 57]. However, PrEP uptake among women remains low [9]. Patient-provider communication may be a concern. Medical mistrust among Black women has been associated with poor communication with health care providers regarding sexual health and HIV prevention needs. In a cross-sectional survey of more than 500 HIV-negative Black women, Tekeste et al. noted that higher levels of medical mistrust were associated with lower comfort discussing PrEP with a provider [58].

Based upon these and other data, numerous intersecting and co-occurring factors contribute to poor interactions between Black and Latinx individuals at risk or living with HIV and their health care providers. These include medical mistrust, homonegativity, suboptimal cross-cultural communication, racism, and discrimination. Language discordance between patients and providers is an additional barrier to patient-provider interactions. More than 25 million people in the US report limited English proficiency, and more than one in six individuals who are newly diagnosed with HIV is non-US born [59, 60]. Furthermore, in recent years, the number of new HIV diagnoses has increased among Latinx MSM [61]. Among Latinx individuals, patient-provider language discordance has been identified as a significant barrier to uptake of HIV services including HIV testing, PrEP, and engagement in care [62, 63]. Among Black individuals, non-US-born men and women from sub-Saharan Africa and the Caribbean have higher rates of new HIV diagnosis and also experience language barriers in accessing HIV-related services [64–66].

Several strategies to improve patient-provider interactions have been described, most of which focus on communication. The dominant theoretical framework for patient-provider communication is "patient-centered." Patient-centered communication is focused on understanding patients as unique individuals whose views, perspectives, and beliefs are central to addressing health care concerns [67]. Including phrases such as "tell me more about what is worrying you" or "what do you believe is the cause of the problem you describe" in interviews are methods to elicit patient-centered perspectives. "Sharing power," which emphasizes the partnership between patients and health care providers and allows for patient control, has also been described. Sharing power helps patients make decisions that are informed and concordant with their goals and values [68]. Enhancing patients' comprehension and retention of what has been said by asking the patient about their understanding is another approach to improve communication. This can be done using the "teach back" approach by asking "Does that make sense to you?" or requesting that the patient repeat the agreed upon treatment plan aloud [69]. Studies specifically focused on communication within HIV care interactions have noted that adherence and antiretroviral therapy counseling are often too brief, highly directive with few open-ended questions, and has little room for patient perspective, desires, and unique needs [70, 71]. To address this concern, Beach et al. developed and tested a brief training based on motivational interviewing principles applied to medication adherence [72]. In a randomized controlled trial, patient-provider interactions in the intervention group included more brainstorming about solutions to adherence, more positive talk, and more probing of patient opinions [72].

The inclusion of nonphysician staff such as nurses, physician assistants, case managers, or peer counselors who may be able to spend additional time with the patient and answer questions may also be useful. The important role that these non-physician staff play in enhancing patient's satisfaction with HIV care is supported in the literature. Patients living with HIV who have a case manager or a primary nurse have been found to be more satisfied with their HIV care [73]. Peer interventions may also improve engagement and retention in primary care among Black and Latinx individuals [74, 75].

Medical and health system mistrust impacts patient-provider communication and is not easily rectifiable [76]. Developing partnerships with community-based organizations (CBOs) within patients' communities may provide patients with trusted linkages to the clinical setting and improve interactions with health care providers [77, 78]. Effective CBO-clinical partnerships can also enhance understanding of patients' lives and increase rapport with highly impacted communities. Improving communication and building relationships with communities may help improve access to care and the experiences that Black and Latinx patients have with the health care system.

For patients with limited English proficiency, medical interpreters are an essential component of care. Linguistically and culturally appropriate patient education materials should be developed and utilized. Additional investment may also be required to expand access to include languages less commonly spoken in the US within clinics where disproportionately high numbers of limited English proficiency African and Caribbean-born patients receive care.

Diversify the HIV Workforce

The landmark Institute of Medicine report "Unequal Treatment: Confronting Racial and Ethnic Disparities in Health Care" highlighted key racial and ethnic disparities in health care outcomes [79]. One of the primary recommendations of that report was to increase the diversity of the health and human services workforce. The call for diversity is inclusive of all cadres of health care providers, including physicians, nurses, social workers, medical assistants, and front desk staff. According to an analysis by the US Department of Health and Human Services (Health Resources and Services Administration), all racial and ethnic minority groups, except for Asians, are underrepresented in health diagnosis and treatment occupations [80]. Evidence suggests that a diverse health care workforce improves health care quality, patient comfort in the health care setting, and patient satisfaction, and is important to achieving health equity [81, 82]. Therefore, the health care workforce, including providers of all categories, should reflect the diversity of patients for which they provide care.

Regarding patient and doctor characteristics, does racial concordance matter? Studies have noted that racial concordance among patients-physicians increases utilization of necessary health services and improves patient-provider interactions [83–85]. However, in a comprehensive literature review, there was inconclusive evidence to support the association between patient-provider racial concordance and improved health outcomes [86]. Of note, this review included a relatively small sample of minority physicians. The authors concluded that further research is needed to understand which health issues and health outcomes may be more sensitive to cultural proximity between patients and providers. Other studies, including a more recent systematic literature review, have clearly demonstrated that racial concordance between patients and providers leads to enhanced patient-provider communication and enhanced uptake of important preventive health interventions [87–89].

HIV care is one of the health issues where workforce diversity is particularly important. In a 2004 study by King et al., patient-provider racial concordance was associated with time to receipt of protease inhibitor (PI) therapy for Black individuals living with HIV [90]. Racial concordance between patient and provider essentially eliminated the disparity in time to receive PIs for Black patients. As previously noted, medical mistrust is a barrier to health care access among patients at risk for or living with HIV. Racial and/or ethnic concordance is important for helping patients understand the health care system, navigate health care resources, and improve access to care. In a cross-sectional survey of individuals living with HIV in New York City, Sohler et al. noted that racial concordance was associated with lower mistrust in the health care system and may overcome barriers to health care access [91].

Efforts are underway to increase the pipeline of racially and ethnically diverse HIV clinical providers, as well as researchers [92–94]. Additional attention should focus on the important role that Black and Latinx health care providers play in improving access to care and overcoming racial and ethnic disparities. No matter how welcoming an HIV care site is, Black and Latinx individuals at risk for or living with HIV may feel even more comfortable if some of the providers are of their own racial and ethnic backgrounds. Employing other staff, such as nurses, case managers, medical assistants, front desk staff, and peer supporters, who reflect the diversity of the patient population is important and improves patient comfortability in care settings. Furthermore, all staff should be trained in structural competency, cultural humility, cross-cultural communication, and best practices regarding patient-centered interactions. All of the aforementioned suggestions will require supportive organizational leadership, training, and changes to hiring and promotion practices.

Summary

Though significant strides have been made, Black and Latinx communities continue to be disproportionately impacted by HIV in the United States. In addition to HIV prevention, care, and treatment interventions specifically targeting HIV, strategies to address the root causes of racial and ethnic inequities will be required to end the epidemic within communities of color. These strategies include increasing structural competency among health care providers, working to improve interactions between Black and Latinx patients and the health care system, and increasing diversity among the HIV services workforce. Implementation will require investments beyond HIV and may have a broader impact on decreasing overall health disparities. Throughout this textbook, chapters describe clinical and public health challenges to ending the HIV epidemic and provide evidence for a greater commitment to achieving health equity.

References

1. Centers for Disease Control and Prevention. HIV surveillance report, 2018 (Preliminary); vol. 30. http://www.cdc.gov/hiv/library/reports/hiv-surveillance.html. Published November 2019. Accessed 4 Apr 2020.
2. Dailey AF, Johnson AS, Wu B. HIV care outcomes among blacks with diagnosed HIV – United States, 2014. MMWR Morb Mortal Wkly Rep. 2017;66(4):97–103.
3. Hoover KW, Hu X, Porter SE, Buchacz K, Bond MD, Siddiqi AE, Haynes SG. HIV diagnoses and the HIV care continuum among women and girls aged ≥13 years-39 states and the District of Columbia, 2015–2016. J Acquir Immune Defic Syndr. 2019;81(3):251–6.
4. Gant Z, Bradley H, Hu X, Skarbinski J, Hall HI, Lansky A, Centers for Disease Control and Prevention (CDC). Hispanics or Latinos living with diagnosed HIV: progress along the continuum of HIV care – United States, 2010. MMWR Morb Mortal Wkly Rep. 2014;63(40):886–90.
5. Chapin-Bardales J, Rosenberg ES, Sullivan PS. Trends in racial/ethnic disparities of new AIDS diagnoses in the United States. Ann Epidemiol. 2017;27(5):329–334.e2.
6. Kanny D, Jeffries WL 4th, Chapin-Bardales J, Denning P, Cha S, Finlayson T, Wejnert C, National HIV Behavioral Surveillance Study Group. Racial/ethnic disparities in HIV pre-exposure prophylaxis among men who have sex with men – 23 urban areas, 2017. MMWR Morb Mortal Wkly Rep. 2019;68(37):801–6.
7. Ojikutu BO, Bogart LM, Higgins-Biddle M, Dale SK, Allen W, Dominique T, Mayer KH. Facilitators and barriers to pre-exposure prophylaxis (PrEP) use among Black individuals in the United States: results from the National Survey on HIV in the Black Community (NSHBC). AIDS Behav. 2018 Nov;22(11):3576–87.
8. Raifman J, Dean LT, Montgomery MC, Almonte A, Arrington-Sanders R, Stein MD, Nunn AS, Sosnowy CD, Chan PA. Racial and ethnic disparities in HIV pre-exposure prophylaxis awareness among men who have sex with men. AIDS Behav. 2019;23(10):2706–9.
9. Huang YA, Zhu W, Smith DK, Harris N, Hoover KW. HIV pre-exposure prophylaxis, by race and ethnicity - United States, 2014-2016. MMWR Morb Mortal Wkly Rep. 2018;67(41):1147–50.
10. Braveman P. What are health disparities and health equity? We need to be clear. Public Health Rep. 2014;129(Suppl 2):5–8.
11. Center for Disease Control and Prevention. Ending the HIV epidemic: a plan for America. Available at: https://www.cdc.gov/endhiv/index.html.

12. Nosyk B, Krebs E, Zang X, et al. 'Ending the Epidemic' will not happen without addressing racial/ethnic disparities in the US HIV epidemic [published online ahead of print, 2020 May 19]. Clin Infect Dis. 2020;ciaa566
13. Buot ML, Docena JP, Ratemo BK, Bittner MJ, Burlew JT, Nuritdinov AR, Robbins JR. Beyond race and place: distal sociological determinants of HIV disparities. PLoS One. 2014;9:e91711.
14. Ransome Y, Kawachi I, Braunstein S, Nash D. Structural inequalities drive late HIV diagnosis: the role of black racial concentration, income inequality, socioeconomic deprivation, and HIV testing. Health Place. 2016;42:148–58.
15. Foley JD, Vanable PA, Brown LK, Carey MP, DiClemente RJ, Romer D, Valois RF. Depressive symptoms as a longitudinal predictor of sexual risk behaviors among African-American adolescents. Health Psychol. 2019;38(11):1001–9.
16. Mimiaga MJ, Reisner SL, Grasso C, Crane HM, Safren SA, Kitahata MM, Schumacher JE, Mathews WC, Mayer KH. Substance use among HIV-infected patients engaged in primary care in the United States: findings from the Centers for AIDS Research Network of Integrated Clinical Systems cohort. Am J Public Health. 2013;103(8):1457–67.
17. Bogart LM, Wagner G, Galvan FH, Banks D. Conspiracy beliefs about HIV are related to antiretroviral treatment nonadherence among African-American men with HIV. J Acquir Immune Defic Syndr. 2010;53(5):648–55.
18. Singer M, Clair S. Syndemics and public health: reconceptualizing disease in bio-social context. Med Anthropol Q. 2003;17:423–41.
19. Powell JA. Structural racism: building upon the insights of John Calmore. North Carolina Law Review. 2008;86:791–816.
20. Structural Racism. Available at: https://www.racialequitytools.org/resourcefiles/Definitions-of%20Racism.pdf. Accessed on: 4 Apr 2020.
21. Freeman R, Gwadz MV, Silverman E, Kutnick A, Leonard NR, Ritchie AS, Reed J, Martinez BY. Critical race theory as a tool for understanding poor engagement along the HIV care continuum among African American/Black and Hispanic persons living with HIV in the United States: a qualitative exploration. Int J Equity Health. 2017;16(1):54.
22. Williams DR, Collins C. Racial residential segregation: a fundamental cause of racial disparities in health. Public Health Rep. 2001;116(5):404–16.
23. Ibragimov U, Beane S, Adimora AA, Friedman SR, Williams L, Tempalski B, Stall R, Wingood G, Hall HI, Johnson AS, Cooper HLF. Relationship of racial residential segregation to newly diagnosed cases of HIV among Black heterosexuals in US metropolitan areas, 2008–2015. J Urban Health. 2019;96(6):856–67.
24. Ojikutu BO, Bogart LM, Mayer KH, Stopka TJ, Sullivan PS, Ransome Y. Spatial access and willingness to use pre-exposure prophylaxis among Black/African American individuals in the United States: cross-sectional survey. JMIR Public Health Surveill. 2019;5(1):e12405.
25. Fennie KP, Lutfi K, Maddox LM, Lieb S, Trepka MJ. Influence of residential segregation on survival after AIDS diagnosis among non-Hispanic blacks. Ann Epidemiol. 2015;25(2):113–9, 119.e1.
26. Dunlap E, Johnson BD. The setting for the crack era: macro forces, micro consequences (1960–1992). J Psychoactive Drugs. 1992;24(4):307–21.
27. Walker LS, Mezuk B. Mandatory minimum sentencing policies and cocaine use in the U.S., 1985–2013. BMC Int Health Hum Rights. 2018;18(1):43.
28. Ojikutu BO, Srinivasan S, Bogart LM, Subramanian SV, Mayer KH. Mass incarceration and the impact of prison release on HIV diagnoses in the US South. PLoS One. 2018;13(6):e0198258.
29. Wohl DA. HIV and mass incarceration: where infectious diseases and social justice meet. N C Med J. 2016;77(5):359–64.
30. Nijhawan AE. Infectious diseases and the criminal justice system. Am J Med Sci. 2016;352(4):399–407.
31. Wise A, Finlayson T, Nerlander L, Sionean C, Paz-Bailey G, NHBS Study Group. Incarceration, sexual risk-related behaviors, and HIV infection among women at increased risk of HIV infection, 20 United States cities. J Acquir Immune Defic Syndr. 2017;75(Suppl 3):S261–7.

32. Khan MR, Doherty IA, Schoenbach VJ, Taylor EM, Epperson MW, Adimora AA. Incarceration and high-risk sex partnerships among men in the United States. J Urban Health. 2009;86(4):584–601.
33. Philbin MM, Kinnard EN, Tanner AE, Ware S, Chambers BD, Ma A, Fortenberry JD. The association between incarceration and transactional sex among HIV-infected young men who have sex with men in the United States. J Urban Health. 2018;95(4):576–83.
34. Wingood GM, DiClemente RJ. The influence of psychosocial factors, alcohol, drug use on African-American women's high-risk sexual behavior. Am J Prev Med. 1998;15:54–9.
35. Baseman J, Ross M, Williams M. Sale of sex for drugs and drugs for sex: an economic context of sexual risk behavior for STDs. Sex Transm Dis. 1999;26:444–9.
36. Tortu S, McCoy HV, Beardsley M, Deren S, McCoy CB. Predictors of HIV infection among women drug users in New York and Miami. Women Health. 1998;27:191–204.
37. Falck RS, Wang J, Carlson RG, Siegal HA. Factors influencing condom use among heterosexual users of injection drugs and crack cocaine. Sex Transm Dis. 1997;24:204–10.
38. Metzl JM, Hansen H. Structural competency: theorizing a new medical engagement with stigma and inequality. Soc Sci Med. 2014;103:126–33.
39. Hansen H, Metzl J. Structural competency in the U.S. healthcare crisis: putting social and policy interventions into clinical practice. J Bioeth Inq. 2016;13(2):179–83.
40. Hardeman RR, Medina EM, Kozhimannil KB. Structural racism and supporting Black lives – the role of health professionals. N Engl J Med. 2016;375(22):2113–5.
41. 2017 Consumer Health Care Priorities Study: what patients and doctors want from the Health Care System. Available at: http://accountablecaredoctors.org/wp-content/uploads/2017/11/capp-research_what-patients-and-doctors-want.pdf. Accessed on 8 Apr 2020.
42. Clever SL, Jin L, Levinson W, Meltzer DO. Does doctor–patient communication affect patient satisfaction with hospital care? Results of an analysis with a novel instrumental variable. Health Serv Res. 2008;43(5 Pt 1):1505–19.
43. Chang CS, Chen SY, Lan YT. Service quality, trust, and patient satisfaction in interpersonal-based medical service encounters. BMC Health Serv Res. 2013;13:22.
44. Haskard Zolnierek KB, DiMatteo MR. Physician communication and patient adherence to treatment: a meta-analysis. Med Care. 2009;47(8):826–34.
45. Stone VE, Weissman JS, Cleary P. Satisfaction with ambulatory care of persons with AIDS: predictors of patient ratings of quality. J Gen Intern Med. 1995;10:239–45.
46. Cargill VA, Stone VE. HIV/AIDS: a minority health issue. Med Clin North Am. 2005;89:895–912.
47. Ingersoll KS, Heckman CJ. Patient-clinician relationships and treatment system effects on HIV medication adherence. AIDS Behav. 2005;9(1):89–101.
48. Dang BN, Westbrook RA, Black WC, Rodriguez-Barradas MC, Giordano TP. Examining the link between patient satisfaction and adherence to HIV care: a structural equation model. PLoS One. 2013;8(1):e54729.
49. Zhang C, McMahon J, Leblanc N, Braksmajer A, Crean HF, Alcena-Stiner D. Association of medical mistrust and poor communication with HIV-related health outcomes and psychosocial wellbeing among heterosexual men living with HIV. AIDS Patient Care STDs. 2020;34(1):27–37.
50. Carey JW, Carnes N, Schoua-Glusberg A, Kenward K, Gelaude D, Denson D, Gall E, Randall LA, Frew PM. Barriers and facilitators for clinical care engagement among HIV-positive African-American and Latino men who have sex with men. AIDS Patient Care STDs. 2018;32(5):191–201.
51. Squires KE, Hodder SL, Feinberg J, Bridge DA, Abrams S, Storfer SP, Aberg JA. Health needs of HIV-infected women in the United States: insights from the women living positive survey. AIDS Patient Care STDs. 2011;25(5):279–85.
52. Quinn K, Dickson-Gomez J, Zarwell M, Pearson B, Lewis M. "A gay man and a doctor are just like, a recipe for destruction": how racism and Homonegativity in healthcare settings influence PrEP uptake among young Black MSM. AIDS Behav. 2019;23(7):1951–63.

53. Calabrese SK, Earnshaw VA, Krakower DS, Underhill K, Vincent W, Magnus M, Hansen NB, Kershaw TS, Mayer KH, Betancourt JR, Dovidio JF. A closer look at racism and heterosexism in medical students' clinical decision-making related to HIV pre-exposure prophylaxis (PrEP): implications for PrEP education. AIDS Behav. 2018;22(4):1122–38.
54. Ayhan CHB, Bilgin H, Uluman OT, Sukut O, Yilmaz S, Buzlu S. A systematic review of the discrimination against sexual and gender minority in health care settings. Int J Health Serv. 2020;50(1):44–61.
55. Poteat T, Wirtz AL, Reisner S. Strategies for engaging transgender populations in HIV prevention and care. Curr Opin HIV AIDS. 2019;14(5):393–400.
56. Rutledge R, Madden L, Ogbuagu O, Meyer JP. HIV risk perception and eligibility for pre-exposure prophylaxis in women involved in the criminal justice system. AIDS Care. 2018;30(10):1282–9.
57. Flash CA, Stone VE, Mitty JA, et al. Perspectives on HIV prevention among urban black women: a potential role for HIV pre-exposure prophylaxis. AIDS Patient Care STDS. 2014;28(12):635–642.
58. Tekeste M, Hull S, Dovidio JF, Safon CB, Blackstock O, Taggart T, Kershaw TS, Kaplan C, Caldwell A, Lane SB, Calabrese SK. Differences in medical mistrust between black and white women: implications for patient-provider communication about PrEP. AIDS Behav. 2019;23(7):1737–48.
59. US Census Bureau. Language spoken at home: 2018 American community survey 1-year estimates. Accessed 9 Apr 2020. https://data.census.gov/cedsci/table?q=B16&d=ACS%201-Year%20Estimates%20Detailed%20Tables&tid=ACSDT1Y2018.B16002
60. Kerani RP, Johnson AS, Buskin S, Rao D, Golden MR, Hu X, Hall I. The epidemiology of HIV in people born outside the United States, 2010–2014. CROI. 2017. Abstract #851.
61. Centers for Disease Control and Prevention. HIV surveillance supplemental report: estimated HIV incidence and prevalence in the United States 2010–2016. 2019;24(1). Available at: https://www.cdc.gov/hiv/pdf/library/reports/surveillance/cdc-hivsurveillance-supplemental-report-vol24-1.pdf. Accessed 8 Apr 2020.
62. Guilamo-Ramos V, Thimm-Kaiser M, Benzekri A, Chacón G, López OR, Scaccabarrozzi L, Rios E. The invisible US Hispanic/Latino HIV crisis: addressing gaps in the national response. Am J Public Health. 2020;110(1):27–31.
63. Ojikutu BO, Mazzola E, Fullem A, Vega R, Landers S, Gelman RS, Bogart LM. HIV testing among Black and Hispanic immigrants in the United States. AIDS Patient Care STDs. 2016;30(7):307–14.
64. Demeke HB, Johnson AS, Wu B, Nwangwu-Ike N, King H, Dean HD. Differences between U.S.-Born and Non-U.S.-born Black adults reported with diagnosed HIV infection: United States, 2008–2014. J Immigr Minor Health. 2019;21(1):30–8.
65. Okoro ON, Whitson SO. Sexual health, HIV care and pre-exposure prophylaxis in the African immigrant population: a needs assessment. J Immigr Minor Health. 2020;22(1):134–44.
66. DeRigne L, Choi JJ, Barsky AE, Albertini V. Reaching Haitian Americans living with HIV/AIDS: met and unmet health care needs. J HIV AIDS Soc Serv. 2012;11(4):388–405.
67. Hashim MJ. Patient-centered communication: basic skills. Am Fam Physician. 2017;95(1):29–34.
68. Stacey D, Hill S, McCaffery K, Boland L, Lewis KB, Horvat L. Shared decision-making interventions: theoretical and empirical evidence with implications for health literacy. Stud Health Technol Inform. 2017;240:263–83.
69. Yen PH, Leasure AR. Use and effectiveness of the teach-back method in patient education and health outcomes. Fed Pract. 2019;36(6):284–9.
70. Wilson IB, Laws MB, Safren SA, Lee Y, Lu M, Coady W, Skolnik PR, Rogers WH. Provider-focused intervention increases adherence-related dialogue but does not improve antiretroviral therapy adherence in persons with HIV. J Acquir Immune Defic Syndr. 2010;53(3):338–47.
71. Barfod TS, Hecht FM, Rubow C, Gerstoft J. Physicians' communication with patients about adherence to HIV medication in San Francisco and Copenhagen: a qualitative study using grounded theory. BMC Health Serv Res. 2006;6:154.

72. Beach MC, Roter DL, Saha S, Korthuis PT, Eggly S, Cohn J, Sharp V, Moore RD, Wilson IB. Impact of a brief patient and provider intervention to improve the quality of communication about medication adherence among HIV patients. Patient Educ Couns. 2015;98(9):1078–83.
73. Effect of case managers on the care of patients with HIV infection. Ann Intern Med. 2001;135(8 Pt 1):S-46.
74. Senn TE, Braksmajer A, Coury-Doniger P, Urban MA, Rossi A, Carey MP. Development and preliminary pilot testing of a peer support text messaging intervention for HIV-infected Black men who have sex with men. J Acquir Immune Defic Syndr. 2017;74 Suppl 2:S121–7.
75. Cabral HJ, Davis-Plourde K, Sarango M, Fox J, Palmisano J, Rajabiun S. Peer support and the HIV continuum of care: results from a multi-site randomized clinical trial in three urban clinics in the United States. AIDS Behav. 2018;22(8):2627–39.
76. Rolfe A, Cash-Gibson L, Car J, Sheikh A, McKinstry B. Interventions for improving patients' trust in doctors and groups of doctors. Cochrane Database Syst Rev. 2014;3:CD004134.
77. Clement ME, Okeke NL, Munn T, Hunter M, Alexis K, Corneli A, Seña AC, McGee K, McKellar MS. Partnerships between a university-affiliated clinic and community based organizations to reach Black men who have sex with men for PrEP care. J Acquir Immune Defic Syndr. 2018;77(2):e25–7.
78. Shapatava E, Rios A, Shelley G, Milan J Jr, Smith S, Uhl G. Community-based organization adaptations to the changing HIV prevention and care landscape in the Southern United States. AIDS Educ Prev. 2018;30(6):516–27.
79. Smedley BD, Stith AY, Nelson AR, editors. Institute of Medicine, Committee on Understanding and Eliminating Racial and Ethnic Disparities in Health Care, Board on Health Sciences Policy. Unequal treatment: confronting racial and ethnic disparities in health care. Washington: National Academies Press; 2003.
80. U.S. Department of Health and Human Services, Health Resources and Services Administration, National Center for Health Workforce Analysis. Sex, race, and ethnic diversity of U.S, Health Occupations (2011–2015). Rockville; 2017.
81. Cohen JJ, Gabriel BA, Terrell C. The case for diversity in the health care workforce. Health Aff (Millwood). 2002;21(5):90–102.
82. Wakefield M. Improving the Health of the Nation: HRSA's mission to achieve health equity. Public Health Rep. 2014;129(Suppl 2):3–4.
83. LaVeist TA, Nuru-Jeter A, Jones KE. The association of doctor–patient race concordance with health services utilization. J Public Health Policy. 2003;24(3–4):312–23.
84. Ma A, Sanchez A, Ma M. The impact of patient-provider race/ethnicity concordance on provider visits: updated evidence from the Medical Expenditure Panel Survey. J Racial Ethn Health Disparities. 2019;6(5):1011–20.
85. Cooper-Patrick L, Gallo JJ, Gonzales JJ, et al. Race, gender, and partnership in the patient–physician relationship. JAMA. 1999;282(6):583–9.
86. Meghani SH, Brooks JM, Gipson-Jones T, Waite R, Whitfield-Harris L, Deatrick JA. Patient–provider race-concordance: does it matter in improving minority patients' health outcomes? Ethn Health. 2009;14(1):107–30.
87. Shen MJ, Peterson EB, Costas-Muñiz R, Hernandez MH, Jewell ST, Matsoukas K, Bylund CL. The effects of race and racial concordance on patient-physician communication: a systematic review of the literature. J Racial Ethn Health Disparities. 2018;5:117–40.
88. Saha S, Beach MC. Impact of physician race on patient decision-making and ratings of physicians. J Gen Intern Med. 2020;35(4):1084–91. https://doi.org/10.1007/s11606-020-05646-z.
89. Alsan M, Garrick O, Graziani G. Does diversity matter for health? Experimental evidence from Oakland. Am Econ Rev. 2019;109(12):4071–111.
90. King WD, Wong MD, Shapiro MF, Landon BE, Cunningham WE. Does racial concordance between HIV-positive patients and their physicians affect the time to receipt of protease inhibitors? J Gen Intern Med. 2004 Nov;19(11):1146–53.

91. Sohler NL, Fitzpatrick LK, Lindsay RG, Anastos K, Cunningham CO. Does patient-provider racial/ethnic concordance influence ratings of trust in people with HIV infection? AIDS Behav. 2007;11(6):884–96. Epub 2007 Mar 10.
92. Singh U, Levy J, Armstrong W, Bedimo R, Creech CB, Lautenbach E, Popovich KJ, Snowden J, Vyas JM, Infectious Diseases Society of America, HIV Medicine Association, and Pediatric Infectious Diseases Society. Policy recommendations for optimizing the infectious diseases physician-scientist workforce. J Infect Dis. 2018;218(suppl_1):S49–54.
93. Stoff DM. Enhancing diversity and productivity of the HIV behavioral research workforce through research education mentoring programs. AIDS Behav. 2019;23(10):2889–97.
94. Macias Gil R, Hardy WD. Spectrum of diversity in today's infectious diseases workforce: it's much broader and brighter than you think. J Infect Dis. 2019;220(Suppl 2):S42–9.

Chapter 2
Epidemiology of HIV Infection in Communities of Color in the United States

Victoria A. Cargill and Florence M. Momplaisir

Introduction

Over the last decade and a half, acquired immunodeficiency syndrome (AIDS) has been transformed from a fatal disease to a chronic, manageable condition, mainly due to the introduction of highly effective combination antiretroviral therapy [1]. In addition, better prevention and management of HIV-associated opportunistic infections enhances the sustained and robust immune responses generated by powerful therapies with convenient dosing schedules – all of which factor significantly into this transformation. However, these critical transformations in HIV care and management have not been achieved nor translated consistently and across all population groups and geographic areas. Although the course of HIV infection has been changed due to better therapies and earlier diagnosis, numerous barriers remain to HIV testing, linkage to care, care engagement, and retention [2, 3]. To achieve an AIDS-free generation, HIV prevention, testing, care linkage, engagement, and retention are critical for maximizing the health of the individual living with HIV as well as for the many public health benefits for the wider community.

V. A. Cargill (✉)
HIV/STD Services and Community Risk Reduction, Baltimore City Health Department, Baltimore, MA, USA
e-mail: victoria.cargill@baltimorecity.gov

F. M. Momplaisir
Department of Medicine, University of Pennsylvania Perelman School of Medicine, Philadelphia, PA, USA
e-mail: florence.momplaisir@pennmedicine.upenn.edu

© Springer Nature Switzerland AG 2021
B. O. Ojikutu, V. E. Stone (eds.), *HIV in US Communities of Color*,
https://doi.org/10.1007/978-3-030-48744-7_2

Epidemiology of HIV Infection in Communities of Color

Changing Definitions

While a detailed discussion of HIV surveillance methods is beyond the scope of this chapter, it is important to understand changes in the HIV surveillance and to briefly review HIV surveillance in the United States, as from this derives vital snapshots of the HIV epidemic across populations and geographic regions. In 2006, the Centers for Disease Control and Prevention (CDC) issued significantly updated HIV testing recommendations that were designed to: (1) reduce the numbers of people with undiagnosed HIV infection; (2) reduce the stigma and barriers associated with testing by promoting universal HIV testing – representing a shift from testing only those who were perceived to be at "high risk" for HIV infection. Shifting to such opt-out testing (meaning the individual is notified that testing will be performed as part of routine testing unless he/she chooses to decline such testing) was recommended after the continued lack of progress in preventing sexual transmission of HIV infection for which screening – at that– time was inconsistently performed [4]. Given findings that most individuals significantly reduce their sexual risk behaviors once aware of their HIV infection, and the clear need to decrease annual HIV transmissions, HIV screening through opt-out testing was recommended [5]. In this way, diagnosis of HIV infection could be enhanced, HIV prevention counseling and linkage to HIV care for those that test positive facilitated, and the testing process destigmatized [6–8].

In addition to this push for enhanced HIV testing, the HIV surveillance case definitions changed. In 2008, for adults and adolescents (i.e., persons aged >13 years), the human immunodeficiency virus (HIV) infection classification system and the surveillance case definitions for HIV infection and acquired immunodeficiency syndrome (AIDS) were revised and combined into a single case definition for HIV infection. The data in this chapter will be drawn from the years after the change in HIV testing and HIV case surveillance for ease of comparison [9].

Overview of the HIV Epidemic in Communities of Color

With more than three dozen individual and combination therapies for the management of HIV infection, greater control of viral replication with immune reconstitution has resulted, transitioning it to a chronic disease requiring ongoing management. The introduction of novel powerful classes of drugs, such as, integrase inhibitors, post attachment inhibitors, and pharmacokinetic enhancers has made the therapeutic armamentarium quite robust but without (1) knowledge of one's HIV status, (2) linkage to HIV care, (3) engagement and retention in HIV care, (4) receipt of antiretroviral therapy (ART), and (5) adherence to ART, control of the HIV epidemic will remain elusive. For communities of color, the decrement in each step of HIV care engagement provides additional opportunities for ongoing transmission of HIV infection.

An estimated 1.2 million people age 13 and older were living with HIV infection in the United States at the end of 2015, including an estimated 162,500 (14.5%) persons whose HIV infection had not been diagnosed [10, 11]. Of those living with HIV infection, the highest prevalence was among blacks followed by persons of mixed race, followed by Latinos. Latinos had the highest rate of undiagnosed infection, followed by blacks [10]. Despite these higher rates, between 2010 and 2015 the annual HIV infection rate declined 8% with decreases in all groups *except* two of note – gay and bisexual black and Latino men. In those two population groups, the HIV rates increased 4% and 14%, respectively [11].

At the end of 2015, an estimated 468,800 black adults and adolescents were living with HIV infection; of these, 15.1% had not been diagnosed. Blacks accounted for 41.8% of the persons living with diagnosed or undiagnosed HIV infection in 2015, over two-thirds of whom were male. The HIV prevalence rate for blacks in 2015 was 7.3 times the rate for whites, and the HIV prevalence rate for black males was 2.3 times that for black females. At year-end 2015, the highest percentage of black males living with diagnosed infection, by transmission category, was that among those with infection attributed to injection drug use (95.2%), but the percentage of black males living with diagnosed HIV infection increased among those aged 13–24 years and those with infection attributed to male-to-male sexual contact (Fig. 2.1). In contrast to males, the percentage of black females living with diagnosed HIV infection in 2015, compared with 2010, remained stable. By transmission category, the highest percentage of black females living with diagnosed HIV infection was among those with infection attributed to injection drug use (95.7%). Overall, the percentage of blacks living with diagnosed HIV infection in 2015, compared with 2010, decreased [11]. Reasons for this decline are not completely clear; however, for black women, it appears that improved health care access, socioeconomic status, and reduction in drug use may have contributed to the decline in this

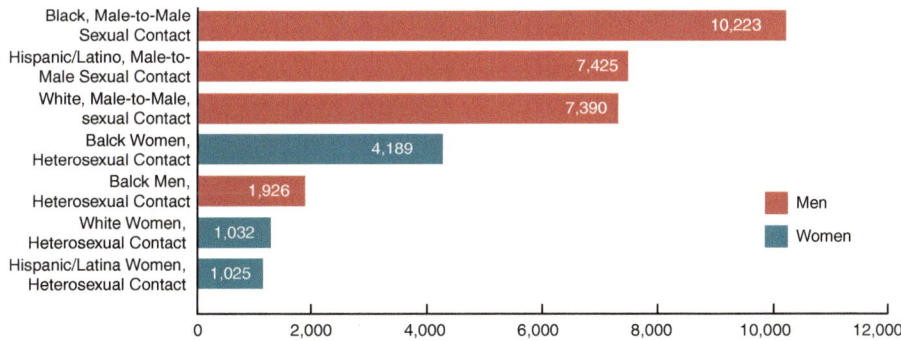

Fig. 2.1 New HIV diagnoses in the United States and dependent areas for the most-affected subpopulations, 2016. Subpopulations representing 2% or less of all people who received an HIV diagnosis in 2016 are not represented in this chart. (Source: CDC. Diagnoses of H IV infection in the United States and dependent areas, 2016. HIV Surveillance Report 2017;28)

population group [12]. These gains, however, may be short-lived given data on accepting and declining HIV testing for Southern black women. Perceptions of the negative consequences of a positive HIV test result, as well as privacy concerns, can offset intent to test for HIV and must be mitigated to continue ongoing HIV testing [13].

For Latino adult and adolescents an estimated 252,400 were living with HIV infection at the end of 2015, including 16.5% whose infection was undiagnosed. Latinos were 22.5% of those estimated to be living with diagnosed or undiagnosed HIV infection at the end of 2015, the majority of whom were male (81.6%). The HIV prevalence rate for Latinos was 3.0 times the rate for whites, and the prevalence rate for Latino males was 4.4 times that of Latina females. Unlike blacks the percentage of Hispanics/Latinos living with diagnosed HIV infection between 2010 and 2015 remained stable, but the percentage of Latino males living with diagnosed HIV infection in 2015, compared with 2010, increased among those aged 13–24 years. In contrast to males, the percentage of Latino females living with diagnosed HIV infection in 2010 and 2015 remained stable [10, 11].

In 2016, the highest rate of HIV diagnoses was among persons aged 25–29, and for race/ethnicity the highest rate was among blacks (43.6%), followed by Latinos(17.0%), persons of multiple races (12.9), and American Indians/Alaska native (10.2%) [11]. From 2011 to 2015, the annual number and rate of infections classified as Stage 3 (or AIDS) declined among all population groups. However, despite these decreases, disparities between racial/ethnic groups persisted in 2016 with the highest rates remaining among blacks (21.1%), followed by persons of mixed race (9.7%) and Latinos (7.2%) [11].

Disparities in HIV Mortality

Disparities in HIV mortality parallel the disparities in HIV infection. Between 1999 and 2015 blacks and Latinos, like their white counterparts experienced a decline in all-cause mortality (Fig. 2.2), however, the mortality rate for persons of mixed race increased [11]. Although HIV-associated deaths declined in every age category – except for those age 65 and older for blacks, when compared to whites – significant disparities with respect to survival were found at every age category [14]. These data corroborate similar findings in a data analysis of deaths from infectious diseases in US counties between 1980 and 2014. Of the infectious diseases analyzed, including lower respiratory illness, diarrheal diseases, meningitis, hepatitis, HIV, and tuberculosis, HIV infection had the widest disparity in county mortality rates [15]. The highest mortality rates were concentrated in counties in the southeastern region of the United States and nationally mortality increased from 1980 to 2014 [15]. Interestingly, HIV mortality shifted during this time period from the more affluent counties of the West Coast to the poorest counties of the South, suggesting the treatment access and advances may not have been as consistently available to the poorer counties in the South [15]. This implication is supported by the data of

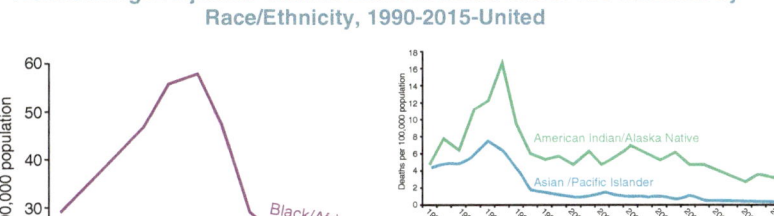

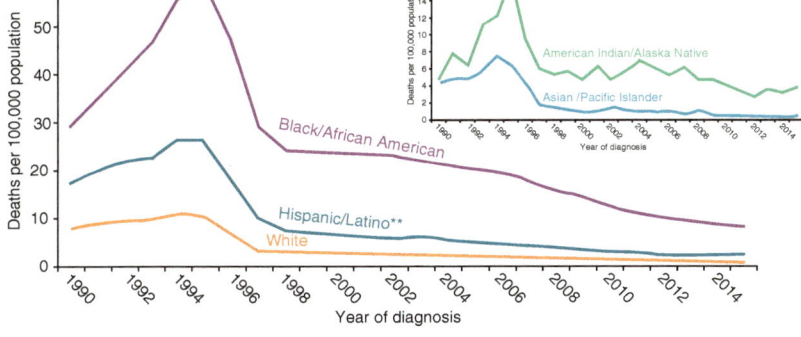

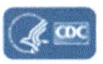

Note.For comparison with date for 1999 and later years, for 1987-1998 were modified to account for ICD-9 rules.
*Standard age distributions of 2000 US population.
**Hispanic/Latinos can be of any race

Fig. 2.2 Trends in age-adjusted annual rates of death due to HIV infection by race/ethnicity, 1990–2015 in the United States. (Source: stacks.cdc.gov › view › cdc › cdc_58351_DS1)

Cunningham et al. who note that blacks had significantly lower educational attainment and home ownership and almost twice the proportion of households below the poverty level compared with whites across the life span. In addition, the authors note that blacks were more likely to report not being able to see a doctor because of cost – although interestingly the percentages of blacks and whites who reported having a personal doctor or health care provider were approximately equal. Other social determinants such as lower educational attainment, lower rates of home ownership, and almost twice the proportion of households living below the poverty level and unemployed were noted in blacks compared to whites in all age groups [14].

Geographic Disparities

As with mortality, HIV infection is not evenly distributed geographically in the United States. Estimated HIV prevalence between 2010 and 2015 demonstrated marked variation in prevalence by region with the highest rates of HIV prevalence occurring in the South and the Northeast [11]. In 2011, eight of the ten states with the highest HIV prevalence were in the Southern United States, where 37% of the US population at the time resided but which accounted for 49% of the HIV diagnoses that year [16]. In addition to the highest diagnoses of HIV infection that year, the South also reported the highest HIV reported morbidity and mortality in the United States that year. As with other studies of this geographic region, this was found to be associated with high levels of poverty, HIV-related stigma, and prevalent STD infection [16].

This geographic disparity can be found across transmission categories in addition to race and ethnicity, although not as prominently. Combining data from the National HIV Surveillance System (NHSS) and estimates of men who have sex with men (MSM) population size in the United States, Rosenberg et al. estimated that among black MSM, the diagnosed HIV prevalence for that population group was more than twice that of MSM in general; however, when examining prevalence by US census regions, black MSM HIV prevalence was the lowest in the Midwest and the highest in the Northeast. However, HIV prevalence among MSM by state demonstrates the highest prevalence states were in the South (Mississippi and South Carolina). Similarly, the states with the highest annual rate of new HIV infections was also in the South, with the highest state rates being in Arkansas and South Carolina [17].

Latino MSM were like their black MSM counterparts; the highest prevalence of diagnosed HIV infection was in the Northeast, due to particularly high prevalence rates in New York and New Jersey. Mississippi was the only other state with a similar HIV prevalence among Latino MSM. As with HIV prevalence, the highest rates of new diagnoses were found in the Northeast and the Mississippi Delta region [17].

Among those with injection drug use (IDU) as a transmission category, in 2015 over three-fourths of the diagnoses of HIV occurred in urban areas [18]. However, a rural outbreak of HIV infection in 2015 was a sentinel warning of the propensity for HIV infection to travel along existing social and injection networks in rural areas. The outbreak occurred among injection partners who heretofore were considered low risk for HIV infection; however, they injected illicit opioids, often sharing injection equipment and with significant numbers of injections per day (range 4–15), and a range of injecting partners from one to six [19]. Since the initial reporting of this outbreak in Indiana, this same phenomenon has been repeated in rural areas around the country as was predicted [20].

The co-occurrence of similar social determinants of health as have been found in the high HIV prevalence Southern states is worth noting – the county had significant unemployment, high rates of undereducation (almost one-quarter had not completed high school), limited health care access, and lower life expectancy [19].

Disparities in HIV Testing and Late Testing

HIV testing is an important first step in the HIV care engagement cascade. Without awareness of one's HIV status, engagement and retention in care, which includes management of comorbid conditions and treatment with effective ART, all the necessary prevention interventions do not occur. This is an important step with significant ramifications for the individual, as well as the community including achieving optimum HIV outcomes for the individual and control of the epidemic for the community.

In 2013, an analysis of CDC-funded health departments and community-based organizations (CBOs) that provided HIV testing and HIV-related services in the

United States demonstrated that blacks accounted for 45% of all CDC-funded HIV testing events, the largest proportion of any racial/ethnic group. Blacks were almost half of the testing events among females and 54.5% of the testing events in the South. Among MSM, 23.3% of the testing events were among black MSM [21]. Blacks accounted for 54.9% of all new positives in this 2013 analysis, with over two-thirds of these new positives in the South and almost 70% (68.9%) of the new positives among women. Black MSM accounted for 37.3% of the new positives among blacks [21]. Analyzing the same 2013 data, Krueger et al. found that in 2013, among persons who received a CDC-funded HIV test, 21.4% were Latino and over half of the tests were conducted in the South. Of those newly diagnosed with a CDC-funded test kit, 19.7% were Latino, which is lower than the national figure [22].

More recently, data from the RADAR cohort study comparing individual and network factors among young men who have sex with men (YMSM) found that black YMSM had higher prevalence rates of HIV compared to white and Hispanic YMSM. Although black YMSM had lower rates of sexual risk behaviors and more lifetime HIV tests, there were higher rates of stigma, trauma, prior childhood sexual abuse, and cannabis use [23].

Adolescents and young adults need HIV testing if sexually active and yet are not as engaged in HIV testing as their adult counterparts. The Youth Risk Behavior Survey (YRBS) and Behavior Risk Factor Surveillance System (BRFSS) data provide a rich resource for analysis of testing behavior. Between 2005 and 2013, no change in HIV testing prevalence was found with only 22% of high school students who had ever had sexual intercourse reporting ever being tested for HIV infection. Slightly more than one-quarter (27%) of young adult males report ever being HIV tested. HIV testing among young adult females during the same time period declined [24].

At the opposite end of the age spectrum, older adults may also forego HIV testing, despite CDC recommendations that routine HIV testing include those up to age 64. Data from the NHBSS from 2003 to 2010 demonstrated an increase in HIV testing in this population immediately after the guideline release, with a slow downward trend except for blacks. Testing increased over time among non-Latino blacks only [25].

HIV prevalence rates among transgender individuals (individuals whose sex assigned at birth does not match their current gender identity or expression) in the United States remains high. Based on data from the US NHSS from 2009 to 2014, 2351 new infections were diagnosed among transgender individuals, 84% of whom were transgender women and 15.4% were transgender men (0.7% had an additional gender identity) [26]. Of the transgender women, half (50.8%) were black, and 29.3% were Latino. These transgender women were young, diagnosed at age 34 or younger (72.9%), with a significant proportion residing in the South (42.8%) at the time of diagnosis. The predominant risk category was sexual transmission (86.8%) and nearly one-fifth (17.4%) were diagnosed with stage 3 infection (AIDS) within 3 months of testing, meaning late diagnosis [26].

Like transgender women, over half of transgender men diagnosed with HIV infection in this time period were black, and 15.2% were Latino. Over half of the

newly diagnosed transgender men were aged 34 or younger (53.5%), and the majority resided in the South (53.5%) at the time of diagnosis [26].

HIV Care Continuum

Just as HIV testing is the key to tracking the emerging trends in the HIV epidemic
by region, population group, and reported risk behavior(s), it is equally important
for demarcating the starting point for tracking the movement of persons living with
HIV infection through the various phases of HIV care engagement – HIV testing,
awareness of HIV status, referral to care, linkage to care, care engagement, and
retention in care. The benefits of highly active antiretroviral therapy, prevention and
management of opportunistic infections, as well as the management of all comorbid
conditions require a series of important steps after an HIV test has been identified
as positive. A decade ago such a spectrum of HIV care engagement was presented
and six key stages along the spectrum were identified: (1) unaware of HIV infection,
(2) aware of HIV infection but not engaged in care, (3) receiving some medical care
but not in HIV care, (4) entered HIV care but lost to follow-up, (5) cyclic or intermittent HIV care user, and (6) fully engaged in HIV care [27]. For all the benefits of
the advances in HIV care and therapy to be realized, the infected individual must be
aware of the infection, be referred to HIV care, be engaged in regular and ongoing
HIV care management, and be adherent with effective ART [28].

The key downstream effects of effective ART adherence and control of the HIV
viral load have been well documented, including decreased transmission to partners, decreased community viral load, and overall reduction in new HIV infections
[29–32]. Thus far from being a model in isolation, quantifying the continuum of
HIV care from pre-awareness of HIV infection to successful HIV care engagement
and retention (all the steps identified by Gardner et al.) provides vital information
needed to achieve the ultimate goal of control and prevention of HIV infection [33].

For example, in 2011, data derived from the US NHSS and the Medical
Monitoring Project (MMP) were used to estimate the number of persons in the
United States diagnosed with HIV infection, living with HIV, engaged in HIV care,
and prescribed antiretroviral therapy. At that time an estimated 1.2 million persons
were living with HIV infection in the United States; of these an estimated 86% were
diagnosed with HIV, 40% were engaged in HIV medical care, 37% were prescribed
ART, and 30% achieved viral suppression. The prevalence of viral suppression varied depending upon age [34].

Identification of the effect of attrition at each stage, and the effect of this attrition
upon HIV transmission, morbidity and mortality is an important component of HIV
control and prevention. At stage 1, those unaware of their HIV status can continue
to engage in behavior(s) that transmit HIV infection and other sexually transmitted
infections placing themselves and others at risk [35]. Similarly, those aware of their

HIV infection but not engaged in care (stage 2) are not receiving important therapies that will not only provide immune reconstitution and reduce HIV-associated morbidity and mortality, but also decrease transmission of HIV infection to others [36]. Those receiving some form of medical care but not HIV care, those who enter HIV care and are lost to follow-up, and those with cyclic or intermittent HIV care represent a significant proportion of those living with HIV infection in the United States.

The HIV Cascade and Blacks

The HIV treatment cascade also varies by age, race, risk behavior, and sexual orientation. Data from the NHSS and the MMP were both used to determine the HIV treatment cascade for US blacks. These data from 2010 and 19 reporting jurisdictions were as follows: for the 8261 blacks diagnosed with HIV infection in 2010, 74.9% were linked to care by 3 months or more after the diagnosis, with a slightly greater portion of females (81.3%) compared to males (72.3%). Age also played a significant role in linkage to care with those ages 13–24 representing the population with the highest number of diagnoses of any age group but the lowest rates of care linkage (68.8%) [37]. For those blacks age 13 years or older living with diagnosed HIV at the end of 2010, 48.0% were retained in care, with a lower percentage in males (46.5%) compared to females (50.9%). In this defined population, those age 25–34, followed by those age 13–24 had the lowest care retention rates. Finally, of those blacks age 18 or greater and living with diagnosed HIV infection by end of 2010, 46.2% had a prescription for ART. A higher percentage of females (50.8%) than males (43.7%) had ART prescriptions, and the prevalence of prescriptions for ART increased by age with a more than doubling of the prevalence between age group 13 and 24 (20.8%) compared to those over 55 years of age (57.4%) [37].

Age and race are not the only factors affecting the HIV care cascade. Transmission category also appears to affect the cascade. For blacks diagnosed with HIV in 2010, those with the lowest linkage to care were those black males with HIV infection attributed to male-to-male sexual contact. Whether diagnosed with HIV infection in 2010 or living with HIV infection by the end of 2010, the group with the lowest percentage retained in care was among males with infection attributed to injection drug use (IDU). This same population had the lowest prevalence of ART prescription [37].

Closer examination of the challenges faced by young black MSM (YBMSM) suggests that it is the intersection of individual barriers and social determinants that impact care engagement; thus, more culturally and contextually responsive care is needed. A randomized trial, health Mpowerment enrolled 465 YBMSM ages 18–30 years, of whom 193 identified as HIV positive [38]. Returning for care visits was associated with insurance, college education, no methamphetamine, or recent marijuana use. The majority of the participants in the trial reported medication adherence; however, those with depressive symptoms had almost 5 times the odds of reporting less adherence. Viral suppression was associated with disclosure to sexual partners [38].

Age interacts with race as an additional factor influencing the HIV treatment cascade with significant ramifications for black adolescents and young adults. Compared with their adult counterparts, for the same year 2010, HIV infections in youth ages 13–24 increased, accounting for 25.7% of new infections – a significant proportion of these attributable to the marked increase in HIV infection among young black MSM [39]. Blacks accounted for 57% of these new infections [3]. More recent data from the 2017 Youth Risk Behavior Surveillance System demonstrates among currently sexually active adolescents 53.8% reported that either they or their partner had used a condom during their last sexual intercourse [40]. Despite this increase in condom use, HIV testing among adolescents and young adults must be accessible to provide information about HIV status and begin the process of linking adolescents to care. In 2010, only 40% of the HIV-infected youth were aware that they were living with HIV infection. More recently venue-based testing has been shown to improve HIV testing rates and can enhance linkage to care and focus group data has provided some guidance for approaching youth for testing [41]. This focus group derived guidance includes discretion, incentivizing HIV testing, and candid discussions about the need for HIV testing [42].

The HIV Care Cascade and Latinos

Kaiser-Permanente, the second largest provider of integrated HIV care services in the United States [43], examined cascade performance over time and by age, sex, and race/ethnicity in their medical program in eight states and the District of Columbia, for patients age 13 and older between 2010 and 2012 [44]. Measuring linkage, care retention, ART prescription, and viral suppression, Latinos were found to have greater retention for all years measured, compared to blacks [44]. These Kaiser findings vary slightly from those reported by the CDC, using the NHSS data to describe HIV care outcomes among Latinos in the US Hispanics or Latinos for persons age 13 years and older reported through December 2016. Using the data from 38 reporting jurisdictions, stage of disease at diagnosis and linkage to care were assessed among Latinos who received a diagnosis of HIV infection during 2015. Of the 6707 Latinos diagnosed in 2015, almost one-quarter (23.1%) were diagnosed as stage 3 (AIDS) or late diagnosis, and for an additional 18.8% the stage was unknown [45]. While linkage to and retention in care was similar for both males and females, males had lower levels of viral suppression than their female counterparts. The lowest levels of care and viral suppression consistently were among males with a transmission category of injection drug use, and heterosexual women had the highest levels of care engagement and viral suppression [45].

HIV Care Cascade in Marginalized Populations

Transgender individuals are well known to be at increased risk for HIV infection, at levels many times that of the general population. Risks for transgender PLWH go beyond HIV risk behaviors and extend to decreased care engagement, disparities in antiretroviral administration, and poorer viral suppression [46]. Denson and colleagues reported HIV risk behaviors, testing behaviors, and health care use among black and Latina transgender women in three cities: Chicago, Houston, and Los Angeles [47]. In their sample of 227 transgender women, over half (58%) had taken an HIV test in the last year, and over 80% had accessed primary health care in the last year despite 62% indicating lack of health insurance. HIV-associated risk behaviors remained high with almost half experiencing condomless anal sex in the antecedent year [47]. A combination of factors including lack of insurance, poverty, stigma, and drug use lead to high prevalence rates of HIV infection in this population and will thwart HIV care engagement and viral suppression efforts without more targeted and sustained interventions. Transgender women appear to have worse antiretroviral adherence than their cis-gender male and female counterparts [48], and they also seemed to be less likely to receive ART [49]. With higher viral loads, higher rates of morbidity and mortality, and lower rates of care engagement and testing, transgender individuals appear to be among the most in need of sustained intervention for HIV care engagement along the entire spectrum [50].

Incarcerated persons in need of HIV care also find themselves in a maze of care options found and lost, depending upon their status as being incarcerated, released, or in between. Data extracted from meta-analysis would suggest that of those inmates who reported being HIV positive, a range of 48–72% reported visiting an HIV provider before incarceration [51]. HIV engagement improved substantially with incarceration, with approximately 54% on average receiving ART before incarceration which increased to an average of 65% during incarceration. Unfortunately, with release ART receipt consistently decreased significantly, on average to 37%. Virologic suppression, as would be expected, decreased markedly as well from 40% to 21% after release. This decline in virologic control after release has significant consequences for both the individual and the community, outlined well by Loeliger et al., including mortality. In their study of the Connecticut correctional system, 14% of inmates released from prison between 2007 and 2014 died, with a standardized mortality ratio (SMR) higher than that for the general US population [52]. HIV infection, HIV comorbidities, and substance abuse–related conditions were among the primary causes of death. In addition to the disproportionate representation of some populations in incarceration settings compared to others (blacks versus whites), the break in viral suppression, with rebound viremia and viral activation, has adverse consequences for the individual and the community to which the individual returns, which in this setting is already disproportionately affected by HIV [53]. The gaps in care linkage, retention, and engagement for the many populations discussed here must be effectively addressed if control of the epidemic is to move from conjecture to reality.

Linkage to Care Disparities in Communities of Color

Linkage to medical care after an HIV diagnosis is essential for timely initiation of ART and entry into life-saving treatment. Linkage to care is also necessary to assist newly diagnosed individuals to cope with their HIV diagnosis, as well as address any health beliefs which may negatively impact future adherence to ART [54]. To critically assess the public health benefits of timely linkage to care, it is important to know the range of definitions for linkage to care used in the medical literature, which vary from initiating care with an HIV provider within 3 months or within 1 month of HIV diagnosis for newly diagnosed patients or having ≥1 medical visit with an HIV provider for an established patient [44]. This information is most often captured by chart review or by using HIV laboratory data (HIV viral load or CD4 count). The first linkage visit is an important one – allowing the patient to establish a relationship with a health care provider, providing access to clinical and support services (including case management, reproductive health, STI testing, and treatment). It is also where confirmatory HIV testing, HIV resistance testing occurs. The visit following the linkage to care visit is usually dedicated to initiating ART. However, some care delivery models are shifting away from delaying the initiation of ART for the follow-up visit, to initiating ART at the first linkage visit, as results of RCTs show that this approach results in higher retention and rapid viral suppression [55, 56]. Regardless of the approach, at the population level, timely linkage to care can result in reduced HIV transmission, particularly in communities with high HIV prevalence. Several studies have shown that failure of timely linkage to care results in delayed receipt of ART, higher viral load, and a lower CD4 at the time of care engagement [57]. An analysis of HIV surveillance data from New York City confirms this: 44% of individuals with a new HIV diagnosis who initiated care within 3 months of diagnosis achieved viral suppression at 12 months after diagnosis compared to 38% for individuals with delayed linkage to care [58].

Despite the widespread availability of ART and the existence of robust clinical programs, racial disparities continue to exist with blacks experiencing a delay in linkage to care compared to whites. The CDC analyzed data capturing people living with HIV age ≥ 13 years across 33 jurisdictions reported through December 2015; these jurisdictions accounted for 65% of blacks with diagnosed HIV infection at the end of 2013 [59]. Among blacks with HIV infection, they found that 71% (n = 8780) linked to care within 1 month after diagnosis compared with 79% of whites. A higher proportion of females (76%) linked to care compared to males (70%), and the proportion linked increased with increasing age. Young MSM (age 13–24) and people who inject drugs accounted for the lowest percentage of persons linked to care (55%), followed by heterosexual males age 25–34 years old (63%). In 2016, review of the NHSS continued to show this disparity, with linkage to care remaining lower among blacks (71%) and females (75%) compared to other racial/ethnic groups. Latino women had the highest percentage of linkage (77%) to care than all other female racial/ethnic groups [60].

There are multiple barriers to care linkage at the individual, community, and health system levels all of which contribute to the persistence of racial disparities in linkage to care. In 2017, a CDC report documented that blacks with the lowest percentages for linkage to care lived in counties with the lowest education and lowest health insurance coverage; these findings were the same across gender of black race [61]. Other social determinants associated with poor HIV care continuum outcomes include poverty, housing instability, and food insecurity [61]. Addressing social determinants can be challenging; however, integrated approaches that consider individual barriers and social determinants have the greatest potential to reduce race disparities [62]. Studies of newly diagnosed individuals repeatedly demonstrate that timely linkage to care occurred more commonly when individuals were tested at a site that offered co-located medical care compared to sites where people had to be referred for HIV care after testing [63, 64]. Clinics structured to include on-site comprehensive services reduce barriers related to transportation and delays caused by referrals to off-site programs and services. Qualitative interviews of clinic directors and HIV testing agencies reinforced that clinic structure matters: clinic models that meet patient needs by offering comprehensive and coordinated services can positively impact linkage to care (ref) [65].

Successful Interventions to Improve HIV Care Linkage

A robust literature exists of published interventions designed to improve linkage to HIV care. In general, these interventions fall under two major projects: the Antiretroviral Treatment Access Study (ARTAS) and the Health Resources and Services Administration Special Projects of National Significance (HRSA SPNS). Data from a randomized control trial using a time-limited strength-based case management strategy versus standard of care to link newly diagnosed individuals in care provides the strongest evidence for linkage to care [66]. The brief case management intervention consists of five case management sessions in which clients are asked to identify their internal strengths and apply these strengths to acquire needed resources. Participants in the case management intervention had significant higher linkage to care compared to the standard of care arm (78% versus 60%). This brief case management intervention was also found to increase linkage to care in an observational effectiveness study using a real-world setting [67] among patients with low education and unstable housing [68]. Results of qualitative analyses demonstrated that participants in the brief case management intervention expressed increased motivation to be linked to care and felt better able to address barriers to linkage to care [69]. Other HRSA SPNS projects used a variety of interventions to address education and support to mitigate linkage and retention in HIV care. These interventions included but were not limited to intensive case management, peer outreach and navigation, behavioral interventions focused on enhancing motivation, and life skills [70]. These interventions were implemented across diverse populations of people living with HIV including women, MSM, youth, and racial minorities. The successful elements from these interventions appear to stem from strategies focused on relationship building (ref) and need to be adapted to meet the needs and social context of specific populations [71].

ART Initiation and Prescription in Communities of Color

Early in the epidemic, disparities in the prescription of ART was widespread and well documented; however, since then, these disparities have diminished significantly but have not been eliminated [72–74]. Analysis of the prescription data obtained from the Medical Monitoring Project (MMP) between 2009 and 2013 confirms reduction in ART prescription disparities but not elimination. Beer et al. identified several striking findings including, by 2013, the disparity between Hispanic and white ART prescribing had been eliminated, as well as no disparity in Hispanic and white viral suppression among MSM. While the prevalence of ART prescriptions for blacks increased over this time period, and disparities in prescribing disappeared when adjusting for confounding variables, white and black disparities remained for viral suppression [75]. Examining ART prescription data using the California Medicare and Medicaid insurance claims data, Landovitz et al. provide additional insights into these disparities. While ART prescribing was high for this cohort (over 90%), a smaller percentage of Medicare and Medicaid enrollees filled an ART prescription or had a recommended ART regimen. Having more two or more comorbidities also decreased the likelihood of ART prescription as well as utilizing a provider with 5 or fewer HIV patients in their caseload [76].

Combinations of age, race, and sexual risk also appear to affect ART receipt and duration of viral suppression. The data from the North American AIDS Cohort Collaboration on Research and Design (NA-ACCORD) identified black MSM, especially as they grew older, as having less viral suppression than their white counterparts [77]. When measuring time spent on ART and time spent virally suppressed, the study found that black men who have sex with women spent less time on ART and virally suppressed compared to white males of the same age and category. Finally, Hispanic females spent more time in care and virally suppressed than their white females of the same age. Data from these studies and others identify key junctures where targeted interventions can decrease this disparity and enhance time in care, ART receipt, and by extension viral suppression and decreased transmission risk.

Successful Interventions to Improve ART Initiation

Rapid ART initiation interventions at point of care, as well as theory-based interventions have been used in the United States to improve early uptake of ART among underserved populations (ref) [78, 79]. A randomized control trial from San

Francisco showed that same day initiation of ART is feasible with the implementation of a "same day initiation" protocol using a multidisciplinary team to address barriers to ART initiation (insurance coverage and other barriers), provide patient education, and initiate ART on the day of the first visit (ref) [79]. The Rapid ART Program for Individuals with an HIV Diagnosis (RAPID) protocol consists of having same-day access to an HIV provider, an accelerated insurance approval process, initiating ART with pre-approved regimens with high barrier to resistance and low community-level resistance (i.e., tenofovir disoproxil plus emtricitabine and dolutegravir or a boosted protease inhibitor) provided in a 5-day starter pack, and having the patient take their first ART dose while in the clinic. Patients received a follow-up phone call a week later to inquire about ART adherence and side effects. A total of 86 patients enrolled in the study, 39 in the RAPID intervention arm and 47 in the standard of care arm. All patients were uninsured, most were male, non-white and many reported homelessness, major mental health disorders and substance abuse. All (100%) of the patients in RAPID initiated ART, 95% of them initiated ART within 24 hours, compared to only 81% of patients who initiated ART in the standard of care arm (p = 0.003). However, patients in the intervention arm experienced minor toxicity at a higher rate (5% versus 0% in the standard of care arm). Theory-based interventions have been used successfully to improve ART initiation. In two HIV clinics in the Southern United States, a brief video incorporating prevention messages into dramatic soap-opera style content was shown in waiting rooms to encourage treatment initiation, medication adherence, and retention in care (ref) [78].The video depicted characters modeling behaviors to overcome barriers to care. The quasi-experimental study design showed an overall increase of 10% in HIV treatment initiation (p < 0.01) and an overall improvement of 6% (p < 0.01) in viral suppression, although with mixed results across sites.

Care Retention and Achieving Viral Suppression

Disparities in Care Retention and Achieving Viral Suppression

Viral suppression has significantly improved in the United States due to both the universal use of ART regardless of CD4 count and the availability of newer ART regimens with lower side-effect profiles and higher barriers to resistance [80, 81]. In addition, U=U public campaigns have galvanized the HIV community to promote ART adherence for the health benefits of individuals living with HIV and their sex partners. U=U refers to the concept that if an individual with HIV is Undetectable, he or she is Untransmittable, as evidenced by numerous RCT and observational studies [82–84]. Despite these advances, significant racial disparities in retention in HIV care and viral suppression remain. For blacks diagnosed with HIV by the end of 2013, only 53% were retained in care the following year and only 48% were virally suppressed [59]. The percentage retained and suppressed was significantly higher among whites (58% and 62%, respectively). Retention was lower among black individuals aged 13–34 and within that age group, black men with injection drug use or heterosexual contact as the cause of HIV infection had the lowest percentage of retention in care (38% and 39%, respectively). Black women were more likely to be retained in care (55%) and suppressed (50%) compared to black men; however, young black females aged 13–24 with HIV infection from injection drug use had the lowest level of viral suppression (30%). Young black men (aged 13–24) with HIV infection from heterosexual contact had the second lowest percentage of viral suppression (31%) (ref) [59]. In 2015, retention in HIV medical care continued to be lower among black males (54%) than all other male racial/ethnic groups; the same was true of viral suppression (53%) (ref) [60].

One of the benefits of using HIV surveillance data to evaluate HIV care continuum outcomes is the ability to describe patterns of HIV care across diverse settings in "real-world" situations. Other cohorts have reported higher rates of retention in HIV care and viral suppression among blacks but even in these settings, racial disparities in retention and viral suppression persist. For example, the average percentage retained in care from 2010 to 2013 among Kaiser Permanente health system was similar among blacks (81%) compared to whites (79%), but viral suppression was substantially lower among blacks (77%) compared to whites (89%) (ref) [44].

Geographic variation in retention in care and viral suppression exists across the United States, but even across these wide geographic areas, blacks are less likely to be retained and virally suppressed compared to whites. An analysis of 78,993 adults with HIV receiving care in 12 clinical cohorts of the NA-ACCORD showed that in 2010 [77], the percent of person-years successfully retained for black individuals was 78% in the Midwest, 77% in the Northeast, 71% in the South, and 68% in the West [81]. These percentages were consistently higher across all four geographic areas for white individuals: they were 83%, 80%, 77%, and 71% in the Midwest, Northeast, South, and West, respectively. The South and West exhibit lower levels of retention in care compared to the Northeast and the West, most likely reflecting regional policies and the existing health care infrastructure within these regions. Nevertheless, the persistently lower retention of blacks across all geographic areas raises the issue of structural racism in the United States.

Key Factors/Challenges in Achieving Viral Suppression

Issues related to lack of economic opportunity and racial segregation across zip codes affect social and sexual networks, HIV risk, and HIV care continuum outcomes for people living with HIV. In 2015, blacks with the lowest percentage of viral suppression lived in counties with the lowest health insurance coverage and Latinos with the lowest percentage of viral suppression lived in counties with the highest vacant housing unit (ref) [60]. Socioeconomic differences are accentuated in the South, where counties with high HIV prevalence among women are also counties predominated by poverty, low median income, and low education; these counties also are mostly populated by blacks [85]. Intersecting with poverty, housing instability, substance abuse, mental health, stigma, and sexual violence are also contributors of poor viral suppression (ref) [86–89]. Identifying the differential impact that any of these factors have on poor retention or poor viral suppression remains challenging, but some investigators have attempted to do so. An analysis from a multiregional cohort of people living with HIV showed that individuals with a substance use disorder had a nine percentage-point decrease in retention in HIV care [90]. An alternative and more holistic approach is to consider that social determinants and individual-level barriers usually overlap and act synergistically to negatively affect retention in care and viral suppression. Many in public health use a syndemic approach to understand how co-occurring morbid conditions (or co-occurring epidemics) contribute to the persistence of racial disparities in HIV care continuum outcomes (ref) [91, 92]. It is important to consider such approaches for the development of effective and comprehensive interventions targeting disproportionately affected racial minorities.

Successful Interventions to Improve Viral Suppression

There have been many interventions tested and implemented across the United States to improve retention in care and viral suppression; however, there evaluations to assess the impact of these interventions on reducing racial disparities is needed. At the health system level, coordinated and positive messaging on the advantages of being retained in care can yield improvement in clinic attendance [93]. Even low effort interventions can yield great dividends – Gardner reported an intervention that used educational brochures and posters in the examination rooms and waiting rooms displaying information on the value of clinic attendance; clinic staff and providers also verbally reinforced the core of these messages. Using this approach, clinic attendance significantly increased in the post-intervention year compared to the pre-intervention year [95]. Receiving appointment reminders, calls after missed visits, and meeting with a clinic interventionalist can also improve visit attendance [94]. Providers who use a compassionate approach to care, who treat patients with dignity and respect, and take the time to listen have a positive impact in adherence to ART and retention in HIV care [95]. A meta-analysis of 207 studies reported that trust and satisfaction with providers was one of the factors significantly associated with adherence to ART [96]. Among African-Americans, this relationship might even be more impactful because of the already existent racial disparities in health care provision and of mistrust in the medical infrastructure [97]. Among Latinos living with HIV addressing cultural themes, such as centrality of family (*familismo*), masculinity (*machismo*), and trusting relationships (*confianza*) can play a role in ART to adherence [98].

Interventions aimed at addressing social determinants, particularly housing instability, to enhance retention in care and viral suppression have shown mixed results. Results of randomized control trials demonstrated no significant effect of housing assistance on HIV care retention and ART adherence [86]. However, when coupled with case management, there is a positive effect on ART adherence and viral suppression: 36% of homeless individuals who received this blended intervention achieved viral suppression compared to 19% in the usual care arm [99]. Other interventions aimed at improving food insecurity and transportation show encouraging results with improved retention in care and ART adherence [87]. The benefit of financial incentives to mitigate the socioeconomic barriers and encourage positive care seeking behaviors remains inconclusive – with no impact on linkage to care and small but positive impact on continuity of care and viral suppression. In the HIV Prevention Trial Network (HPTN) 065, continuity of care, defined as having a CD4 or VL during at least 4 of the prior 5 calendar quarters, was 9% higher in the financial incentive arm compared to the standard of care arm. Viral suppression, defined as a VL < 400 copies/ml using the most recent VL, was 5% higher in the intervention arm. These differences, although small in percentage point, can have a larger impact in reducing HIV transmissions at the population level.

Interventions focused on enhancing personal contact and providing support either through peers, patient navigation, or case management have shown a positive impact on retention in care and viral suppression. For example, the HRSA SPNS peer navigation interventions have shown significant improvement in retention in care and in viral suppression before and after implementing the intervention across several clinics (ref) [100]. Another way to increase personal contact with patients is the use of health technology. Bidirectional laboratory health information exchange allows provider-patient communication to be more efficient and decreases delays related to prescription of ART, and in one study, resulted in increased viral suppression, particularly among blacks (ref) [101]. This is one of the few interventions that have specifically reduced black-white disparity in viral suppression.

Care Retention Challenges in Marginalized and Vulnerable Populations

In 2014, the World Health Organization released new "Consolidated Guidelines on HIV Prevention, Diagnosis, Treatment and Care for Key Populations." These key populations were identified based on their disproportionate risk for HIV infection and because of the inadequacy of care received, resulting in poor health outcomes. They include men who have sex with men, people who inject drugs, people in prisons and other closed settings, sex workers, and transgender people. The World Health Organization also provided guidance on clinical interventions and policies to improve health outcomes for patients falling under these key populations (ref) [102]. Of note, issues related to adolescents took center stage and were addressed in a comprehensive manner in the published guidance. In the United States, racial minorities falling under these key populations suffer from poor HIV-related outcomes and other populations, including women who are pregnant or postpartum, also require attention. We will discuss key issues related to retention and viral suppression among these populations and provide examples of interventions that have proven to be efficacious among these groups.

Vulnerable Populations

Men Who Have Sex with Men

For population such as young black MSM, MSM of color in general, and transgender of color, linking and engaging in care is inconsistent with the result disparity in HIV outcomes such as viral suppression and HIV morbidity and mortality. Multiple interventions have been created and tested to address the needs of these populations. In 2005, HRSA developed a national initiative focused on YMSM of color. One intervention, In Style, targeted black and Latino YMSM to diagnose and engage those testing HIV positive in HIV primary care. Overall 63% were retained in care (defined as one visit every 4 months) compared to the 3 years prior to the intervention [103]. Clues for retention in care have been identified from other studies; feeling respected in care and receiving services from the clinic [104].

More recently, use of technology holds promise to increase HIV testing and referral. In one intervention, All About Me, black MSM and transwomen completed a computerized baseline assessment and are then linked to receive HIV testing recommendations. To date, 92% of participants enrolled have been retained offering additional possibilities for reaching and engaging this population [105]. However, the challenge continues to be to identify the drivers, when studies repeatedly demonstrate less receipt of ART for black MSM as captured by Hoots and colleagues [106]. In analyzing the NHSS data, black MSM were consistently less likely to obtain ART even after controlling for other predictors of low access to ART such as less education, poverty, and lack of health insurance [107]. Given variations by geography and population characteristic, effective interventions are still sorely needed. Simplicity, despite these nuances, may result in more effective messaging. Herbst and colleagues in a pilot study, Men4Men, the majority of HIV positive black MSM reported increased intention to use ART and almost one-quarter indicated that the benefit of ART to their partners was new [108]. The need for intervention to increase care engagement and ART adherence remains significant.

Transgender Populations

Transgender individuals have much higher risk of HIV infection than the general population, especially transgender women, but effective interventions to promote HIV care engagement, retention, and treatment adherence are few. Identifying correlates of HIV treatment adherence and engagement is one way to determine those factors that promote care engagement. Although limited by a heavy dependence upon self-report, Sevelius and colleagues identified factors including older age and abstinence from alcohol as associated with self-reported ART adherence, as was being in a relationship [109]. However, the HIV treatment cascade for transgender individuals begins with missed opportunities for testing, before moving into poor retention in care and low rates of ART initiation [110]. In a cohort of predominantly black and Latina transgender women, several key factors were identified as being essential for engaging and retaining these individuals in care: (1) a welcoming clinic environment that is respectful to transgender patients, (2) having some control with respect to medications and decisions made about them with respect to their effects upon their body; (3) fear of stigma and loss of confidentiality, and (4) unmet needs whether related to housing or substance use, or simply competing priorities, this was an important component as well [110]. Finally, the HRSA SPNS project Enhancing Engagement and Retention in Quality HIV Care for Transgender Women of Color Initiative in 2012 funded five demonstration projects around the country that provide direct medical care, as well as four community sites that do not provide direct services but partnered with local clinical settings [111]. The interventions provided ranged from peer support, to trans affirming care to peer navigation and wrap-around services. While the final outcomes and evidence-based recommendations are forthcoming, the interventions offered are informed by focus groups, community consultations, and observational data reported around the United States.

Adolescents and Young Adults Living with HIV

In the United States, adolescents living with HIV fall into two major categories: children who were perinatally infected and are now reaching adolescence or early adulthood, and adolescents who acquired HIV behaviorally, either through unprotected sex or through injection drug use. The majority of infections (80%) are now occurring among young people aged 20–24, not among neonates, and the majority of these new infections are among young men who have sex with men [112]. (ref) The challenges regarding adherence to ART and viral suppression often differ among youth who were perinatally versus behaviorally infected. Youth with perinatal HIV often develop multi-class resistance to ART due to life-long exposure to multiple regimens and have advanced HIV disease by the time they reach adolescence [113]. Regardless of the mode of HIV transmission, adolescents are at risk of poor adherence to ART. During adolescence, the brain is developing, and this period of physical and sexual maturation can often be associated with disinhibition [114] resulting in more risk taking [115, 116]. In addition, adolescents want to blend with their peers and dislike being perceived as "different." For these reasons, adolescents are much less likely to be retained in HIV care or adherent to ART. A review of the published literature from the United States show that only 43% of youth, aged 13–29, are retained in care and only 54% are virally suppressed [3]. In these studies, black and Latino adolescents tend to do worse compared to white adolescents [3, 117, 118]. Adolescent-focused interventions repeatedly demonstrate that those with youth friendly services have higher retention in HIV care [119, 120]. In an analysis of HIV Research Network (HIVRN) clinics serving close to 700 youth living with HIV, youth friendly clinics were defined based on their youth friendly related educational materials and services, having a youth friendly waiting area, the use of technology for communication, their proximity to public transportation, having flexible hours for appointments, and having providers trained in adolescent medicine. As is the case with the adult population, having access to intensive case management is a critical factor to keeping youth engaged in care and helping with the transition to adult HIV services [121].

The transition from pediatric to adult HIV is a time when many adolescents or young adults disengage in HIV care [122, 123]. Pediatric clinics are usually structured to be a "one-stop-shop" model, where adolescents or young adults receive coordinated HIV and intensive social support. The care structure in the adult clinics can be more variable and is not always well equipped to meet the needs of adolescents or young adults with HIV. Youth with perinatal HIV, in particular, who receive care in a pediatric HIV clinic since childhood, form strong bonds with providers and clinic staff; a transition of care can be traumatic to them. This can be compounded by the fact that adolescents or young adults with HIV are at higher risk for cognitive impairment, have issues related to socioeconomic and health insurance status, and have specific needs related to sexuality, reproductive health, and gender identity that adult clinics are not always ready to handle. The US Department of Health and Human Services has published recommendations for promoting a successful transition from pediatric/adolescent to adult HIV care, and the recommendations are listed in Table 2.1.

People Who Inject Drugs

Interventions in the United States have reduced but not eliminated racial disparities with respect to HIV infection among people who inject drugs. According to the NHSS, HIV incidence has decreased among people who inject drugs but racial inequities persist with a black-to-white PWID diagnosis ratio of 2 to 1 [124]. Many studies show that blacks engage in less high-risk behaviors compared to whites [125–127] but remain disproportionately affected by HIV, highlighting the potential significance of one's peer network and community HIV prevalence. For example, data from HIV Prevention Trial Network 037 show that needle sharing was twice as low in black networks of people who inject drugs compared with white networks of people who inject drugs, but black networks had disproportionately high prevalence of HIV. Other contributors for racial disparities include having less access to HIV care and being less likely to receive ART compared to other populations [128, 129]. In addition, the criminalization of drug use and suppressive policies toward blacks has had a negative impact on access to HIV care and HIV treatment. To keep people

Table 2.1 US Department of Health and Human Services recommendations for promoting successful transition of HIV-infected children and adolescents from pediatric/adolescent to adult care

Developing an individualized transition plan to address comprehensive care needs, including medical, psychosocial, and financial aspects of transitioning
Optimizing provider communication between adolescent clinics and adult clinics
Identifying adult care providers who are willing to care for adolescents and young adults
Addressing patient and family resistance to transition of care caused by lack of information, concerns about stigma or risk of disclosure, and differences in practice styles
Helping youth develop life skills, including counseling them on the appropriate use of a primary care provider and how to manage appointments; the importance of prompt symptom recognition and reporting; and the importance of self-efficacy in managing medications, insurance, and assistance benefits
Identifying an optimal clinic model based on specific needs (i.e., simultaneous transition of mental health and/or case management versus a gradual phase-in)
Implementing ongoing evaluation to measure the success of a selected clinic model
Engaging adult and adolescent care providers in regular multidisciplinary case conferences
Implementing interventions that may improve outcomes, such as support groups and mental health consultation
Incorporating a family planning component into clinical care
Educating HIV care teams and staff about transitioning

Source: Panel on Antiretroviral Guidelines for Adults and Adolescents. (2019). Guidelines for the use of antiretroviral agents in HIV-1-infected adults and adolescents

who inject drugs retained in HIV care and suppressed, close coordination of HIV treatment with substance use disorders treatment programs is needed. HIV clinics must be structured to meet the multidisciplinary needs of people who inject drugs and provide comprehensive care without stigmatization. Strategies that have been shown to promote medication adherence among people who inject drugs include modified directly observed therapy [130, 131] and other adherence support mechanisms. For example, HPTN 074 demonstrated that integrated systems navigation and psychosocial counseling have a positive impact on HIV outcomes (ART use and viral suppression) and also helps to support medication-assisted-treatment uptake, and lowers mortality for people who inject drugs [132].

People in Prisons and Other Closed Settings

The United States has the largest population of incarcerated individuals in the world, and incarceration rates are mostly concentrated in communities of color with blacks being disproportionately affected (Fig. 2.3a, b) [133]. The incarceration rate of blacks for drug charges is almost 6 times that of whites, although blacks and whites use drugs at similar rates [134]. British sociologist Stanley Cohen uses the moral panic theory to explain this phenomenon, and which posits outcomes when a socio-politically weaker group is assigned unwarranted blame and stigma [135]. The

Fig. 2.3 (**a**) World incarceration rates and (**b**) disproportionate impact of drug laws on black and Latino communities. (Source: Drug Policy Alliance. The Drug War, Mass Incarceration and Race. January 25, 2018)

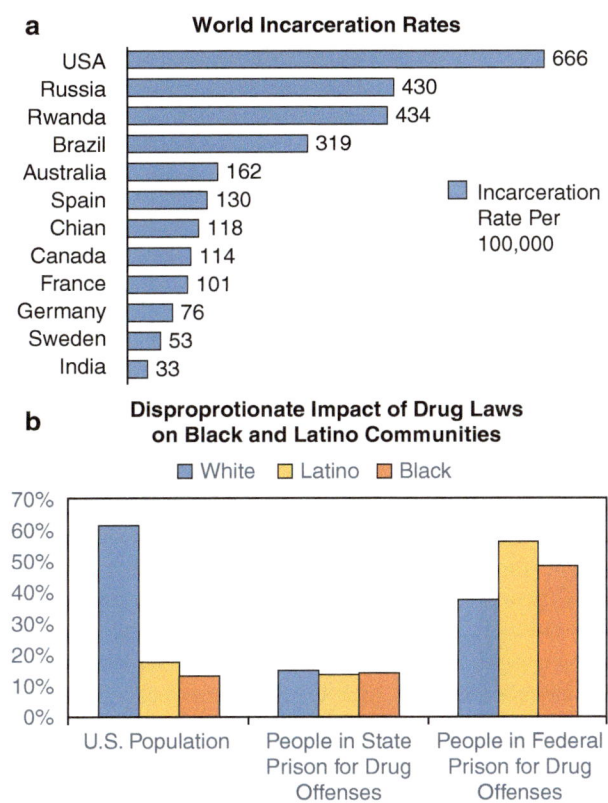

a **World Incarceration Rates**

USA — 666
Russia — 430
Rwanda — 434
Brazil — 319
Australia — 162
Spain — 130
Chian — 118
Canada — 114
France — 101
Germany — 76
Sweden — 53
India — 33

Incarceration Rate Per 100,000

b **Disproprotionate Impact of Drug Laws on Black and Latino Communities**

White Latino Black

U.S. Population | People in State Prison for Drug Offenses | People in Federal Prison for Drug Offenses

result is implementation of policies that foster social injustice and discrimination. The declaration of the federal war on drugs, with passage of the federal Controlled Substances Act Title II of the Comprehensive Drug Abuse Prevention and Control Act of 1970, is one such example: this Act mandated a highly disproportionate 100-to-1 sentencing for crack cocaine, predominantly used by communities of color, versus powder cocaine (more heavily used by Caucasians) offenses. This resulted in a disproportionate amount of incarceration rate among blacks, feeding into the cycle of poverty, which in turn is strongly associated poor health outcomes, including poor HIV outcomes for people living with HIV.

The transition period following incarceration is associated with significant disruptions in HIV care: timely linkage to HIV care often does not occur and even after linkage, people who were recently incarcerated experience poor retention in HIV care [136, 137]. According to a systematic review, only 30% of individuals are retained in HIV care in the post-incarceration period [138]. These poor outcomes seem to affect both men and women, but women particularly are vulnerable post-release with poor rates of engagement in HIV care, poor adherence to ART, and low levels of viral suppression [139]. Multi-level interventions providing social support, housing assistance, health insurance, and re-integration in one's community hold promise in improving HIV outcomes. A randomized control trial showed that a peer navigation intervention, providing social support, empowerment against stigma and discrimination, and HIV knowledge, resulted in higher viral suppression of men and transgender women, compared to transitional case management. This effect was sustained 12 months post-incarceration [140].

Women of Color and Those Who Are Pregnant or Postpartum

Nationally, black women account for 61% of new cases of HIV among women, though they represent only 13% of the American population [141]. Although new infections among women are declining, in 2015, the HIV diagnosis rate was 16 and 3 times higher among black women and Latina, respectively, than among white women [142]. Young reproductive age women are significantly affected: nearly one-third of new infections (29%) occur among those aged 25–44, and 22% among women aged 13–24. The Southern United States is now the epicenter of the nation's HIV epidemic and women in southern states have among the highest incidence of HIV among women of all regions of the country [85]. Women living with HIV who become pregnant face significant challenges remaining adherent to their ART and engaging in HIV care in the postpartum period [143, 144]. During pregnancy, guidelines recommend a high level of care engagement, suggesting monthly visits up to 28 weeks, biweekly visits up to 36 weeks, and weekly visits thereafter. For pregnant women, these visits provide opportunities to optimize HIV treatment and minimize the risk of perinatal HIV transmission. In addition, the universal use of ART during pregnancy and other clinical recommendations have resulted in a significant decline of perinatal transmission from 30% in the pre-ART era to less than 2% in 2013 [145]. Despite this success, perinatal transmission remains ten times higher among black compared to white women [141] and rates of retention in care and viral suppression are extremely poor postpartum. A retrospective cohort analysis in Philadelphia, Pennsylvania, of deliveries from 2005 to 2011, found that only 39% of women were retained in HIV care during the first year following delivery and that number had dropped to 25% at year two [144]. Analyses conducted in the South show similar rates of poor retention, ranging from 37% in Mississippi (1999–2006) [146] to 46% in Atlanta (2011–2015) [147]. More importantly, a substantial number of women experience mortality postpartum: 12% (68/549) of women who delivered in Mississippi (2002–2014) died within 5 years of delivery, and the major cause of death was AIDS (73%) [148, 149]. These preventable deaths occur among young women who are mothers, caregivers, and valued members of their community. There is an urgent need to improve health outcomes of women in the postpartum period and capitalize on the fact that during pregnancy, levels of care engagement are high. Interventions aimed at improving retention in HIV care and viral suppression in the postpartum period have the potential to improve the quality of life of the new mother and her newborn who depends on her for healthy development.

The Way Forward

Increase Awareness and Uptake of Existing Prevention Modalities

From the beginning, a strong emphasis on prevention has been a key strategy for reducing the number of new cases in the epidemic and this continues. Prevention remains an essential component of the National HIV/AIDS Strategy, updated for 2020, which includes reducing the number of new HIV infections as a key indicator [150]. The prevention toolkit has expanded significantly beyond condoms to include the following: (1) pre-exposure and post-exposure prophylaxis; (2) education and behavior change tools; (3) male and female condoms; (4) HIV testing and status awareness; (5) effective antiretroviral therapy; (6) male circumcision, (7) topical microbicides, (8) long-acting antiretrovirals NS, and (9) antiretroviral laced vaginal rings. However, without increased scale up, awareness of and education about these tools, disparities will remain. Multiple studies have demonstrated the gap in knowledge about PrEP among significant populations at risk for HIV infection [151–153]. Expanding both the reach and the penetration of HIV prevention services into communities and populations disproportionately affected by the HIV epidemic will be critical. To do this effectively, it will be important to not only understand those factors associated with increased risk of HIV infection but also those factors that impede and facilitate seeking and obtaining routine HIV testing. These studies can identify not only the gaps, but ways to address these important gaps in HIV testing [154]. This is a key indicator in the National HIV/AIDS Strategy updated for 2020, that 90% of people living with HIV are aware of their serostatus.

Enhancing Access to Care and Treatment Services

HIV testing without linkage to care and an array of HIV management and care services is of limited value. Understanding and addressing the individual and macrostructural barriers to HIV testing and care engagement will not only help move individuals through the many and important steps in the spectrum of HIV testing and care engagement, but also increase access to those tools that empower them to reduce transmission to others. Wilton et al. identified a clear need for culturally competent services, as well as for services and linkages to care from correctional institutions for black MSM. For many populations overrepresented in the HIV statistics, it is not just the remediation of structural barriers, but also obtaining the skills necessary to navigate complex systems of care to achieve successful engagement [155, 156] and retention.

Addressing the Role of the Social Determinants of Health

If there is one theme throughout this chapter, it is the undeniable and unrelenting ongoing effect of the intersection of the many social determinants of health – poverty, undereducation, homelessness, lack of insurance – on increased risk of HIV infection, increased incidence rates of HIV infection, and increased morbidity and mortality from HIV infection [157–159]. These factors overlap and affect the outcomes of a range of diverse health conditions from sexually transmitted infections to reproductive health, maternal health outcomes, and more [160–162]. HIV disparities specifically and health disparities in general are a true social justice issue [163], such that remediation of these issues extends far beyond the reaches of HIV science and will require a reconceptualization of our society, justice, and what truly defines public health for all [164].

Research and Evidence Base

It is clear from the disproportionate impact of HIV and its attendant consequences on communities of color in general and specific subpopulations such as MSM and transgender, that a robust and evidence-based inventory of interventions is sorely needed. An inventory alone will be insufficient, there must also be wide dissemination of these effective interventions, especially to those organizations that interface with – and more importantly are trusted by – the target populations [165]. This would include YMSM, transgender men and women, and substance-using populations. Successful interventions have emerged in the literature with more on the horizon, making this an important pipeline to nurture and grow [111]. From biomedical interventions to health system navigation to coping with stigma, evidence-based effective interventions at every step of the HIV care engagement spectrum will be critical for decreasing the annual numbers of new HIV infections.

In summary, the HIV epidemic in communities of color represents an ongoing critical public health need that has emerged from a confluence of social, biological, and political factors. The significant impact of the social determinants of health on HIV risk behavior and HIV acquisition cannot be dismissed, and the impact of incarceration upon the epidemic in communities of color cannot be ignored. The longstanding and ongoing effect of these factors upon HIV outcomes including care engagement and morbidity and mortality require a robust public health response that engages partners at the local, community, state, federal, academic, and political levels. HIV infection may be the spotlight under which a number of social injustices and inequities are highlighted – but with collaborations and concerted action at all levels decreased transmissions can be achieved moving us ever forward toward the day of an AIDS-free generation.

References

1. Scandlyn J. When AIDS became a chronic disease. West J Med. 2000;172(2):130–3.
2. Arnold EA, Rebchook GM, Kegeles SM. 'Triply cursed': racism, homophobia and HIV-related stigma are barriers to regular HIV testing, treatment adherence and disclosure among young black gay men. Cult Health Sex. 2014;16(6):710–22. https://doi.org/10.1080/1369105 8.2014.905706.
3. Zanoni BC, Mayer KH. The adolescent and young adult HIV cascade of care in the United States: exaggerated health disparities. AIDS Patient Care STDs. 2014;28(3):128–35.
4. Branson BM, Handsfield HH, Lampe MA, Janssen RS, et al. Revised recommendations for HIV testing of adults, adolescents, and pregnant women in health-care settings. MMWR. 2006;55(RR14):1–17. https://www.cdc.gov/mmwr/preview/mmwrhtml/rr5514a1.htm.
5. Branson BM, Ibid. 2006.
6. Marks G, Crepaz N, Senterfitt JW, Janssen RS. Meta-analysis of high-risk sexual behavior in persons aware and unaware they are infected with HIV in the United States: implications for HIV prevention programs. J Acquir Immune Defic Syndr. 2005;39:446–53.
7. Beckwith CG, Flanigan TP, del Rio C, et al. It is time to implement routine, not risk-based, HIV testing. Clin Infect Dis. 2005;40:1037–40.
8. Bozzette SA. Routine screening for HIV infection---timely and cost-effective. N Engl J Med. 2005;352:620–1.
9. Schneider E, Whitemore S, Glynn MK, Dominguez K, et al. Surveillance case definitions for HIV infection among adults, adolescents, and children aged <18 months and for HIV infection and AIDS among children aged 18 months to <13 years – United States, 2008. MMWR. 2008;57(RR10):1–8. https://www.cdc.gov/mmwr/preview/mmwrhtml/rr5710a1.htm.
10. Centers for Disease Control and Prevention. Estimated HIV incidence and prevalence in the United States, 2010–2015. HIV Surveillance Supplemental Report. 2018;23(1). http://www.cdc.gov/hiv/library/reports/hiv-surveillance.html. Published March 2018. Accessed 10-16-2018.
11. Centers for Disease Control and Prevention. Diagnoses of HIV infection in the United States and dependent areas, 2016. Centers for Disease Control and Prevention. HIV Surveillance Report. 2016; vol. 28. http://wwwcdcgov/hiv/library/reports/hiv-surveillancehtml Published November 2017. Last accessed 12 Sept 2018.
12. Ivy W, Ngwangwu-Ike N, Paz-Bailey G. Reductions in HIV diagnoses among African American women: a search for explanations. J Acquir Immune Defic Syndr. 2017;75(Suppl 3):S253–60.
13. Cheong C, Tucker JA, Chandler SD. Reasons for accepting and declining free HIV testing and counseling among young African American women living in disadvantaged southern urban communities. AIDS Patient Care STDs. https://doi.org/10.1089/apc.2018.0090.
14. Cunningham TO, Croft JB, Liu Y, Lu H, et al. Vital signs: racial disparities in age-specific mortality among blacks or African Americans — United States, 1999–2015. MMWR. 2017;66(17):444–56.
15. el Bcheraoui C, Mokdad AH, Dwyer-Lindgren L, Bertozzi-Villa A, et al. Trends and patterns of differences in infectious disease mortality among US counties, 1980–2014. JAMA. 2018;319(12):1248–60.
16. Reif SS, Whetten K, Wilson ER, McAllaster C, et al. HIV/AIDS in the Southern USA: a disproportionate epidemic. AIDS Care. 26(3):351–9.
17. Rosenberg ES, Purcell DW, Grey JA, Hankin-Wei A, et al. Rates of prevalent and new HIV diagnoses by race and ethnicity among men who have sex with men, U.S. states, 2013–2014. Ann Epidemiol. 2018; https://doi.org/10.1016/j.annepidem.2018.04.008.

18. Burnett JC, Broz D, Spiller MW, Wejnert C, Paz-Bailey G. HIV infection and HIV-associated behaviors among persons who inject drugs — 20 cities, United States, 2015. MMWR. 2018;67(1):23–8.
19. Conrad C, Bradley HM, Broz D, Buddha W, et al. Community outbreak of HIV infection linked to injection drug use of oxymorphone — Indiana, 2015. MMWR Morb Mortal Wkly Rep. 2015;64(16):443–4.
20. Van Handel MM, Rose CE, Hallisey EJ, Kolling JL, et al. County-level vulnerability assessment for rapid dissemination of HIV or HCV infections among persons who inject drugs, United States. J Acquir Immune Defic Syndr. 2016;73(3):323–31.
21. Seth P, Walker T, Hollis N, Figueroa A, Belcher L. HIV testing and service delivery among blacks or African Americans — 61 health department jurisdictions, United States, 2013. MMWR Morb Mortal Wkly Rep. 2015;64(4):87–90.
22. Krueger A, Dietz P, Van Handel M, Belcher L, et al. Estimates of CDC-funded and national HIV diagnoses: a comparison by demographic and HIV-related factors. AIDS Behav. 2016;20:2961–5.
23. Mustanski B, Morgan E, D'Aquila R, Birkett M, et al. Individual and network factors associated with racial disparities in HIV among young men who have sex with men: results from the Radar Cohort Study. J Acquir Immune Defic Syndr. 2018; https://doi.org/10.1097/QAI.0000000000001886. [Epub ahead of print].
24. Van Handel M, Kann L, Olsen EO, Dietz P. HIV testing among US high school students and young adults. Pediatrics. 2016;137(2):e20152700.
25. Ford CL, Mulatu MS, Godette DC, Gaines TL. Trends in HIV testing among U.S. older adults prior to and since release of CDC's routine HIV testing recommendations: National Findings from the BRFSS. Public Health Rep. 2015;130:514–25.
26. Clark H, Babu AS, Wiewel EW, Opoku J, Crepaz N. Diagnosed HIV infection in transgender adults and adolescents: results from the National HIV Surveillance System, 2009–2014. AIDS Behav. 2017;21:2774–83.
27. Eldred L, Malitz F. Introduction to the supplemental issue on the HRSA SPNS outreach initiative. AIDS Patient Care STDS. 2007;21(Suppl 1):S1–2.
28. Gardner EM, McLees MP, Steiner JE, del Rio C, Burman WJ. The spectrum of engagement in HIV care and its relevance to test-and-treat strategies for prevention of HIV infection. CID. 2011;52:793–800.
29. Eshleman SH, Hudelson SE, Redd AD, Swanstrom R, et al. Treatment as prevention: characterization of partner infections in the HIV prevention trials network 052 trial. J Acquir Immune Defic Syndr. 2017;74(1):112–6.
30. Das M, Chu PL, Santos GM, Scheer S, Vittinghoff E, et al. Decreases in community viral load are accompanied by reductions in new HIV infections in San Francisco. PLoS One. 2010;5(6):e11068.
31. Montaner JSG, Lima VC, Harrigan PR, Lourenc L, et al. Expansion of HAART coverage is associated with sustained decreases in HIV/AIDS morbidity, mortality and HIV transmission: the "HIV treatment as prevention" experience in a Canadian setting. PLoS One. 2014;9(2):e87872.
32. Sheehan DM, Fennie KP, Mauck DE, Maddox L, et al. Retention in HIV care and viral suppression: individual- and Neighborhood-level predictors of racial/ethnic differences, Florida, 2015. AIDS Patient Care STDs. 2017;31(4):167–75.
33. Giordano TP. The HIV treatment cascade – a new tool in HIV prevention. JAMA Intern Med. 2015;175(4):596–7. https://doi.org/10.1001/jamainternmed.2014.8199.
34. Bradley H, Hall I, Wolitski RJ, Van Handel MM, et al. Vital signs: HIV diagnosis, care, and treatment among persons living with HIV — United States, 2011. MMWR. 2014;63(47):1113–7.
35. Skarbinski J, Rosenberg E, Paz-Bailey G, et al. Human immunodeficiency virus transmission at each step of the care continuum in the United States. JAMA Intern Med. 2015;175(4):588–96.

36. Hull M, Montaner J. Antiretroviral therapy: a key component of a comprehensive HIV pre-vention strategy. Curr HIV/AIDS Rep. 2011;8:85–93.
37. Whiteside YO, Cohen SM, Bradley H, Skarbinski J, et al. Progress along the continuum of HIV care among blacks with diagnosed HIV – United States 2010. MMWR. 2014;63(5):85–9.
38. Hightow-Weidman L, LeGrand S, Choi SK, Egger J, et al. Exploring the HIV continuum of care among young black MSM. PLoS One. 2017;12(6):e0179688.
39. Whitmore SK, Kann L, Prejean J, Koenig LJ, et al. Vital signs: HIV infection, testing, and risk behaviors among youths — United States. MMWR. 2012;61(47):971–6.
40. Kann L, McManus KL, Harris WA, Shanklin SL, Flint KH, Queen B, et al. Youth risk behav-ior surveillance – United States, 2017. MMWR Surveill Summ. 2018;67(8):1–114.
41. Camacho-Gonzalez AF, Gillespie SE, Thomas-Seaton L, Frieson K, et al. The Metropolitan Atlanta community adolescent rapid testing initiative study: closing the gaps in HIV care among youth in Atlanta, Georgia, USA. AIDS. 2017;31(Suppl 3):S267–75.
42. Murray A, Hussen SA, Toledo L, Thomas-Seaton L, Gillespie S. Optimizing community-based HIV testing and linkage to care for young persons in Metropolitan Atlanta. AIDS Patient Care STDs. 2018;32(6):234–40.
43. Kaiser Permanente Research Brief – HIV/AIDS. 2018. https://share.kaiserpermanente.org/wp-content/uploads/2018/07/research_brief_hiv_aids_20180709.pdf.
44. Hornberg MA, Hurley LB, Klein DB, Towner WJ, et al. The HIV care cascade measured over time and by age, sex, and race in a large national integrated care system. AIDS Patient Care STDs. 2015;29(11):582–90.
45. Gantt Z, Dailey A, Hu X, Satcher-Johnson A. HIV care outcomes among Hispanics or Latinos with diagnosed HIV infection — United States, 2015. MMWR. 2017;66(40):1065–72.
46. Baral SD, Poteat T, Stromdahl S, et al. Worldwide burden of HIV in transgender women: a systematic review and meta-analysis. Lancet Infect Dis. 2013;13(3):214–22.. https://doi.org/10.1016/S1473-3099(12)70315-8
47. Denson DJ, Padgett PM, Pitts N, Paz-Bailey G, et al. Health care use and HIV-related Behaviors of black and Latina transgender women in 3 US Metropolitan areas: results from the transgender HIV behavioral survey. J Acquir Immune Defic Syndr. 2017;75:S268–75.
48. Sevelius J, Carrico A, Johnson M. Antiretroviral therapy adherence among transgen-der women. J Assoc Nurses AIDS Care. 2010;21(3):256–64. https://doi.org/10.1016/j.jana.2010.01.005.
49. Melendez R, Exner T, Ehrhardt A, et al. Health and health care among male-to-female trans-gender persons who are HIV positive. Am J Public Health. 2005;95:5–7.
50. Sevelius JM, Patouhas E, Keatley JG, Mallory O, et al. Barriers and facilitators to engage-ment and retention in care among transgender women living with human immunodeficiency virus. Ann Behav Med. 2014;47(1):5–16. https://doi.org/10.1007/s12160-013-9565-8.
51. Iroh PA, Mao H, Nijhawan AE. The HIV care cascade before, during, and after incarceration: a systematic review and data synthesis. Am J Public Health. 2015;105(7):e5–e16.
52. Loeliger KB, Altice FL, Ciarleglio MM, Rich KM, et al. All-cause mortality among people with HIV released from an integrated system of jails and prisons in Connecticut, USA, 2007-14: a retrospective observational cohort study. Lancet HIV. 2017; https://doi.org/10.1016/S2352-3018(18)30175-9.
53. Wohl DA, Rosen DL. Inadequate HIV care after incarceration: case closed. Lancet HIV. 2018;5(2):e64–5.
54. Bogart LM, et al. Medical mistrust among social network members may contribute to anti-retroviral treatment nonadherence in African Americans living with HIV. Soc Sci Med. 2016;164:133–40.
55. Hoenigl M, et al. Rapid HIV viral load suppression in those initiating antiretroviral therapy at first visit after HIV diagnosis. Sci Rep. 2016;6:2947.
56. Koenig SP, et al. Same-day HIV testing with initiation of antiretroviral therapy ver-sus standard care for persons living with HIV: a randomized unblinded trial. PLoS Med. 2017;14(7):e1002357.

57. Mugavero MJ, Amico KR, Horn T, Thompson MA. The state of engagement in HIV care in the United States: from cascade to continuum to control. CID. 2013;57(8):1164–71.
58. Robertson MK, et al. Linkage and retention in care and the time to HIV viral suppression and viral rebound–New York City. AIDS Care. 2015;27(2):260–7.
59. Dailey AF, Satcher Johnson A, Wu B. HIV care outcomes among blacks with diagnosed HIV — United States, 2014. MMWR Morb Mortal Wkly Rep. 2017;66(4):97–103.
60. Centers for Disease Control and Prevention. Social determinants of health among adults with diagnosed HIV infection, 2016. Part B: county-level social determinants of health and selected care outcomes among adults with diagnosed HIV infection—39 states and the District of Columbia. HIV Surveillance Supplemental Report. 2018;23(No. 6, pt B). http://www.cdc.gov/hiv/library/reports/hiv-surveillance.html. Published October 2018.
61. Centers for Disease Control and Prevention. Social determinants of health and selected HIV care outcomes among adults with diagnosed HIV infection in 37 states and the District of Columbia, 2015. HIV Surveillance Supplemental Report. 2017;22(4). http://www.cdc.gov/hiv/library/reports/hiv-surveillance.html.
62. Storholm ED, Bogart LM, Mutchler MG, Klein DJ, et al. Antiretroviral adherence trajectories among black Americans living with HIV. AIDS Behav. 2018; https://doi.org/10.1007/s10461-018-2303-2. [Epub ahead of print].
63. Torian LV, Wiewel EW, Liu KL, Sackoff JE, Frieden TR. Risk factors for delayed initiation of medical care after diagnosis of human immunodeficiency virus. Arch Intern Med. 2008;168:1181–7.
64. Hightow-Weidman LB, Jones K, Wohl AR, et al. Early linkage and retention in care: findings from the outreach, linkage, and retention in care initiative among young men of color who have sex with men. AIDS Patient Care STDs. 2011;25(suppl 1):S31–8.
65. Bauman LJ, Braunstein S, Calderon Y, Chhabra R, et al. Barriers and facilitators of linkage to HIV primary care in New York City. J Acquir Immune Defic Syndr (1999). 2013;64(0 1):S20–6.
66. Gardner LI, Metsch LR, Anderson-Mahoney P, Loughlin AM, Del Rio C, Strathdee S, Sansom SL, Siegal HA, Greenberg AE, Holmberg SD. Efficacy of a brief case management intervention to link recently diagnosed HIV-infected persons to care. AIDS. 2005;19(4):423–31.
67. Craw JA, Gardner LI, Marks G, et al. ARTAS II: brief strengths-based case management promotes entry into HIV medical care: results of the antiretroviral treatment access study-II. J Acquir Immune Defic Syndr. 2008;47:597–606.
68. Gardner LI, Marks G, Craw J, Metsch L, Strathdee S, Anderson-Mahoney P, del Rio C. Demographic, psychological, and behavioral modifiers of the antiretroviral treatment access study (ARTAS) intervention. AIDS Patient Care STDs. 2009;23(9):735–42.
69. Parnell H, Berger M, Gichance M, et al. Lost to care and back again: patient and navigator perspectives on HIV care re-engagement. AIDS Behav. 2017; https://doi.org/10.1007/s10461-017-1919-y.
70. Rajabiun S, Cabral H, Tobias C, Relf M. Program design and evaluation strategies for the Special Projects of National Significance Outreach Initiative. AIDS Patient Care STDs. 2007;21(S1):1–9.
71. Liau A, Crepaz N, Lyles CM, Higa DH, Mullins MM, DeLuca J, Petters S, Marks G. Interventions to promote linkage to and utilization of HIV medical care among HIV-diagnosed persons: a qualitative systematic review, 1996–2011. AIDS Behav. 2013;17(6):1941–62.
72. Anderson RM, Bozzette SM, Shapiro MR, et al. Access of vulnerable groups to antiretroviral therapy among persons in care for HIV disease in the U.S. Health Serv Res. 2000;35(2):389–416.
73. Gebo KA, Fleishman JA, Conviser R, et al. Racial and gender disparities in receipt of highly active antiretroviral therapy persist in a multistate sample of HIV patients in 2001. J Acquir Immune Defic Syndr. 2005;38(1):96–103.

74. Cunningham WE, Mardson LW, Andersen RM, et al. Prevalence and predictors of highly active antiretroviral therapy use in patients with HIV infection in the United States. J Acquir Immune Defic Syndr. 2000;25(2):115–23.
75. Beer L, Bradley H, Mattson CL, Johnson CH, et al. Trends in racial and ethnic disparities in antiretroviral therapy prescription and viral suppression in the United States, 2009-2013. J Acquir Immune Defic Syndr. 2016;73(4):446–53.
76. Landovitz RJ, Desmond KA, Leibowitz AA. Antiretroviral therapy: racial disparities among publicly insured Californians with HIV. J Health Care Poor Underserved. 2017;28(1):406–29.
77. Desir FA, Lesko CR, Moore RD, Horberg MA, et al. One size fits (n)one: the influence of sex, age, and sexual human immunodeficiency virus (HIV) acquisition risk on racial/ethnic disparities in the HIV care continuum in the United States. CID. 2018; https://doi.org/10.1093/cid/ciy556.
78. Neumann MS, Plant A, Margolis AD, Borkowf CB, et al. Effects of a brief video intervention on treatment initiation and adherence among patients attending human immunodeficiency virus treatment clinics. PLoS One. 2018;13(10):e0204599. https://journals.plos.org/plosone/article?id=10.1371/journal.pone.0204599#references.
79. Pilcher CD, Ospina-Norvell C, Dasgupta A, Jones D, et al. The effect of same-day observed initiation of antiretroviral therapy on HIV viral load and treatment outcomes in a US public health setting. J Acquir Immune Defic Syndr. 2017;74(1):44–51.
80. Branson BM, et al. Revised recommendations for HIV testing of adults, adolescents, and pregnant women in health-care settings. Morb Mortal Wkly Rep Recomm Rep. 2006;55(14):1–17.
81. Rebeiro PF, Gange SJ, Horberg MA, Abraham AG, Napravnik S, Samji H, Yehia BR, Althoff KN, Moore RD, Kitahata MM, Sterling TR. Geographic variations in retention in care among HIV-infected adults in the United States. PLoS One. 2016;11(1):e0146119.
82. Grinsztejn B, Hosseinipour MC, Ribaudo HJ, Swindells S, Eron J, Chen YQ, Wang L, Ou SS, Anderson M, McCauley M, Gamble T. 2014. Effects of early versus delayed initiation of antiretroviral treatment on clinical outcomes of HIV-1 infection: results from the phase 3 HPTN 052 randomised controlled trial. Lancet Infect Dis. 2014;14(4):281–90.
83. Rodger A, Bruun T, Cambiano V, Vernazza P, et al. HIV transmission risk through condomless sex if HIV+ partner on suppressive ART: PARTNER study. 21st Conference on retroviruses and opportunistic infections, 3–6 March 2014. Boston; 2014.
84. Grulich AE, Bavinton BR, Jin F, Prestage G, et al. HIV transmission in male serodiscordant couples in Australia, Thailand and Brazil [Poster Number 1019LB]. 22nd Conference on retroviruses and opportunistic infections. Seattle;, 2015.
85. Breskin A, Adimora A, Westreich D. Women and HIV in the United States. PLoS One. 2017;12(2):e0172367.
86. Wolitski RJ, Kidder DP, Pals SL, et al. Randomized trial of the effects of housing assistance on the health and risk behaviors of homeless and unstably housed people living with HIV. AIDS Behav. 2010;14:493–503.
87. Cantrell RA, Sinkala M, Megazinni K, et al. A pilot study of food supplementation to improve adherence to antiretroviral therapy among food-insecure adults in Lusaka, Zambia. J Acquir Immune Defic Syndr. 2008;49:190–5.
88. Andersen M, Hockman E, Smereck G, et al. Retaining women in HIV medical care. J Assoc Nurses AIDS Care. 2007;18:33.
89. Lipira L, Williams EC, Huh D, Kemp C, et al. HIV-related stigma and viral suppression among African-American women: exploring the mediating roles of depression and ART non-adherence. AIDS Behav. 2018 Oct 20; https://doi.org/10.1007/s10461-018-2301-4. [Epub ahead of print].
90. Hartzler B, Dombrowski JC, Williams JR, Crane HM, Eron JJ, Geng EH, Mathews C, Mayer KH, Moore RD, Mugavero MJ, Napravnik S. Influence of substance use disorders on 2-year HIV care retention in the United States. AIDS Behav. 2018;22(3):742–51.

91. Mustanski B, Garofalo R, Herrick A, Donenberg G. Psychosocial health problems increase risk for HIV among urban young men who have sex with men: preliminary evidence of a syndemic in need of attention. Ann Behav Med. 2007;34(1):37–45.
92. Sullivan KA, Messer LC, Quiinlivan EB. Substance abuse, violence, and HIV/AIDS (SAVA) syndemic effects on viral suppression among HIV positive women of color. AIDS Patient Care STDs. 2015;9(S1):S42–8.
93. Gardner LI, Marks G, Craw JA, Wilson TE, et al. A low-effort, clinic-wide intervention improves attendance for HIV primary care. CID. 2012;55(8):1124–34. https://doi.org/10.1093/cid/cis623.
94. Gardner LI, Giordano TP, Marks G, Wilson TE, Craw JA, Drainoni ML, Keruly JC, Rodriguez AE, Malitz F, Moore RD, Bradley-Springer LA. Enhanced personal contact with HIV patients improves retention in primary care: a randomized trial in 6 US HIV clinics. CID. 2014;59(5):725–34.
95. Beach MC, Keruly J, Moore RD. Is the quality of the patient-provider relationship associated with better adherence and health outcomes for patients with HIV? JGIM. 2006;21(6):661–5. https://doi.org/10.1111/j.1525-1497.2006.00399.x.
96. Langebeek N, Gisolf EH, Reiss P, Vervoort SC, et al. Predictors and correlates of adherence to combination antiretroviral therapy (ART) for chronic HIV infection: a meta-analysis. BMC Med. 2014;12:142.
97. Bogart LM, Wagner G, Galvan FH. Conspiracy beliefs about HIV are related to antiretroviral treatment nonadherence among African American men with HIV. J Acquir Immune Defic Syndr. 2010;53(5):648–55.
98. Levison JH, et al. "Where it falls apart": barriers to retention in HIV care in Latino immigrants and migrants. AIDS Patient Care STDs. 2017;31(9):394–405.
99. Buchanan D, Kee R, Sadowsi LS. Garcia. The health impact of supportive housing for HIV positive homeless patients: a randomized control trial. Am J Public Health. 2009;99(Suppl 3):S675–80.
100. Bradford JB, Coleman S, Cunningham W. HIV system navigation: an emerging model to improve HIV care access. AIDS Patient Care STDs. 2007;21(suppl 1):S49–58.
101. Cunningham WE, et al. Effects of a laboratory health information exchange intervention on antiretroviral therapy use, viral suppression, and racial/ethnic disparities. JAIDS. 2017;75(3):290–8.
102. Lall P, Lim SH, Khairuddin N, Kamarulzaman A. An urgent need for research on factors impacting adherence to and retention in care among HIV-positive youth and adolescents from key populations. J Int AIDS Soc. 2017;18:19393.
103. Hightow-Weidman LB, Justin C, Smith EV, Matthews D, et al. Keeping them in "STYLE": finding, linking, and retaining young HIV-positive black and Latino men who have sex with men in care. AIDS Patient Care STDs. 2011;25(1):37–45.
104. Magnus M, Jones K, Phillips G, Binson HW, et al. Characteristics associated with retention among African American and Latino adolescent HIV-positive men: results from the outreach, care, and prevention to engage HIV-seropositive young MSM of color special project of National Significance Initiative. JAIDS J Acquir Immune Defic Syndr. 2010;53(4):529–36.
105. Koblin B, Hirshfield S, Chaisson MA, Wilton L, et al. Intervention to match young black men and transwomen who have sex with men or transwomen to HIV testing options (all about me): protocol for a randomized controlled trial. JMIR Res Protoc. 2017;6(12):e254.
106. Hoots BE, Finlayson TJ, Wejnert C, Paz-Bailey G, NHBS Study Group. Updated data on linkage to HIV care and antiretroviral treatment among men who have sex with men—20 cities, United States. J Infect Dis. 2017;216:808–12.
107. Vermund SH. The continuum of HIV Care in the Urban United States: black men who have sex with men (MSM) are less likely than white MSM to receive antiretroviral therapy. J Infect Dis. 2017;216(7):790–4.

108. Herbst JH, Mansergh PN, Denson D, et al. Effects of brief messages about antiretroviral therapy and condom use benefits among black and Latino MSM in three U.S. cities. J Homosex. 2018;65(2):154–66.
109. Sevelius JM, Saberi P, Johnson MO. Correlates of antiretroviral adherence and viral load among transgender women living with HIV. AIDS Care. 2014;26(8):976–82.
110. Sevelius JM, Patouhas E, Keatley JG, Johnson MO. Barriers and facilitators to engagement and retention in care among transgender women living with human immunodeficiency virus. Ann Behav Med. 2014;47(1):5–16.
111. Rebchook G, Keatley J, Contreras R, Perloff J, Molano LF, Reback CJ, et al. The transgender women of color initiative: implementing and evaluating innovative interventions to enhance engagement and retention in HIV care. Am J Public Health. 2017;107(2):224–9.
112. Centers for Disease Control and Prevention. HIV among youth. https://www.cdc.gov/hiv/group/age/youth/index.html. Last accessed 28 Oct 2018.
113. Agwu AL, Fairlie L. Antiretroviral treatment, management challenges and outcomes in perinatally HIV-infected adolescents. J Int AIDS Soc. 2013;16:18579.
114. Arnett JJ. Emerging adulthood: the winding road from the late teens through the twenties. New York: Oxford University Press; 2004.
115. Blanton RE, Levitt JG, Thompson PM, Narr KL, Capetillo-Cunliffe L, Nobel A, et al. Mapping cortical asymmetry and complexity patterns in normal children. Psychiatry Res Neuroimaging. 2001;107(1):29–43.
116. Toga AW, Thompson PM, Sowell ER. Mapping brain maturation. Trends Neurosci. 2006;29(3):148–59.
117. Prejean J, Song R, Hernandez A, Ziebell R, Green T, Walker F, et al. Estimated HIV incidence in the United States, 2006–2009. PLoS One. 2011;6(8):e17502.
118. Millett GA, Peterson JL, Flores SA, Hart TA, Jeffries WL, Wilson PA, et al. Comparisons of disparities and risks of HIV infection in black and other men who have sex with men in Canada, UK, and USA: a meta-analysis. Lancet. 2012;380(9839):341–8.
119. Lee L, Yehia BR, Gaur AH, Rutstein R, Gebo K, Keruly JC, et al. The impact of youth-friendly structures of care on retention among HIV-infected youth. AIDS Patient Care STDs. 2016;30(4):170–7.
120. Fortenberry JD, Koenig LJ, Kapogiannis BG, Jeffries CL, Ellen JM, Wilson CM. Implementation of an integrated approach to the national HIV/AIDS strategy for improving human immunodeficiency virus care for youths. JAMA Pediatr. 2017;171(7):687–93.
121. Panel on Antiretroviral Guidelines for Adults and Adolescents. Guidelines for the use of antiretroviral agents in adults and adolescents living with HIV. Department of Health and Human Services. Available at http://www.aidsinfo.nih.gov/ContentFiles/AdultandAdolescentGL.pdf. Accessed 29 Mar 2018.
122. Cervia JS. Easing the transition of HIV-infected adolescents to adult care. AIDS Patient Care STDs. 2013;27(12):692–6.
123. Dowshen N, D'Angelo L. Health care transition for youth living with HIV/AIDS. Pediatrics. 2011;128(4):762–71.
124. Mitsch AJ, Hall HI, Babu AS. Trends in HIV infection among persons who inject drugs: United States and Puerto Rico, 2008–2013. Am J Public Health. 2016;106(12):2194–201.
125. Hallfors DD, Iritani BJ, Miller WC, Bauer DJ. Sexual and drug behavior patterns and HIV and STD racial disparities: the need for new directions. Am J Public Health. 2007;97(1):125–32.
126. Burnett JC, Broz D, Spiller MW, Wejnert C, Paz-Bailey G. HIV infection and HIV-associated behaviors among persons who inject drugs – 20 cities, United States, 2015. MMWR Morb Mortal Wkly Rep. 2018;67(1):23–8.
127. Des Jarlais DC, Bramson HA, Wong C, Gostnell K, Cepeda J, Arasteh K, et al. Racial/ethnic disparities in HIV infection among people who inject drugs: an international systematic review and meta-analysis. Addiction. 2012;107(12):2087–95.
128. Lucas GM, Gebo KA, Chaisson RE, Moore RD. Longitudinal assessment of the effects of drug and alcohol abuse on HIV-1 treatment outcomes in an urban clinic. AIDS. 2002;16(5):767–74.

129. Wolfe D, Carrieri MP, Shepard D. Treatment and care for injecting drug users with HIV infection: a review of barriers and ways forward. Lancet. 2010;376(9738):355–66.
130. Milloy MJ, Kerr T, Bangsberg DR, Buxton J, Parashar S, Guillemi S, et al. Homelessness as a structural barrier to effective antiretroviral therapy among HIV-seropositive illicit drug users in a Canadian setting. AIDS Patient Care STDs. 2012;26(1):60–7.
131. Macalino GE, Hogan JW, Mitty JA, Bazerman LB, Delong AK, Loewenthal H, et al. A randomized clinical trial of community-based directly observed therapy as an adherence intervention for HAART among substance users. AIDS. 2007;21(11):1473–7.
132. Miller WC, Hoffman IF, Hanscom BS, Ha TV, Dumchev K, Djoerban Z, et al. A scalable, integrated intervention to engage people who inject drugs in HIV care and medication-assisted treatment (HPTN 074): a randomised, controlled phase 3 feasibility and efficacy study. Lancet. 2018;392(10149):747–59.
133. Wildeman C, Wang EA. Mass incarceration, public health, and widening inequality in the USA. Lancet. 2017;389(10077):1464–74.
134. Substance Abuse and Mental Health Services Administration. Summary of the effects of the 2015 National Survey on drug use and health questionnaire redesign: implications for data users. CBHSQ Methodology Report. Rockville: Center for Behavioral Health Statistics and Quality, Substance Abuse and Mental Health Services Administration; 2016.
135. Eversman MH, Bird JD. Moral panic and social justice: a guide for Analyzing social problems. Soc Work. 2017;62(1):29–36.
136. Costa M, Montague BT, Solomon L, Sammartino C, Gutman R, Zibman C, et al. Assessing the effect of recent incarceration in prison on HIV care retention and viral suppression in two states. J Urban Health. 2018;95(4):499–507.
137. Centers for Disease Prevention and Control. HIV among incarcerated populations. http://www.cdc.gov/hiv/group/correctional.html. Accessed: 1 June 2016.
138. Iroh PA, Mayo H, Nijhawan AE. The HIV care cascade before, during, and after incarceration: a systematic review and data synthesis. Am J Public Health. 2015;105(7):e5–16.
139. Erickson M, Shannon K, Sernick A, Pick N, Ranville F, Martin RE, et al. Women, incarceration and HIV: a systematic review of HIV treatment access, continuity of care and health outcomes across incarceration trajectories. AIDS. 2019;33(1):101–11.
140. Cunningham WE, Weiss RE, Nakazono T, Malek MA, Shoptaw SJ, Ettner SL, et al. Effectiveness of a peer navigation intervention to sustain viral suppression among HIV-positive men and transgender women released from jail: the LINK LA randomized clinical trial. JAMA Intern Med. 2018;178(4):542–53.
141. CDC. CDC fact sheet: HIV among women. 2014. http://www.cdc.gov/hiv/risk/gender/women. Last accessed Feb 2015.
142. CDC. CDC fact sheet: new HIV infections in the United States. 2016. https://www.cdc.gov/nchhstp/newsroom/docs/factsheets/new-hiv-infections-508.pdf. Last accessed Feb 2018.
143. Nachega JB, Uthman OA, Anderson J, Peltzer K, Wampold S, Cotton MF, et al. Adherence to antiretroviral therapy during and after pregnancy in low-income, middle-income, and high-income countries: a systematic review and meta-analysis. AIDS. 2012;26(16):2039–52.
144. Adams JW, Brady KA, Michael YL, Yehia BR, Momplaisir FM. Postpartum engagement in HIV care: an important predictor of long-term retention in care and viral suppression. Clin Infect Dis. 2015;61(12):1880–7.
145. Taylor AW, Nesheim SR, Zhang X, Song R, FitzHarris LF, Lampe MA, et al. Estimated perinatal HIV infection among infants born in the United States, 2002–2013. JAMA Pediatr. 2017;171(5):435–42.
146. Rana AI, Gillani FS, Flanigan TP, Nash BT, Beckwith CG. Follow-up care among HIV-infected pregnant women in Mississippi. J Women's Health. 2010;19(10):1863–7.
147. Meade CM, Badell M, Hackett S,Mehta CC, Haddad LB, Camacho-Gonzalez A, Ford J, Hostad MM, Armstrong WS and Sheth AN. HIV Care Continuum Among Post Partum Women Living in Atlanta. Infect Dis Obstet Gynecol. 2019;2019:8161495. Published 2019 Feb 14. https://doi.org/10.1155/2019/8161495.

148. Rana A JK, Lanier C, Nash B, Zlotnick C, Wingood G, Mena L, Konkle-Parker D, Wilson I. High mortality among HIV-infected women following delivery in Mississippi. In: 12th International conference on HIV treatment and prevention adherence. Miami; 2017.
149. Rana AI JK, Lanier C, Nash B, Zlotnick C, Wingood G, Mena L, Konkle-Parker D, Wilson IB. High mortality and low rates of long term engagement in care following delivery among HIV infected women in Mississippi (oral presentation). In: 11th International conference on HIV treatment and prevention adherence. Ft. Lauderdale; 2016.
150. The National HIV/AIDS Response Overview. https://www.hiv.gov/federal-response/national-hiv-aids-strategy/overview. Last accessed 1 Nov 2018.
151. Walters SM, Reilly KH, Neaigus A, Braunstein S. Awareness of pre-exposure prophylaxis (PrEP) among women who inject drugs in NYC: the importance of networks and syringe exchange programs for HIV prevention. Harm Reduct J. 2017;14(1):40.
152. Johnsen LE, Thimm MA, Singer JM, Page KR. P2.24 Awareness and interest in pre-exposure prophylaxis (PREP) among patients receiving services at a public sexually transmitted diseases (STD) clinic in a high prevalence urban setting. Sex Trans Infect. 2017;93(Suppl 2):A79.72–A79.
153. Chapman Lambert C, Marrazzo J, Amico KR, Mugavero MJ, Elopre L. PrEParing women to prevent HIV: an integrated theoretical framework to PrEP black women in the United States. J Assoc Nurses AIDS Care. 2018;29(6):835–48.
154. Gwadz M, Cleland CM, Kutnick A, Leonard NR, Ritchie AS, Lynch L, et al. Factors associated with recent HIV testing among heterosexuals at high risk for HIV infection in New York City. Front Public Health. 2016;4:76.
155. Levy ME, Wilton L, Phillips G 2nd, Glick SN, Kuo I, Brewer RA, et al. Understanding structural barriers to accessing HIV testing and prevention services among black men who have sex with men (BMSM) in the United States. AIDS Behav. 2014;18(5):972–96.
156. Yehia BR, Stewart L, Momplaisir F, Mody A, Holtzman CW, Jacobs LM, et al. Barriers and facilitators to patient retention in HIV care. BMC Infect Dis. 2015;15:246.
157. Centers for Disease Control and Prevention. Social determinants of health and selected HIV care outcomes among adults with diagnosed HIV infection in 37 states and the District of Columbia, 2015. HIV Surveillance Supplemental Report. 2017;22(No. 4). http://wwwcdc-gov/hiv/library/reports/hiv-surveillancehtml. Published October 2017. Accessed 22 Oct 2018.
158. Wolitski RJ, Kidder DP, Pals SL, Royal S, Aidala A, Stall R, et al. Randomized trial of the effects of housing assistance on the health and risk behaviors of homeless and unstably housed people living with HIV. AIDS Behav. 2010;14(3):493–503.
159. Desir FA, Lesko CR, Moore RD, Horberg MA, Wong C, Crane HM, et al. One size fits (n) one: the influence of sex, age, and sexual human immunodeficiency virus (HIV) acquisition risk on racial/ethnic disparities in the HIV care continuum in the United States. Clin Infect Dis. 2019;68(5):795–802.
160. Tabler J, Mykyta L, Schmitz RM, Kamimura A, Martinez DA, Martinez RD, et al. Social determinants of sexual behavior and awareness of sexually transmitted infections (STI) among low-income HIV+ or STI at-risk hispanic residents receiving care at the U.S.-Mexico Border. J Community Health. 2019;44(1):127–36.
161. Garrido M, Sufrinko N, Max J, Cortes N. Where youth live, learn, and play matters: tackling the social determinants of health in adolescent sexual and reproductive health. Am J Sex Educ. 2018;13(1):1–14.
162. Howland R, Angley M, Won SH, Searing H, Wilcox W. A population-based study of severe maternal morbidity in New York City, 2008–2012 [30C]. Obstet Gynecol. 2016;127:34S.
163. Pellowski JA, Kalichman SC, Matthews KA, Adler N. A pandemic of the poor: social disadvantage and the U.S. HIV epidemic. Am Psychol. 2013;68(4):197–209.
164. De Cock KM, Simone PM, Davison V, Slutsker L. The new global health. Emerg Infect Dis. 2013;19(8):1192–7.
165. Poteat T, Wirtz AL, Radix A, Borquez A, Silva-Santisteban A, Deutsch MB, et al. HIV risk and preventive interventions in transgender women sex workers. Lancet. 2015;385(9964):274–86.

Chapter 3
PrEP and the Black Community

Dawn K. Smith and M. Keith Rawlings

Background

Nearly four decades after recognition of the HIV epidemic in the United States, significant progress has been made in the diagnosis of HIV infection and its treatment resulting in marked decreases in mortality overall. At the same time, despite prevention efforts, the annual number of new HIV diagnoses has stalled in recent years and the disproportionate share of new HIV diagnoses among African-American/black persons (hereafter called black) has not changed. In 1984, 25% of all reported AIDS cases including gay, bisexual, and other men who had sex with men (MSM), persons who had injected drugs (PWID), hemophiliacs, and Haitians were blacks as were 37% of persons not in a recognized risk group [2]. In 2017, of 38,739 new HIV diagnoses in the United States, 43% (16,694) were among black adults and adolescents while blacks composed 13% of the US population in 2017 [3]. Blacks had disproportionate numbers of new HIV diagnoses overall and among MSM, women, and PWID (Table 3.1).

A new HIV prevention method was proven highly effective in 2010 for MSM and in 2012 for heterosexually active adults and for PWID. Preexposure prophylaxis (PrEP) consists of taking a daily pill with the fixed-dose combination of either tenofovir disoproxil fumarate (TDF) and emtricitabine (FTC [Truvada]) or tenofovir alafenamide (TAF) and FTC (Descovy).

In clinical trials, Truvada has been shown to be safe, have few side effects, and to reduce the risk of sexual acquisition by up to 99% if taken with high adherence. Efficacy in PWID was >70% with high adherence. Based on these findings, in 2012

D. K. Smith
Division of HIV/AIDS Prevention, National Center for HIV/AIDS, STD, Viral Hepatitis, and TB Prevention, Centers for Disease Control and Prevention, Atlanta, GA, USA

M. K. Rawlings (✉)
ViiV Healthcare, Research Triangle Park, Durham, NC, USA
e-mail: Keith.m.rawlings@viivhealthcare.com

© Springer Nature Switzerland AG 2021
B. O. Ojikutu, V. E. Stone (eds.), *HIV in US Communities of Color*,
https://doi.org/10.1007/978-3-030-48744-7_3

Table 3.1 New HIV diagnoses, the United States and dependent areas, 2017

	Number (column %): all race/ethnicities	Number (row %): Black
Total	38,739 (100%)	16,694 (43%)
MSM	25,748 (70%)	9807 (38%)
Women	7401 (19%)	4397 (59%)
PWID	3602 (9%)	1697 (47%)

Source: https://www.cdc.gov/hiv/pdf/library/reports/surveil-lance/cdc-hiv-surveillance-report-2017-vol-29.pdf

the FDA approved a PrEP indication for Truvada. In 2019, the US Preventive Services Task Force recommended Truvada for PrEP be offered to persons at substantial risk of HIV acquisition with an "A" grade [4]. Following the first FDA approval, CDC issued clinical guidelines for PrEP use in 2014 and updated them in 2017 [5].

In 2019, a double-blinded, randomized, active control study of adult men who have sex with men (MSM) and transgender women (TGW) found that Descovy was noninferior to Truvada for PrEP. Based on the trial population, the FDA granted an indication in at-risk adults and adolescents (≥ 35 kg) to reduce the risk of sexually acquired HIV-1 infection, excluding individuals at risk from receptive vaginal sex. HIV-1-negative status must be confirmed immediately prior to initiation. DESCOVY FOR PrEP™ is not indicated in individuals at risk of HIV-1 from receptive vaginal sex because effectiveness in this population has not been evaluated.

In the years since 2010, efforts have been made to accelerate PrEP use in all populations who would benefit from it. However, while the number of persons prescribed PrEP has steadily increased, significant racial disparities in PrEP use quickly became apparent and have persisted. CDC estimated in 2015 that 1.1 million people have indications for PrEP use of whom 44% are non-Hispanic blacks, 25% are Hispanic, and 26% are non-Hispanic whites [6]. However, a recent analysis of national PrEP prescription data found that 14.9% of PrEP prescriptions initiated in 2017 were to black persons, 15.3% to Hispanic persons, and 64.0% to white persons [7].

To significantly expand PrEP use among black men and women with indications for its use, a more fully informed understanding of racially and culturally specific constraints to completing the several steps in the continuum of PrEP care must be addressed in order to achieve its full prevention potential.

Knowledge of HIV Status

In prior years, HIV testing has been focused on black and Hispanic MSM primarily for the purpose of identifying persons with HIV infection so they could initiate treatment, both for the benefit of their own health and to reduce the likelihood of transmission to others. People living with HIV who are adherent to antiretroviral (ARV) medications and are virally suppressed pose effectively no risk of HIV transmission to the sexual partners. However, viral suppression rates differ by race/ethnicity. The CDC estimated that in 2015, overall, 51% of all persons living with HIV in the United States (whether infection was diagnosed or undiagnosed) achieved viral suppression, and that blacks had the lowest rate at 46% [8].

While increased efforts have been successful in mitigating disparities in testing, rates remain too low for all racial/ethnic populations. PrEP is only indicated for persons without HIV infection, so increasing HIV testing frequency among persons with risk for HIV acquisition, in whom testing is recommended at least annually, is an important first step. For persons who test negative, it is an opportunity to educate about and offer PrEP. This is especially the case for partner services testing conducted with sexual contacts of persons with HIV or another sexually transmitted infection (STI).

In a partner services study of HIV testing conducted among sexual partners of persons with newly diagnosed HIV infection in 55 jurisdictions, 37.6% of male and 25.4% of female partners with test results were newly diagnosed with HIV infection. Since all were at risk of HIV infection due to sex with a partner newly diagnosed with HIV, approximately two-thirds of men and three-quarters of women who tested HIV negative had indications for PrEP use. Black partners were 1.5 times more likely to test HIV positive than non-Hispanic white partners, male partners were 1.8 times more likely to test positive than female partners, and partners in the South were 2.2 times more likely to test positive than partners in the Midwest [9].

A recent pooled analysis was conducted with 2016 and 2017 data from the nationally representative Behavioral Risk Factor Surveillance System (BRFSS) to examine HIV testing frequency in the 57 jurisdictions that are the initial focus for a federal HIV initiative. Among persons aged ≥18 years who reported HIV risk behaviors (that would indicate utility of PrEP if HIV negative), nationally, 64.8% had ever been tested for HIV infection and 29.2% in the past year. By current recommendations, all persons with risk behaviors should be tested at least annually. In the 50 local jurisdictions that account for nearly half of the HIV burden in the United States, only 34.3% of those with risk behaviors were tested in the past year. In seven states with significant rural epidemics, 18% of those residing in rural areas and 29.0% of those in urban areas were tested in the past year [10].

A meta-analysis of HIV testing patterns among black MSM reported in studies published during 1996–2018 found high lifetime HIV testing (88.2%) but lower annual testing (recent testing, 67.4%) or frequent testing (42.4% every 3–6 months) [11].

As new modalities of STI testing are becoming available, a focus group study asked 36 young black MSM in Alabama to consider the various options. Interestingly, they preferred STI testing in clinical settings performed by clinical staff although they wanted a variety of locations to be available to them (e.g., private doctors, STI clinics, community health centers). While they felt urine samples were easiest and less painful, they trusted blood results more. Home testing was negatively perceived because of concerns about both privacy and accuracy [12]. This is relevant to PrEP care because of the frequent STI testing recommended for PrEP patients. A similar study about preferences of black MSM for HIV testing alternatives would be useful.

Awareness and Knowledge of PrEP

Awareness is the lowest level of knowledge about PrEP, that is, does the person know that an HIV prevention method called PrEP exists [13]. Higher levels of knowledge about PrEP are required to make an informed decision about whether and where to seek PrEP or whether to begin using it. Yet we have the most data for black men and women about their awareness and very little data about any higher level of PrEP knowledge. To our knowledge, no published studies have examined the health information networks of black men and women by which PrEP information could most efficiently be disseminated.

"One Thousand Strong" a longitudinal study of a national panel of HIV-negative gay and bisexual men in the United States reported that of 995 men, 7.6% of whom were black, 65% reported HIV risk behaviors that indicate use of PrEP would be beneficial. Men were asked about PrEP using the framework of the stages of change trans-theoretical model, and 53% were in pre-contemplation, 23% were contemplating PrEP use, 11% were planning to initiate PrEP, and only 4% were taking PrEP medication [14]. In the American Men's Internet Survey (AMIS) conducted during 2014–2015, 63.1% of 333 black men surveyed were aware of PrEP, 68.3% were willing to use PrEP, and 7.5% had used PrEP in the past year [15].

In a survey of 1615 black adult MSM and 58 TGW in New York City, who were HIV negative by self-report (6.6% of whom subsequently tested HIV positive), the respondents were asked questions about PrEP, HIV stigma, and HIV risk behavior. Participants' median age was 40 years, 59.9% identified as bisexual, 23.6% as homosexual, and 13.0% as heterosexual. Among the respondents, 54.8% were homeless and 71.3% were unemployed. Participants reported health provider mistrust and low stigma toward persons with HIV. Overall, only 18.2% were aware of PrEP with a gradual increase over the years of recruitment from 15.5% in 2012 to 28.3% in 2015. In multivariate analysis, men who identified as gay were 2.5 times more likely and those identifying as "other/unknown" sexual orientation were 2.9 times more likely to be aware of PrEP than men who identified as heterosexual. Other independent predictors of PrEP awareness were less education, higher number of sexual partners, more HIV tests in the prior year, younger age, and more problematic alcohol or substance use [16].

Questions about HIV, HIV testing, and PrEP were included in a countywide survey with purposive sampling during a testing initiative in Durham County, NC, during 2015–2016. In this survey, 75% of the 139 respondents were black. No difference in PrEP awareness was seen among black respondents compared with other race/ethnicities. Overall, 38% of respondents were aware of PrEP, including 63% of black MSM. In multivariate analysis, MSM were 5.6 times more likely to be aware of PrEP than were other respondents [17].

A focus group study with 25 young black MSM in Alabama asked about risk perception, stigmas, and PrEP. Five main themes emerged: (1) stigma about race and sexual orientation, (2) absence of community discussion about sexual health and HIV prevention, (3) stigma in the black community about PrEP, (4) limited information about PrEP side effects, and (5) low personal perceived risk of HIV acquisition or need for PrEP [18].

Findings from a 2013 focus group study conducted with 144 women in 6 US cities, 92% of whom were black, reported that few were aware of PrEP prior to study introduction. Many had had an HIV test (59.6%) and many expressed willingness to discuss PrEP with their health care providers. Barriers to PrEP use mentioned were stigma associated with HIV medication, some indication of medical mistrust although many felt they had a good relationship with their own primary care provider (PCP), and few raised cost as a concern. They expressed concern that taking a daily pill would be hard given competing priorities of daily life and were interested in other modalities that may become available (e.g., injectable PrEP) [19].

HIV-negative respondents in the National HIV Behavioral Surveys were asked questions about awareness and use of PrEP. In the MSM survey conducted in 23 cities in 2017, 78.3% of black MSM had heard of PrEP, and 18.8% had ever taken it. In the heterosexual survey conducted in 17 cities in 2016, 7.1% of black men and women had heard of PrEP and 0.2% had ever taken it. In the 2015 survey with PWID in 20 cities, 7.7% of black men and women had heard of PrEP, and 0.2% had ever used it [20].

A variety of approaches have been undertaken to increase awareness of PrEP, with most focused on MSM broadly, and few focused on black MSM, PWID, or heterosexual women and men. These include media campaigns, network interventions, social media, mobile apps, and CBO education efforts. Examples of efforts featuring black men and women are a web-based video https://www.youtube.com/watch?v=mLZsTRPe4uA&feature=youtu.be and the women's campaign https://sexualbeing.org/get-involved/prep-for-her/ designed by the Washington DC Health Department, a national commercial for "Truvada for PrEP" produced by Gilead Sciences https://www.youtube.com/watch?v=6GEOB9aplh0, and Chicago's PrEP4Love campaign https://prep4love.com/about.html. However, no studies have examined the reach and scale of such approaches that would be needed to significantly scale up PrEP use in the large population with indications [21].

Seeking and Obtaining PrEP

For persons who are aware of PrEP, perceived risk of HIV acquisition and resulting perceived need for PrEP is important. However, knowledge of where to obtain PrEP and receiving services from an informed and unbiased provider is also necessary. All of these issues are contributing to the current low use of PrEP by black men and women who have indications for its use.

Interest in the use of PrEP is usually reported as "willingness." However, willingness must be distinguished from demand as indicated by actual initiation of PrEP use. Willingness is often measured with PrEP presented as a hypothetical intervention or without respondents having knowledge of significant aspects of PrEP use. Understanding the requirements for PrEP care (e.g., indications, daily pill-taking, quarterly visits for HIV testing and clinical follow-up, and paperwork for financial coverage) is important context for people to consider when deciding if they are willing or reluctant to initiate PrEP. In addition, "demand" for PrEP implies a perceived need for (additional) HIV protection. A qualitative study of 29 young black MSM in Atlanta offered PrEP reported that their perceived need for PrEP was low even among men who met the indications criteria in the PrEP guidelines [22].

Yet studies have shown that black MSM [18, 22] and women [23, 24] often underestimate their risk of HIV acquisition when compared to behavioral risk criteria. Few studies have examined their understanding of the prevalence of HIV infection in their communities [25] and the role it plays in the increased risk of HIV acquisition. Expressed willingness to take PrEP has varied across studies and subgroups.

In a survey of 225 women in 3 southern states (83% of whom were black), only 11% had heard of PrEP and only 1 had ever taken it. However once informed about PrEP, among those with HIV risk behavior indications for it, 88% expressed willingness to take it [23].

In an urban family clinic in Philadelphia, of 389 women surveyed (65% of whom were black), only 27% had heard of PrEP, 57% indicated they would take it, and 64% felt comfortable discussing it with their health care provider [26].

Black women when interested in PrEP may be discouraged from initiating it by peers with HIV infection [27] or encouraged when female peers are using PrEP [28]. Trust in one's primary health care provider has been shown to predict willingness to discuss and use PrEP [29]. Women are more likely to initiate PrEP if their health care providers recommend it [28].

Ojikutu and colleagues compared reported PrEP use among 308 black men and 479 black women in the National Survey on HIV in the Black Community (NSHBC), a nationally representative sample, to geographic distribution of PrEP providers listed on the PrEP locator website (www.PrEPlocator.org). Among respondents, 23% reported HIV risk behavior, of whom 40.8% were willing to use PrEP (compared to 26% of all persons surveyed). Willingness to use PrEP was associated with being in an area with higher PrEP clinic density but 38% of those surveyed lived >1 hour's driving time from a PrEP clinic [30].

In an analysis of the Veterans Health Administration (VHA) data, among the 39% of charts with documentation of the type of initiation, 85% of PrEP discussions were initiated by the patient. Infectious disease specialists were the most common PrEP prescribers (69%), while primary care providers (PCPs) (13%) and infectious disease pharmacists (7%) prescribed PrEP less often [31].

A widely reported study of 115 medical students reported apparent bias against prescribing PrEP to black MSM [32], but a further mediation analysis of this data showed no evidence for racial bias but did find evidence for an indirect effect of heterosexism [33]. It is not known if the same results would be found in practicing clinicians rather than medical students.

A survey of PCPs in North Carolina found that a lack of knowledge about PrEP was reported by 60% and that PrEP prescribing was low (17%) although it increased among those who attended offered training sessions (35%) [34].

In a 2017 survey of PCPs in six southern jurisdictions where high number of black men and women at substantial risk for HIV acquisition reside, 52.3% of providers reported having never heard about or having little knowledge of PrEP. Only 22.1% had had a patient request PrEP and only 18.1% had prescribed PrEP [35].

Studies in both South Carolina [36] and New York City [37] have shown that health care providers miss many opportunities to provide PrEP to persons with bacterial STIs, many of whom are black, to prevent incident HIV infections.

A national online survey of family planning providers conducted in 2015 found that among 342 potential prescribers who responded, only 38% correctly defined PrEP; only 36% had seen any PrEP guidelines; and 87% wanted education about PrEP [38].

Training options that have been proven effective in increasing PCP knowledge about prescribing PrEP include tele-mentoring [39], public health detailing, and offering continuing medical education (CME) online. However, no published studies have examined the effect of these methods on increasing PrEP provision to black men and women.

While efforts to provide cultural competency training to health care providers are commonly recommended, both to address race/ethnicity and sexual orientation biases, none of the curricula have yet demonstrated significant impact in any area of health care and no impact studies have been published specifically for PrEP. Delivery of this kind of training is time consuming and not widely accepted by clinicians [40].

Taking PrEP

Once prescribed PrEP, adherence to medication dosing is a prerequisite to achieving protection. Studies have shown that missed daily doses are more forgiving for anal sex (e.g., MSM) than for penile-vaginal sex. MSM who take four or more of seven daily doses per week have full protection [41] while women need to take six of seven daily doses [42] to sustain fully protective drug levels. Measuring adherence to PrEP is challenging because self-report has been shown to overestimate adherence when compared to objective measures like dried blood spot analysis of drug levels. Yet, in clinical practice, only self-report and frequency of refills are available. Equally important is continuing PrEP throughout periods of risk for HIV acquisition (persistence).

The HIV Prevention Trials Network (HPTN) study 073 recruited 226 black MSM in Los Angeles, Washington DC, and Chapel Hill, NC, between 2013 and 2015, offered them PrEP, provided supportive services, and followed them with clinical monitoring. Among the men, 79% initiated PrEP, and of these 64% had biologic measures indicating high adherence (≥4 doses per week) at 26 weeks of observation. Only reporting condomless anal sex with an HIV-positive sex partner or casual partners of unknown HIV status was independently associated with initiating PrEP in multivariate analysis. Independent predictors of adherent use were older age, knowing a male partner taking PrEP before having sex, and feeling that they had enough money. As a result, HIV incidence among PrEP users was 2.9 per 100 person years vs. 7.7 in the non-PrEP users. All seroconversions among PrEP users were associated with having discontinued PrEP or having no/low drug levels indicating inadequate adherence to achieve protection [43].

The US Veterans Health Administration (VHA) has gradually scaled up PrEP provision from 27 patients who initiated in 2012–2013 to 691 in 2016–2017. Among VHA patients, 91% were male, which is similar to the national estimate of 97% of PrEP patients in 2017. Of 688 PrEP prescriptions in 2016 (both initiations and continuations), 23% were for black patients while blacks comprised 12% of the VHA population in 2016 [44]. Adherence to PrEP in the first year was found to be high for VHA patients with the median having refills that covered >74% of days (equivalent to >5 doses of the 7 prescribed per week). In multivariate analysis, higher adherence was associated with male sex, older age, white race, and having diabetes. However, 44% of patients discontinued PrEP during the first year, and discontinuations were more common among younger, black, and female PrEP users [45]. In another analysis of the VHA PrEP data from 2012 to 2016, 20% of PrEP patients were black, 75.9% were MSM, 8.7% were bisexual men, 7.6% were heterosexual men, 2.3% were heterosexual women, 0.6% were transgender, and 0.9% were PWID. PrEP initiations were concentrated in 3 states, including 27% in California, 8.6% in Florida, and 7.6% in Texas, all states with large black populations [31].

Data from a chart review of 267 PrEP patients in Providence, RI, St. Louis, MO, and Jackson, MS, reported that black MSM who initiated PrEP had an 87% reduced odds of persistence at 3 months compared to those of any other race/ethnicity and among those continuing at 3 months, a 26% reduced odds of persistence at 3 months [46].

In a retrospective cohort analysis of persons receiving PrEP in a large health care system in New York City, 23% of whom were black, persistence did not differ by race/ethnicity or a variety of demographic and social factors assessed. Retention was lower in patients <30 years of age, those who initiated PrEP in a sexual health clinic, and those who were given prescriptions on the same day they were assessed for indications. Overall, 68% of patients were retained at the first follow-up visit but only 34% by the third quarterly follow-up visit [47].

Both adherence and persistence have been shown to be particularly low among black adolescents and young adults [48]. In an open-label study of 200 young MSM 18–22 years of age at enrollment, and 55% of whom were black, 56% had protective drug levels on dried blood spots at 4 weeks of follow-up but only 34% at 48 weeks. Median drug levels for black participants were not protective at all time points. By 48 weeks, 29% of all young men in the study had been lost to follow-up or had withdrawn from the study [49].

No published data are yet available about PrEP adherence or persistence among PWID in the United States. To begin that conversation, Bazzi conducted a systematic review of facilitators for and barriers to antiretroviral therapy (ART) adherence in PWID [50]. They found that younger age, female sex, non-white race/ethnicity, and competing social needs (e.g., homelessness, unemployment, low education) were barriers. Enablers included a good provider-patient relationship, use of medication-assisted therapy (MAT), and social support.

Event-Driven PrEP

Although not recommended in CDC PrEP guidelines or FDA approved, event driven, non-daily dosing of TDF/FTC has been proven effective in French MSM [51]. Although trials did not include American MSM of any race/ethnicity, it has been adopted as an alternative strategy in IAS-USA guidelines [52] and those in New York State and San Francisco. This regimen, sometimes called "2-1-1" dosing, entails taking 2 doses in the 2–24 hours before sex, followed by a dose 24 hours later, and then a final dose 48 hours later. This regimen is intended for MSM who have sex infrequently enough that periodic dosing may be preferred to daily use. This regimen has not been studied in heterosexual men and women or in PWID and the pharmacokinetics suggest it is unlikely to be effective in these populations unlike in MSM [53]. The HPTN 067/ADAPT study examined adherence to daily vs. two non-daily dosing schedules among 176 MSM in Harlem, New York, of whom 59% were black. Many MSM had difficulty anticipating sex as required for appropriate use of a "2-1-1" regimen. Adherence measured by hair and blood drug levels showed that more sex acts were covered with protective levels of medication among those using daily dosing than either of the non-daily regimens [54–56]. Given the high risk of HIV acquisition faced by black MSM, daily PrEP should be recommended for most to offer the highest level of protection.

Future PrEP Modalities

While daily oral medication is the only FDA-approved form of PrEP currently, studies are underway to assess the safety and HIV prevention effectives of antiretroviral medications delivered by injection every few months (cabotegravir), vaginal rings that would be changed monthly (dapivirine, TDF), and subdermal implants that may deliver medication at protective levels for 6–12 months (islatravir, TAF). If and when any of these new PrEP methods are FDA approved in the next few years, PrEP use will increase as persons who prefer these modalities have access to non-pill options.

Getting to Equitable Impact

Increasing adherent, persistent PrEP use in black men and women with indications for its use is imperative. The lifetime risk for HIV acquisition for those uninfected at age 18 is 1 in 97 among black heterosexual men, 1 in 54 among black heterosexual women, 1 in 11 among black male PWID, 1 in 7 among black female PWID, and 1 in 2 among black MSM [57]. And despite the availability of effective treatment, HIV was in the top ten causes of death in 2015 for black women aged 20–54 [58] and black men aged 20–64 [59].

A recent study in Australia where rapid scale up of PrEP occurred among MSM, there was a 32% decline in new HIV infections comparing the year after scale-up to the year before it began [60], demonstrating the potential for significant population-level impact with increased PrEP use. However, a model that examined levels of PrEP awareness, uptake, adherence, and retention needed to reduce HIV incidence significantly in black MSM in the United States found that even with levels twice than that seen in white MSM, while a significant reduction among black MSM was predicted, parity in HIV incidence reduction would not be achieved [61].

As the federal initiative "Ending the HIV Epidemic: A Plan for America" gets underway, it will be critical to fully address the glaring inequity in PrEP use by black men and women [62]. If PrEP scale up occurs primarily among white men (as current use is concentrated), it is likely that the disparity in PrEP use among black men and women will increase. Preventing this requires more generalizable research focused on the black community so that findings can be used to deliver PrEP at scale in diverse settings. In addition, rapid assessment methods to understand what is working and what is not can allow for redirection of efforts, and substantially more implementation research is needed to understand how best to address patient, environmental, and health systems issues specific to black men and women at substantial risk of HIV infection [63]. Beyond issues of social justice that are invoked by the current inequity, it will not be possible to achieve the initiative goal of 75% reduction in HIV incidence in 5 years and by at least 90% in 10 years, without markedly increasing PrEP use among black men and women who currently account for nearly half of new HIV infections.

References

1. Fauci AS, Redfield RR, Sigounas G, Weahkee MD, Giroir BP. Ending the HIV epidemic: a plan for the United States. JAMA. 2019;321(9):844–5.
2. Chamberland ME, Castro KG, Haverkos HW, Miller BI, Thomas PA, Reiss R, et al. Acquired immunodeficiency syndrome in the United States: an analysis of cases outside high-incidence groups. Ann Intern Med. 1984;101(5):617–23.
3. Centers for Disease Control and Prevention. Diagnoses of HIV infection in the United States and dependent areas, HIV Surveillance Report, 2017; 29. Retrieved 2 July 2019, from https://www.cdc.gov/hiv/pdf/library/reports/surveillance/cdc-hiv-surveillance-report-2017-vol-29.pdf.
4. US Preventive Services Task Force. Final recommendation statement: prevention of Human Immunodeficiency Virus (HIV) infection: preexposure prophylaxis. [Internet]. 2019. Retrieved 2 July 2019, from https://www.uspreventiveservicestaskforce.org/Page/Document/RecommendationStatementFinal/prevention-of-human-immunodeficiency-virus-hiv-infection-pre-exposure-prophylaxis.
5. Centers for Disease Control and Prevention. US Public Health Service: preexposure prophylaxis for the prevention of HIV infection in the United States—2017 Update: a clinical practice guideline2018. Retrieved 2 July 2019, from https://www.cdc.gov/hiv/pdf/risk/prep/cdc-hiv-prep-guidelines-2017.pdf.
6. Smith DK, Van Handel M, Grey J. Estimates of adults with indications for HIV pre-exposure prophylaxis by jurisdiction, transmission risk group, and race/ethnicity, United States, 2015. Ann Epidemiol. 2018;28(12):850–7.e9.

7. Nguyen C HT, Anderson J, Bush S, Dinh T, McCallister S, Mera R. Utilization of emtricitabine/tenofovir disoproxil fumarate (FTC/TDF) for HIV pre-exposure prophylaxis (PrEP) in the United States by age, gender and ethnicity (2014–2017). 10th IAS conference on HIV science (IAS 2019); Mexico City, 2019.
8. Centers for Disease Control and Prevention. Selected National HIV prevention and care outcomes. 2017. Retrieved 26 July 2019, from https://www.cdc.gov/hiv/pdf/library/slidesets/cdc-hiv-prevention-and-care-outcomes.pdf.
9. Song W, Mulatu MS, Rorie M, Zhang H, Gilford JW. HIV testing and positivity patterns of partners of HIV-diagnosed people in partner services programs, United States, 2013–2014. Public Health Rep. 2017;132(4):455–62.
10. Pitasi MA, Delaney KP, Brooks JT, DiNenno EA, Johnson SD, Prejean J. HIV testing in 50 local jurisdictions accounting for the majority of new HIV diagnoses and seven states with disproportionate occurrence of HIV in rural areas, 2016–2017. MMWR Morb Mortal Wkly Rep. 2019;68(25):561–7.
11. Liu Y, Silenzio VMB, Nash R, Luther P, Bauermeister J, Vermund S, et al. Suboptimal recent and regular HIV testing among black men who have sex with men in the United States: implications from a meta-analysis. J Acquir Immune Defic Syndr. 2019;81(2):125–33.
12. Eaton EF, Austin EL, Dodson CK, Heudebert JP, Muzny CA. Do young black men who have sex with men in the deep south prefer traditional over alternative STI testing? PLoS One. 2018;13(12):e0209666.
13. Trevethan R. Deconstructing and assessing knowledge and awareness in public health research. Front Public Health. 2017;5:194.
14. Parsons JT, Rendina HJ, Lassiter JM, Whitfield TH, Starks TJ, Grov C. Uptake of HIV pre-exposure prophylaxis (PrEP) in a national cohort of gay and bisexual men in the United States: the motivational PrEP cascade. J Acquir Immune Defic Syndr. 2017;74(3):285.
15. Li J, Berg CJ, Kramer MR, Haardörfer R, Zlotorzynska M, Sanchez TH. An integrated examination of county-and individual-level factors in relation to HIV pre-exposure prophylaxis awareness, willingness to use, and uptake among men who have sex with men in the US. AIDS Behav. 2019;23(7):1721–36.
16. Garnett M, Hirsch-Moverman Y, Franks J, Hayes-Larson E, El-Sadr WM, Mannheimer S. Limited awareness of pre-exposure prophylaxis among black men who have sex with men and transgender women in New York city. AIDS Care. 2018;30(1):9–17.
17. Zhang HL, Murthy B, Johnston B, Mortiboy M, Wu J, Samsa GP, et al. Public awareness of HIV pre-exposure prophylaxis in Durham, North Carolina: results of a community survey. N C Med J. 2019;80(1):7–11.
18. Elopre L, McDavid C, Brown A, Shurbaji S, Mugavero MJ, Turan JM. Perceptions of HIV pre-exposure prophylaxis among young, black men who have sex with men. AIDS Patient Care STDs. 2018;32(12):511–8.
19. Auerbach JD, Kinsky S, Brown G, Charles V. Knowledge, attitudes, and likelihood of pre-exposure prophylaxis (PrEP) use among US women at risk of acquiring HIV. AIDS Patient Care STDs. 2015;29(2):102–10.
20. Centers for Disease Control and Prevention. National HIV behavioral surveys – reports. 2019. Retrieved 2 July 2019, from https://www.cdc.gov/hiv/statistics/systems/nhbs/reports.html.
21. Sophus AI, Mitchell JW. A review of approaches used to increase awareness of pre-exposure prophylaxis (PrEP) in the United States. AIDS Behav. 2018:1–22.
22. Lockard A, Rosenberg ES, Sullivan PS, Kelley CF, Serota DP, Rolle C-PM, et al. Contrasting self-perceived need and guideline-based indication for HIV pre-exposure prophylaxis among young, black men who have sex with men offered pre-exposure prophylaxis in Atlanta, Georgia. AIDS Patient Care STDs. 2019;33(3):112–9.
23. Patel AS, Goparaju L, Sales JM, Mehta CC, Blackstock OJ, Seidman D, et al. Brief report: PrEP eligibility among at-risk women in the southern United States: associated factors, awareness, and acceptability. J Acquir Immune Defic Syndr. 2019;80(5):527–32.

24. Sales JM, Sheth AN. Associations among perceived HIV risk, behavioral risk and interest in PrEP among black women in the southern US. AIDS Behav. 2019;23(7):1871–76.
25. Blackstock OJ, Frew P, Bota D, Vo-Green L, Parker K, Franks J, et al. Perceptions of community HIV/STI risk among US women living in areas with high poverty and HIV prevalence rates. J Health Care Poor Underserved. 2015;26(3):811.
26. Koren DE, Nichols JS, Simoncini GM. HIV pre-exposure prophylaxis and women: survey of the knowledge, attitudes, and beliefs in an urban obstetrics/gynecology clinic. AIDS Patient Care STDs. 2018;32(12):490–4.
27. Goparaju L, Experton LS, Praschan NC, Warren-Jeanpiere L, Young MA, Kassaye S. Women want pre-exposure prophylaxis but are advised against it by their HIV-positive counterparts. J AIDS Clin Res. 2015;6(11):1.
28. Wingood GM, Dunkle K, Camp C, Patel S, Painter JE, Rubtsova A, et al. Racial differences and correlates of potential adoption of pre-exposure prophylaxis (PrEP): results of a national survey. J Acquir Immune Defic Syndr. 2013;63(0 1):S95.
29. Braksmajer A, Fedor TM, Chen S-R, Corales R, Holt S, Valenti W, et al. Willingness to take PrEP for HIV prevention: the combined effects of race/ethnicity and provider trust. AIDS Educ Prev. 2018;30(1):1–12.
30. Ojikutu BO, Bogart LM, Mayer KH, Stopka TJ, Sullivan PS, Ransome Y, et al. Spatial access and willingness to use pre-exposure prophylaxis among Black/African American individuals in the United States: cross-sectional survey. J Med Inf Res Public Health. 2019;5(1):e12405.
31. Garner W, Wilson BM, Beste L, Maier M, Ohl ME, Van Epps P. Gaps in preexposure prophylaxis uptake for HIV prevention in the Veterans Health Administration. Am J Public Health. 2018;108(S4):S305–S10.
32. Calabrese SK, Earnshaw VA, Underhill K, Hansen NB, Dovidio JF. The impact of patient race on clinical decisions related to prescribing HIV pre-exposure prophylaxis (PrEP): assumptions about sexual risk compensation and implications for access. AIDS Behav. 2014;18(2):226–40.
33. Calabrese SK, Earnshaw VA, Krakower DS, Underhill K, Vincent W, Magnus M, et al. A closer look at racism and heterosexism in medical students' clinical decision-making related to HIV pre-exposure prophylaxis (PrEP): implications for PrEP education. AIDS Behav. 2018;22(4):1122–38.
34. Clement ME, Seidelman J, Wu J, Alexis K, McGee K, Okeke NL, et al. An educational initiative in response to identified PrEP prescribing needs among PCPs in the Southern US. AIDS Care. 2018;30(5):650–5.
35. Henny KD, Duke CC, Geter A, Gaul Z, Frazier C, Peterson J, et al. HIV-related training and correlates of knowledge, HIV screening and prescribing of nPEP and PrEP among primary care providers in Southeast United States. AIDS Behav. 2017;2019:1–10.
36. Smith DK, Chang M-H, Duffus WA, Okoye S, Weissman S. Missed opportunities to prescribe preexposure prophylaxis in South Carolina, 2013–2016. Clin Infect Dis. 2018;68(1):37–42.
37. Mclaughlin S, Pitts R, Kapadia F, Greene R. Capturing missed opportunities for PrEP prescription in patient diagnosed with other STIs. ST I& HIV World Congress; Vancouver, Canada. Br Med J. 2019;95(Suppl 1):A202.
38. Seidman D, Carlson K, Weber S, Newmann S, Witt J. Family planning providers' knowledge of and attitudes toward preexposure prophylaxis for HIV prevention: a national survey. Contraception. 2015;92(4):411.
39. Wood BR, Mann MS, Martinez-Paz N, Unruh KT, Annese M, Spach DH, et al. Project ECHO: telementoring to educate and support prescribing of HIV pre-exposure prophylaxis by community medical providers. Sex Health. 2018;15(6):601–5.
40. McGregor B, Belton A, Henry TL, Wrenn G, Holden KB. Improving behavioral health equity through cultural competence training of health care providers. Ethn Dis. 2019;29(Suppl 2):359–64.
41. Grant RM, Anderson PL, McMahan V, Liu A, Amico KR, Mehrotra M, et al. Uptake of pre-exposure prophylaxis, sexual practices, and HIV incidence in men and transgender women who have sex with men: a cohort study. Lancet Infect Dis. 2014;14(9):820–9.

42. Cottrell ML, Yang KH, Prince HM, Sykes C, White N, Malone S, et al. A translational pharmacology approach to predicting outcomes of preexposure prophylaxis against HIV in men and women using tenofovir disoproxil fumarate with or without emtricitabine. J Infect Dis. 2016;214(1):55–64.
43. Wheeler DP, Fields SD, Beauchamp G, Chen YQ, Emel LM, Hightow-Weidman L, et al. Pre-exposure prophylaxis initiation and adherence among black men who have sex with men (MSM) in three US cities: results from the HPTN 073 study. J Int AIDS Soc. 2019;22(2):e25223.
44. Chartier M, Gylys-Cowell I, Van Epps P, Beste LA, Ohl M, Lowy E, et al. Accessibility and uptake of pre-exposure prophylaxis for HIV prevention in the veterans health administration. Fed Pract. 2018;35(Suppl 2):S42.
45. van Epps P, Maier M, Lund B, Howren MB, Beck B, Beste L, et al. Medication adherence in a nationwide cohort of veterans initiating pre-exposure prophylaxis (PrEP) to prevent HIV infection. J Acquir Immune Defic Syndr. 2018;77(3):272–8.
46. Chan PA, Mena L, Patel R, Oldenburg CE, Beauchamps L, Perez-Brumer AG, et al. Retention in care outcomes for HIV pre-exposure prophylaxis implementation programmes among men who have sex with men in three US cities. J Int AIDS Soc. 2016;19(1):20903.
47. Zucker J, Carnevale C, Richards P, Slowikowski J, Borsa A, Gottlieb F, et al. Predictors of disengagement in care for individuals receiving pre-exposure prophylaxis (PrEP). JAIDS J Acquired Immune Defic Syndr. 2019;81(4):e104–e8.
48. Arrington-Sanders R, Wilson CM, Perumean-Chaney SE, Patki A, Hosek S. Brief report: role of sociobehavioral factors in subprotective TFV-DP levels among YMSM enrolled in 2 PrEP trials. J Acquired Immune Defic Syndr. 2019;80(2):160–5.
49. Hosek S, Rudy B, Landovitz R, Kapogiannis B, Siberry G, Rutledge B, et al. An HIV pre-exposure prophylaxis (PrEP) demonstration project and safety study for young MSM. J Acquir Immune Defic Syndr. 2017;74(1):21.
50. Bazzi AR, Drainoni M-L, Biancarelli DL, Hartman JJ, Mimiaga MJ, Mayer KH, et al. Systematic review of HIV treatment adherence research among people who inject drugs in the United States and Canada: evidence to inform pre-exposure prophylaxis (PrEP) adherence interventions. BMC Public Health. 2019;19(1):31.
51. Molina J-M, Charreau I, Spire B, Cotte L, Chas J, Capitant C, et al. Efficacy, safety, and effect on sexual behaviour of on-demand pre-exposure prophylaxis for HIV in men who have sex with men: an observational cohort study. Lancet HIV. 2017;4(9):e402–e10.
52. Saag MS, Benson CA, Gandhi RT, Hoy JF, Landovitz RJ, Mugavero MJ, et al. Antiretroviral drugs for treatment and prevention of HIV infection in adults: 2018 recommendations of the International Antiviral Society–USA Panel. JAMA. 2018;320(4):379–96.
53. Anderson PL, García-Lerma JG, Heneine W. Non-daily pre-exposure prophylaxis for HIV prevention. Curr Opin HIV AIDS. 2016;11(1):94.
54. Grant RM, Mannheimer S, Hughes JP, Hirsch-Moverman Y, Loquere A, Chitwarakorn A, et al. Daily and nondaily oral preexposure prophylaxis in men and transgender women who have sex with men: the Human Immunodeficiency Virus Prevention Trials Network 067/ADAPT Study. Clin Infect Dis. 2018;66(11):1712–21.
55. Velloza J, Bacchetti P, Hendrix CW, Murnane P, Hughes JP, Li M, et al. Short and long-term pharmacologic measures of HIV pre-exposure prophylaxis use among high-risk men who have sex with men in HPTN 067/ADAPT. J Acquir Immune Defic Syndr. 2019;82(2):149–58.
56. Mannheimer S, Hirsch-Moverman Y, Franks J, Loquere A, Hughes JP, Li M, et al. Factors associated with sex-related pre-exposure prophylaxis adherence among men who have sex with men in New York City in HPTN 067. J Acquir Immune Defic Syndr. 2019;80(5):551.
57. Hess KL, Hu X, Lansky A, Mermin J, Hall HI. Lifetime risk of a diagnosis of HIV infection in the United States. Ann Epidemiol. 2017;27(4):238–43.
58. National Center for Health Statistics. Leading Causes of Death (LCOD) by age group, black females-United States, 2015. 2018. Retrieved 22 July 2019, from https://www.cdc.gov/women/lcod/2015/black/index.htm.

59. National Center for Health Statistics. Leading Causes of Death (LCOD) by Age Group, Black Males-United States, 2015. 2018. Retrieved 22 July 2019, from https://www.cdc.gov/healthequity/lcod/men/2015/black/index.htm.
60. Grulich AE, Guy R, Amin J, Jin F, Selvey C, Holden J, et al. Population-level effectiveness of rapid, targeted, high-coverage roll-out of HIV pre-exposure prophylaxis in men who have sex with men: the EPIC-NSW prospective cohort study. Lancet HIV. 2018;5(11):e629–e37.
61. Jenness SM, Maloney KM, Smith DK, Hoover KW, Goodreau SM, Rosenberg ES, et al. Addressing gaps in HIV preexposure prophylaxis care to reduce racial disparities in HIV incidence in the United States. Am J Epidemiol. 2018;188(4):743–52.
62. Departnment of Health and Human Services. What is 'ending the HIV epidemic: a plan for America'?. 2019. Retrieved 22 July 2019, from https://www.hiv.gov/federal-response/ending-the-hiv-epidemic/overview.
63. Department of Health and Human Services. Flyer: ending the HIV epidemic: a plan for America. 2019. Retrieved 22 July 2019, from https://files.hiv.gov/s3fs-public/ending-the-hiv-epidemic-flyer.pdf.

Chapter 4
HIV Prevention, Care, and Treatment Among Black Men Who Have Sex with Men (MSM)

Leo Wilton

Introduction

Nearly four decades since the onset of the HIV epidemic, black men who have sex with men (MSM) have been severely affected by HIV burden, indicative of an urgent public health crisis in the United States [1–4]. Within this context, MSM refer to gay, bisexually, and heterosexually identified men who engage in sexual behavior with other men. Current research has shown that a multitude of epidemiologic, structural, and psychosocial factors has contributed to the disparate HIV incidence and prevalence rates of black MSM [2]. Acute HIV infection, a higher prevalence of HIV and other sexually transmitted infections (STIs) within sexual networks, low rates of viral suppression, irregular HIV testing/STI patterns, and undiagnosed and untreated HIV/STI infections have served as key epidemiologic factors that influence HIV/STI vulnerability among black MSM [3–6]. Structural factors that have contributed to HIV-related inequities among black MSM include inadequate access to health care and treatment, socioeconomic factors (being uninsured and underinsured, income and educational inequalities, un-/underemployment, housing, and food instability), incarceration, stigma, discrimination, and immigration status [1, 7–17]. These current trends have been indicative of a persistent increase in the incidence and prevalence of HIV and AIDS among black MSM in the United States.

Building on the current research in this area, the objective of this chapter is to better understand the prevention, care, and treatment considerations for black MSM. Thus, this chapter examines (1) theoretical approaches to HIV prevention with a specific focus on the role of stigma, marginalization, and structural inequalities in black MSM communities; (2) factors associated with HIV prevention in

L. Wilton (✉)
Department of Human Development, College of Community and Public Affairs (CCPA),
State University of New York at Binghamton, Binghamton, NY, USA
e-mail: lwilton@binghamton.edu

© Springer Nature Switzerland AG 2021
B. O. Ojikutu, V. E. Stone (eds.), *HIV in US Communities of Color*,
https://doi.org/10.1007/978-3-030-48744-7_4

black MSM; and (3) psychosocial support and mental health needs in black MSM communities. In particular, culturally-relevant conceptualizations for black MSM that articulate the significance of a paradigm shift in the field of public health that integrates core theoretical premises of interdisciplinarity, intersectionality, and structural inequalities undergird this chapter. Parallel to these fundamental ideas, this work will provide praxis—theoretical applications and strategies for engaging the intersection of race/ethnicity, gender, sexuality, immigration status, and social class—that transcend traditional ways of thinking and focuses on the socio-cultural contexts associated with the HIV epidemic in black MSM communities.

Theoretical Approaches to HIV Prevention in Black MSM Communities

The Role of Stigma, Marginalization, and Structural Inequalities

A key element in addressing HIV-related health disparities for black MSM relates to the development of theoretical frameworks that are grounded within culturally relevant conceptualizations [18]. Within this context, a critical analytic framework for HIV prevention research, including theory, methodologies, and praxis, incorporates a connection to the interface of racial, gender, sexual, and social class politics [19]. Thus, a major part of this work calls for a paradigm shift that links HIV prevention within intersectional and interdisciplinary discourses that correspond with sociocultural factors that are relevant to the life experiences of black MSM. In particular, the concepts of stigma, marginalization, and structural inequalities provide a theoretical framework to examine the complexities of the HIV epidemic, as situated in the everyday lived experiences of black MSM.

Building on the work of Cohen [19], these fundamental ideas provide a conceptual framework for addressing asymmetrical power relationships (i.e., power inequalities) in black communities, including those who incorporate socio-historical and -political experiences of "exclusion and marginalization" based on race/ethnicity, gender, sexuality, and social class. Further, as articulated by Cohen [19], a major component of these critical analyses relates to the duality of examining macro (e.g., external processes) and micro (e.g., internal processes) structures that have an impact on black communities in relation to the HIV epidemic. For example, macro-level processes involve marginalization associated with broader social structures (e.g., structural inequalities based on legal, political, economic, and educational social structures such as institutionalized racism) and micro-level processes that relate to "secondary marginalization" (e.g., based on gender and sexuality) within black communities [19]. Therefore, the integration of transformative discourses in the area of HIV that provide intersectional and interdisciplinary analyses serves as significant interventions in the field of public health. As such, this scholarly work must be at the center of the discourse through incorporating critical, innovative, and transformative analyses that interrogate and challenge hegemonic, Eurocentric, patriarchal, and hetero-normative discourses that pathologize black communities.

In the field of public health, the production of knowledge in HIV prevention research has been based, in part, on epistemological/theoretical frameworks in bio-medical and social science research that have not incorporated critical interdisci-plinary and intersectional approaches in the study of HIV-related health inequities from a health justice standpoint based on a systematic approach for black MSM communities [20]. In particular, the work of Mullings and Schulz [21] is relevant here, and it provides an account of the significance of incorporating intersectional approaches as a mechanism to better understand and to develop theoretical formula-tions that address health disparities within the sociocultural contexts of communi-ties: ". . . . Intersectional theory views race, gender, class [and sexuality] not as fixed and discrete categories or as properties of individuals but as social constructs that both reflect and reinforce unequal relationships between classes, racial groups, gen-ders, [and sexualities]" (p. 373) [21].

Core theoretical paradigms in the areas of public health and social science research that relate to HIV prevention have been primarily based on Western/ Eurocentric theoretical or conceptual frameworks that focus on individual behavior (e.g., social cognitive theoretical frameworks) [20]. As a result, the production of knowledge in HIV prevention research has often been shaped within an insular dis-ciplinary context, thus maintaining a disconnection from transformative scholarly inquiries as well as the sociocultural realities of the lived experiences of black MSM communities. Thus, as situated through an intersectional theoretical conceptualiza-tion, one of the major problematic implications of this logic is that the multiple identities of black MSM (e.g., racial, gender, and sexual identities) have been nega-tively constructed and pathologized through theoretical frameworks that have not adequately integrated the sociohistorical, sociopolitical, socioeconomic, and socio-cultural contexts that have been integral to the cultural specificities of their lived experiences [19].

Another major limitation of the socioeconomic (SES) discourse in public health involves the absence or peripheralization of the socio-historical and -political impact of marginalization based on racial hierarchies in the United States (e.g., institution-alized racism) [22–25]. Historically, several scholars have challenged the hege-monic, Eurocentric theoretical paradigms that have been utilized in research on black communities [25]. For example, the historical legacy of cultural mistrust has been a central theme related to the health experiences (e.g., medical experimenta-tion on black men and black women) of black communities in the United States [26]. A recent significant illustration of medical abuse has been documented in black and Latino/a children living with HIV in foster care in the New York Metropolitan Area. These youth of color were mandated by a child welfare agency to take highly toxic and experimental HIV drug medicines [26]. More specifically, over the years, several scholars have documented the cumulative effects of the Tuskegee Syphilis Experiment that was conducted on black men to study untreated tertiary syphilis in Macon County, Alabama, from 1932 through 1972 by the US Public Health Service [27]. Researchers also have investigated cultural mistrust and cultural beliefs about AIDS-related genocide in black communities [28]. In particular, as black MSM have experienced a significant impact of the HIV epidemic, cultural mistrust and cultural beliefs about genocide have had an impact on HIV prevention as a result of the historical experiences with the medical establishment [29], including the Tuskegee Syphilis Experiment Study [27].

Integrating Interdisciplinary and Intersectional Approaches in Health Disparities

Building on interdisciplinary and intersectional theoretical approaches, an integral component to the study of health inequities in black MSM communities is the incorporation and application of epistemological/theoretical frameworks and methodologies based on cultural studies (e.g., African Diaspora Studies and Caribbean Studies), gender studies, and sexuality studies. One of the objectives in utilizing the scholarly work of these areas in the study of health inequities relates to the development of epistemological/theoretical frameworks that provide the basis for incorporating the socio-historical, -political, -economic, and -cultural contexts that have been integral in black communities. As such, theoretical and methodological approaches based on these scholarly areas work to juxtapose theory and practice that are grounded in culturally relevant conceptualizations, which are fundamental to the lived experiences of black MSM. According to [30], "Central to this intersectional theory is the tenet that racism and sexism, as well as other forms of oppression . . . operate as mutually reinforcing systems of inequality" (p. 371). These areas provide a critical approach to the work on health disparities that engage a critique of service at macro- and micro-levels with respect to the sociopolitical processes that influence structural inequalities in black MSM communities. This paradigm shift has the promise of providing opportunities to engage intellectually rigorous dialogues regarding the centrality of social justice perspectives as well as an interrogation of knowledge to incorporate intersectional and interdisciplinary approaches within the domain of health disparities.

One contemporary illustration of the innovative scholarly research on black MSM communities that incorporates culturally grounded theoretical, methodological, and community-centered approaches has related to research on house ball communities [31, 32]. This research provides originality within the context of integrating intersectional and interdisciplinary perspectives that are integrated into the core of the analysis within the context of HIV prevention. According to the researchers, house ball communities have been conceptualized as a network or group of individuals who are connected through houses, which serve as familial, cultural, and supportive systems (e.g., fictive kin) for MSM of color (with a particular focus on black, Latino/a/x, and trans communities). In this ethnographic investigation, the researchers examined the critical role that house ball communities have served in building home and kinship networks, including a core value of articulating the importance of gender and sexuality expression as an integral part of an individual's racial, gender, and sexual identities [31]. As such, this work is particularly relevant for groups that have experienced multiple forms of marginalization based on the intersection of racial, gender, social class, and heteronormative hierarchies as well as those that manifest in customary HIV prevention interventions developed for black MSM. The findings of this study demonstrated that house ball communities have assumed a salient leadership role in providing HIV prevention "intraventions" (e.g., prevention work that occurs organically within the context of the communities) for groups that often have experienced stigma and discrimination [31]. The implications of this work for providing culturally applicable HIV prevention "intraventions" for black MSM communities represent transformative approaches in the field of public health.

Sociocultural Factors as Innovative Theoretical Frameworks

Connected to stigma, marginalization, and structural inequalities, recent research has examined the effect of sociocultural factors on HIV sexual risk behavior in black MSM [33–35]. In one study, Ayala et al. [33] incorporated the concept of social oppression as a core domain to account, in part, for the disproportionate health-related disparities in HIV based on their work with a probability sample of African American and Latino MSM surveyed from three US cities. The researchers provided an intersectional, tripartite model that found empirical support for the impact of sociocultural factors (e.g., racism, homophobia, and poverty) on HIV sexual risk behavior among the men. The findings from this study demonstrated that social oppression based on racism, poverty, and homophobia related to sexual experiences that provided the context for HIV sexual risk behavior with a serodiscordant or sero-status unknown partner. Specifically, social oppression (e.g., racism, poverty, and homophobia) was mediated through participation in HIV sexual risk behaviors and inadequate social support. Taken together, these research investigations provide theoretical and empirical support in examining the impact of racism, homophobia, and poverty as these intersectional domains manifest in the lives of MSM of color.

Factors Related to HIV Prevention in Black MSM

Preexposure Prophylaxis (PrEP) as Biomedical Prevention in Black MSM

The implementation of HIV antiretroviral medicines as a form of biomedical prevention represents a vital component of the multilevel prevention strategies to modulate HIV acquisition [36]. Randomized clinical trials have demonstrated the efficacy of antiretroviral preexposure prophylaxis (PrEP) in preventing HIV acquisition among men who have sex with men (MSM) [37]. However, limited studies have examined initiation and adherence to PrEP among black MSM in the United States who are disproportionately represented among newly HIV-diagnosed and late to care individuals [38]. The HPTN 073 study, a theoretically and culturally-informed biomedical prevention intervention demonstration project utilizing a client-centered care coordination (C4) model, investigated preexposure prophylaxis (PrEP) initiation, acceptability, and feasibility for black MSM ($N = 226$) in three US cities (Los Angeles, CA; Washington, DC' and Chapel Hill, NC) [39]. Men were offered once daily oral emtricitabine/tenofovir (FTC/TDF) PrEP combined with C4 at no personal cost and were followed for 12 months. The findings from this study demonstrated that 79% ($n = 178$) of participants accepted PrEP. Of these men, 64% demonstrated PrEP adherence at week 26 (the midpoint of the study) based on pharmacokinetic testing. This vanguard study also indicated that greater age, perception of having enough money (rent, food, or utilities), and knowledge of male partner taking PrEP before sex were statistically significantly associated with an increased likelihood of PrEP adherence at week 26. The findings from the HPTN 073 demonstration project suggest that a high level of PrEP initiation was established among at-risk black MSM and the data support the importance of addressing socio-structural and -cultural contextual factors that affect PrEP initiation and adherence among black MSM.

The HIV Care Continuum for Black MSM

One overarching objective of HIV treatment is to achieve viral suppression, which promotes optimal health for people living with HIV or AIDS. Based on empirical research, the Prevention Access Campaign implemented the Undetectable = Untransmissible (U = U concept) framework that maintains that people living with HIV who are taking antiretroviral therapy and have an undetectable viral load and maintain viral suppression cannot transmit the HIV virus to other individuals [40]. In this context, a critical component calls for a strengthening of the steps along the HIV care continuum that facilitate optimal viral suppression: diagnosis, linkage to care, received or retained in care, and viral suppression [41]. Research has observed that black MSM experience significant disparities along the HIV care continuum related to late diagnosis (including acute HIV infection and receiving an advanced HIV disease diagnosis when initially being tested for HIV). Black MSM are less likely to be engaged in care, to have inadequate access to HIV care and treatment, and be virally suppressed in comparison to MSM from other race/ethnicities [42–44]. Furthermore, limited research has focused on the facilitators and barriers to engagement along the HIV care continuum including, but not limited to, multilayered processes connected to socio-structural factors (e.g., poverty, education, employment status, access to health care and treatment [e.g., un-/underinsured], housing and food instability, racialized and sexuality-based stigma and discrimination, and HIV stigma and discrimination) [45]. Taken together, the provision of culturally-informed systems of care for black MSM living with HIV or AIDS is urgently needed to address these disproportionate realities, particularly as early diagnosis and treatment of HIV have predicted increased quality of life for persons living with HIV and AIDS [44]. This dilemma has facilitated a critical void in our understanding of how to leverage biomedical prevention intervention strategies in addressing the HIV epidemic among black MSM who are most at risk for HIV [46].

Building Innovative, Culturally Congruent Research on Black MSM

The development of a systematic base of scientific research in the area of HIV-related health disparities that focuses on black MSM has been germane to addressing the considerable limitations in the field of public health [14]. In this regard, the next steps in the development of scholarly research on HIV-related health disparities among black MSM involves incorporating intersectional and interdisciplinary approaches that are culturally relevant for black MSM [19]. More specifically, as a strategy to develop scholarly research on black MSM that serves to curtail their substantial HIV prevalence rates, researchers from the Black Gay Men's Research Group [38] have posited that a vision for research on black MSM incorporates several guiding principles in the development and implementation of this work: (1) research must be conducted in an efficient manner; (2) research needs to be developed, implemented, and applied principally by black MSM researchers; (3) research needs to examine the cultural complexities and specificities of the intersectional identities of black MSM; (4) research should be funded through a multiplicity of resources that will have a meaningful impact on the state of the AIDS epidemic for black MSM; and (5) research must be conducted in combination with organizations and individuals that are reflective of black MSM.

Contextualizing Sex in Black MSM Communities: The Role of Sexual Contexts and Networks

Research has shown that a number of sexual contexts have contributed to HIV sexual behavior in black MSM over the last few years [47]. Some of these contexts have related to the characteristics of sexual partners, emergence of bareback sex (e.g., the intention to engage in condomless anal intercourse), the use of the Internet in interfacing with sexual partners (e.g., sexual partners in cyberspace), the use of substances (e.g., alcohol and illicit drugs before or during sex), and perceived safer sex strategies (e.g., serosorting, seropositioning, and withdrawal before ejaculation) [47–50]. One of the strengths in conducting formative research on emerging trends and contextual factors associated with HIV sexual risk behavior in black MSM is that the findings can be used to contribute to the current scientific knowledge and the development of efficacious HIV prevention strategies. However, one of the research challenges in this area relates to the need to incorporate culturally appropriate methodologies based on strong collaborations with practitioners affiliated with community-based organizations. This represents a major component of culturally congruent HIV prevention work as communities provide perspectives that are relevant to the experiences of black MSM.

Experiences of Violence in the Context of HIV Prevention for Black MSM Communities

Studies have provided empirical support for examining the relationship between multiplicative forms of violence, including childhood sexual abuse (CSA), intimate partner violence (IPV), and other kinds of victimization in relation to HIV sexual risk behavior [51]. These areas of scholarly inquiry have been significantly understudied in black MSM, although some research has emerged in this area [52]. For example, in a qualitative study of CSA in black MSM, findings indicated a 32% prevalence rate in CSA, based on a sample from three geographic regions in the United States [53]. Also, according to Fields et al. [53], the contexts of CSA involved (1) the experience of CSA from a familial individual (e.g., older male relative); (2) the attribution of "same sex desire" as a result of the experience of CSA; and (3) psychological distress (e.g., depression and suicidality) and substance use due to CSA. In another study, black and Latino gay and nongay identifying MSM who reported histories of CSA, which often were connected to a history of trauma, related to HIV sexual risk behavior [51]. These research investigations provide empirical data for the significance of developing research studies to further examine the social contexts of how the experience of violence serves as a structural determinant to HIV sexual risk behavior. Moreover, the implications of these studies for both medical and mental health providers relate to the development and implementation of mechanisms to assess violence-related experiences, particularly within the context of how these foci relate to HIV prevention.

Substance Use in Relation to HIV Sexual Risk Behavior in Black MSM

Much of the HIV prevention research has demonstrated that the influence of substance use (e.g., alcohol and illicit drugs) has had an impact on HIV sexual risk behavior in MSM [54]. However, a limited number of intra- or within-group studies have specifically examined the relationship between substance use and HIV sexual risk behavior (e.g., UAI) in community-based samples of black MSM [55–57]. In a community-based sample of 481 black gay and bisexual men in the New York Metropolitan Area, the findings showed that the use of alcohol before or during sex was related to relationship status (e.g., having a primary and casual sexual partner), higher income, STI testing history, and a higher number of male sex partners. And, recreational drug use before or during sex was associated with being younger, having a casual sex partner, having an HIV-positive status, and reporting UAI with a male sex partner [58].

The Influence of Immigration on Black MSM and Its Connection to HIV Prevention

The role of immigration status on the sexual health of black MSM has been an understudied domain in HIV prevention research [7, 59–61]. Much of the scholarly work in this area has focused on the experiences of Latino MSM and Asian MSM with a void in studies on Caribbean (e.g., English-speaking) MSM and African MSM [61]. Significantly, the process of immigration has been a critical factor in understanding how cultural worldviews (e.g., cultural values and beliefs) influence sexual attitudes and behavior as well as the impact of social structures on access to health care, including HIV prevention and care, for immigrant groups [7].

This emerging area of research provides considerable implications for increasing the scholarly focus on the experiences and processes associated with immigration for black MSM that explore the complexities of the social contexts of sexuality and how these factors relate to sexual health [59]. In terms of immigration, contextual factors involving identity (e.g., racial, gender, and sexual identities) as well as stigma and discrimination (e.g., based on immigration status) need to be addressed in HIV prevention research and services for black MSM [7]. Indeed, a sustained emphasis on addressing how social structures have an impact on health care inequities for black MSM is critically significant, especially those that examine the role of discrimination based on legal status (e.g., undocumented individuals) in the United States [7]. Also, the development, implementation, and assessment of culturally congruent HIV prevention and testing services (e.g., pre-/post-test counseling), including the provision of linguistically competent services, need to be integrated into HIV prevention and care [62].

Qualitative investigations utilizing ethnographic fieldwork, focus groups, and in-depth interviews need to be conducted to better understand how contextual factors work in the lives of African and Caribbean MSM. For example, qualitative studies need to explore how social constructions of gender and sexuality within culturally relevant frameworks relate to barriers in accessing culturally congruent health care (including HIV prevention and care) [63]. An integral part of this work calls for an examination of how stigma and discrimination (e.g., the intersection of racialized, gender-based, and sexuality-based forms of stigma) relate to the lived experiences of black MSM within inter- and intragroup domains. These methodological approaches will provide critical formative data as a basis for the development of culturally grounded HIV prevention interventions for black MSM that will address HIV-related health disparities.

Psychosocial Support and Mental Health Needs for Black MSM

As the HIV epidemic enters its fourth decade, the current state of scholarly research regarding psychosocial and mental health issues for black MSM is understudied [51, 64]. According to the US Surgeon General's report, people of color have experienced barriers in accessing quality mental health services and care and have not been adequately represented in research in the area of mental health [65]. Similarly, black MSM have reported dissatisfaction with mental health services as a result of structural barriers including but not limited to heterosexism and homophobia [66]. Much of the extant research on the influence of racial/ethnic discrimination on mental health for people of color utilizing population-based studies has found that the experience of racial/ethnic discrimination relates to increased psychological distress for people of color, including diagnosis of major depression, generalized anxiety disorder, and onset of substance use [23]. Similarly, population-based studies of LGBT communities have shown that perceived discrimination (e.g., lifetime and daily discrimination) had a negative impact on their quality of life in addition to increases in current psychological distress and mental health disorders [67]. Other population-based studies have reported a higher prevalence of mental health disorders, suicidal ideation, and substance use among lesbian, gay, and bisexual (LGB) individuals as compared to heterosexual individuals [64]. In this regard, large-scale studies of black MSM are needed to ascertain characteristics of mental health utilization as well as the prevalence of mental health and substance use morbidity.

Building on the work of several scholars, stigma has been a core critical issue for black MSM communities [68]. Specifically, the negotiation of racial, gender, and sexual identities juxtaposed with experiences of individual and institutionalized racism and homophobia has worked as relevant culturally specific psychosocial issues for black MSM [63]. For example, black MSM have to work through the stressors associated with being a black male (e.g., racism, unemployment, incarceration, and health issues) and that of being emotionally and/or sexually attracted to men (e.g., gender role expectations) [69]. A significant part of this work relates to the negotiation of relationships with significant others, including family, friends, and sexual partners. Further, in a qualitative study of black and Latino HIV-positive MSM who reported a history of childhood sexual abuse, the findings showed that the sociocultural context of the men's lives was central to their lived experiences. For example, predominant themes that emerged from the study related to sexual identity; the role of family and cultural expectations regarding children; gender role socialization; influence of substance use; religiosity and spirituality; and HIV-related stigma, marginalization, and barriers to HIV care [70].

Based on the work of Meyer [71], the sociocultural model of minority stress in lesbian, gay, and bisexual (LGB) communities has provided a theoretical framework to examine the relationship between chronic stress and stigmatization, particularly as related to psychosocial distress [71–74]. In particular, through the use of a distal-proximal domain, Meyer [71] posited that the experiences of "minority" stressors for LGB individuals (e.g., expectations of stigma, internalized homophobia, and experiences of prejudice and discrimination) relate to mental health outcomes. As part of minority stress processes, distal refers to experiences of prejudice, discrimination, and violence based on sexual identity and proximal relates to experiences associated with "expectations of rejection, concealment, and internalized homophobia" (p. 248) [71]. In addition, with a specific focus on black MSM, researchers have developed theoretical models to examine the effects of social discrimination (e.g., racism, homophobia, and poverty) in relation to psychological distress and resiliency [75].

The experiences of HIV-related stigma and discrimination both within and external to black MSM communities have served as relevant psychosocial issues for black MSM [10, 14, 76]. Within this context, black MSM living with HIV and AIDS have to negotiate their HIV-positive status involving issues of disclosure to romantic and sexual partners, families, friends, health care providers, as well as significant others [77]. Black MSM living with HIV or AIDS also have to manage the stressors of stigma within black MSM communities (e.g., issues of rejection and discrimination). Therefore, prevention interventions need to address the stigmatization of black MSM living with HIV or AIDS by HIV-negative black MSM.

Summary

Since the onset of the HIV epidemic, black MSM communities have experienced considerable HIV-related health inequities in the United States. There have been significant limitations in the conceptual frameworks utilized in research on HIV-related health inequities for black MSM. Traditional models used in research on HIV-related health disparities have not integrated to a substantial degree culturally relevant conceptualizations at the core of the analyses. Thus, the objective of this chapter was to examine the factors that contribute to the significant incidence and prevalence rates of HIV and AIDS in black MSM communities. In particular, the concepts of stigma, marginalization, and structural inequalities were posed as a theoretical framework to examine HIV-related health disparities in black MSM communities. A basic premise of this work involves a paradigm shift that integrates intersectional and interdisciplinary theoretical and methodological approaches in the study of HIV-related health disparities in black communities. One of the core ideas put forth in the development of this work relates to a focus on the intersection of race, gender, social class, and sexual politics within the context of HIV prevention in black MSM communities.

References

1. Millett GA, Jeffries WL, Peterson JL, et al. Common roots: a contextual review of HIV epidemics in black men who have sex with men across the African diaspora. Lancet (London, England). 2012;380:411–23.
2. Millett GA, Peterson JL, Flores SA, et al. Comparisons of disparities and risks of HIV infection in black and other men who have sex with men in Canada, UK, and USA: a meta-analysis. Lancet (London, England). 2012;380:341–8.
3. Pathela P, Jamison K, Braunstein SL, Schillinger JA, Varma JK, Blank S. Incidence and predictors of HIV infection among men who have sex with men attending public sexually transmitted disease clinics, New York City, 2007-2012. AIDS Behav. 2017;21:1444–51.
4. Singh S, Song R, Johnson AS, McCray E, Hall HI. HIV incidence, prevalence, and undiagnosed infections in U.S. men who have sex with men. Ann Intern Med. 2018;168:685–94.
5. Mannheimer SB, Wang L, Wilton L, et al. Infrequent HIV testing and late HIV diagnosis are common among a cohort of black men who have sex with men in 6 US cities. J Acquir Immune Defic Syndr (1999). 2014;67:438–45.
6. Mayer KH, Wang L, Koblin B, et al. Concomitant socioeconomic, behavioral, and biological factors associated with the disproportionate HIV infection burden among Black men who have sex with men in 6 U.S. cities. PLoS One. 2014;9:e87298.
7. Adekeye OA, Adesuyi BF, Takon JG. Barriers to healthcare among African immigrants in Georgia, USA. J Immigr Minor Health. 2018;20:188–93.
8. Bogart LM, Wagner GJ, Galvan FH, Landrine H, Klein DJ, Sticklor LA. Perceived discrimination and mental health symptoms among black men with HIV. Cultur Divers Ethnic Minor Psychol. 2011;17:295–302.
9. Brewer RA, Magnus M, Kuo I, Wang L, Liu TY, Mayer KH. Exploring the relationship between incarceration and HIV among black men who have sex with men in the United States. J Acquir Immune Defic Syndr (1999). 2014;65:218–25.
10. Cahill S, Taylor SW, Elsesser SA, Mena L, Hickson D, Mayer KH. Stigma, medical mistrust, and perceived racism may affect PrEP awareness and uptake in black compared to white gay and bisexual men in Jackson, Mississippi and Boston, Massachusetts. AIDS Care. 2017;29:1351–8.
11. Eaton LA, Earnshaw VA, Maksut JL, Thorson KR, Watson RJ, Bauermeister JA. Experiences of stigma and health care engagement among Black MSM newly diagnosed with HIV/STI. J Behav Med. 2018;41:458.
12. Irvin R, Wilton L, Scott H, et al. A study of perceived racial discrimination in black men who have sex with men (MSM) and its association with healthcare utilization and HIV testing. AIDS Behav. 2014;18:1272–8.
13. Lassiter JM. Extracting dirt from water: a strengths-based approach to religion for African American same-gender-loving men. J Relig Health. 2014;53:178–89.
14. Levy ME, Wilton L, Phillips G 2nd, et al. Understanding structural barriers to accessing HIV testing and prevention services among black men who have sex with men (BMSM) in the United States. AIDS Behav. 2014;18:972–96.
15. Mena L, Crosby RA, Geter A. A novel measure of poverty and its association with elevated sexual risk behavior among young black MSM. Int J STD AIDS. 2017;28:602–7.
16. Miller RL Jr. Legacy denied: African American gay men, AIDS, and the black church. Soc Work. 2007;52:51–61.
17. Nelson LE, Wilton L, Moineddin R, et al. Economic, legal, and social hardships associated with HIV risk among black men who have sex with men in six US cities. J Urban Health. 2016;93:170–88.
18. Bowleg L, Del Rio-Gonzalez AM, Holt SL, et al. Intersectional epistemologies of ignorance: how behavioral and social science research shapes what we know, think we know, and don't know about U.S. black men's sexualities. J Sex Res. 2017;54:577–603.

19. Cohen CJ. The boundaries of blackness: AIDS and the breakdown of black politics. Chicago: University of Chicago Press; 1999.
20. Bowleg L. Towards a critical health equity research stance: why epistemology and methodology matter more than qualitative methods. Health Educ Behav. 2017;44:677–84.
21. Mullings L, Schulz A. Intersectionality and health: an introduction. New York: Wiley; 2005.
22. Smedley A, Smedley BD. Race as biology is fiction, racism as a social problem is real: anthropological and historical perspectives on the social construction of race. Am Psychol. 2005;60:16–26.
23. Williams DR, Lawrence J, Davis B. Racism and health: Evidence and needed research. Annu Rev Public Health. 2019; 40:105–125.
24. Paradies Y, Ben J, Denson N, et al. Racism as a determinant of health: a systematic review and meta-analysis. PLoS One. 2015;10:e0138511.
25. Williams DR, Cooper LA. Reducing racial inequities in health: using what we already know to take action. Int J Environ Res Public Health. 2019;16:606.
26. Bailey M, Mobley IA, Charles N, et al. Open letter to editors of Journal of the National Medical Association from the black feminist health science studies collective. J Natl Med Assoc. 2019;111:573.
27. Thomas SB, Quinn SC. The Tuskegee Syphilis Study, 1932 to 1972: implications for HIV education and AIDS risk education programs in the black community. Am J Public Health. 1991;81:1498–505.
28. Bogart LM, Dale SK, Christian J, et al. Coping with discrimination among HIV-positive black men who have sex with men. Cult Health Sex. 2017;19:723–37.
29. Magnus M, Franks J, Griffith S, Arnold MP, Goodman K, Wheeler DP. Engaging, recruiting, and retaining black men who have sex with men in research studies: don't underestimate the importance of staffing--lessons learned from HPTN 061, the BROTHERS study. J Public Health Manag Pract. 2014;20:E1–9.
30. Schulz AJ, Freudenberg N, Daniels J. Intersections of race, class, and gender in public health interventions. In AJ Schulz & L Mullings (Eds.), Gender, race, class, and health: Intersectional approaches. New York: John Wiley & Sons, Inc. 2005;371–93.
31. Arnold EA, Bailey MM. Constructing home and family: how the ballroom community supports African American GLBTQ youth in the face of HIV/AIDS. J Gay Lesbian Soc Serv. 2009;21:171–88.
32. Wong JO, Benjamin M, Arnold EA. 'I want the heart of fierceness to arise within us': maintaining public space to promote HIV-related health with House Ball Community members in an era of gentrification. Cult Health Sex. 2019;22:444.
33. Ayala G, Bingham T, Kim J, Wheeler DP, Millett GA. Modeling the impact of social discrimination and financial hardship on the sexual risk of HIV among Latino and black men who have sex with men. Am J Public Health. 2012;102(Suppl 2):S242–9.
34. Choi KH, Han CS, Paul J, Ayala G. Strategies for managing racism and homophobia among U.S. ethnic and racial minority men who have sex with men. AIDS Educ Prev. 2011;23:145–58.
35. Han CS, Ayala G, Paul JP, Boylan R, Gregorich SE, Choi KH. Stress and coping with racism and their role in sexual risk for HIV among African American, Asian/Pacific islander, and Latino men who have sex with men. Arch Sex Behav. 2015;44:411–20.
36. Rolle CP, Rosenberg ES, Luisi N, et al. Willingness to use pre-exposure prophylaxis among black and white men who have sex with men in Atlanta, Georgia. Int J STD AIDS. 2017;28:849–57.
37. Liu AY, Vittinghoff E, von Felten P, et al. Randomized controlled trial of a mobile health intervention to promote retention and adherence to pre-exposure prophylaxis among young people at risk for human immunodeficiency virus: the EPIC study. Clin Infect Dis. 2018;68:2010.
38. Wheeler DP, Lucas J, Wilton L, et al. Building effective multilevel HIV prevention partnerships with Black men who have sex with men: experience from HPTN 073, a pre-exposure prophylaxis study in three US cities. J Int AIDS Soc. 2018;21(Suppl 7):e25180.
39. Wheeler DP, Fields SD, Beauchamp G, et al. Pre-exposure prophylaxis initiation and adherence among black men who have sex with men (MSM) in three US cities: results from the HPTN 073 study. J Int AIDS Soc. 2019;22:e25223.

40. Eisinger RW, Dieffenbach CW, Fauci AS. HIV viral load and transmissibility of HIV infection: undetectable equals untransmittable. JAMA. 2019;321:451–2.
41. Hightow-Weidman L, LeGrand S, Choi SK, Egger J, Hurt CB, Muessig KE. Exploring the HIV continuum of care among young black MSM. PLoS One. 2017;12:e0179688.
42. Chandler CJ, Sang JM, Bukowski LA, et al. Characterizing the HIV care continuum among a community sample of black men who have sex with men in the United States. AIDS Care. 2019;31:816–20.
43. Clement ME, Johnston BE, Eagle C, et al. Advancing the HIV pre-exposure prophylaxis continuum: a collaboration between a Public Health Department and a Federally Qualified Health Center in the Southern United States. AIDS Patient Care STDs. 2019;33:366.
44. Friedman MR, Sang JM, Bukowski LA, et al. HIV care continuum disparities among black bisexual men and the mediating effect of psychosocial comorbidities. J Acquir Immune Defic Syndr (1999). 2018;77:451–8.
45. Nelson LE, McMahon JM, Leblanc NM, et al. Advancing the case for nurse practitioner-based models to accelerate scale-up of HIV pre-exposure prophylaxis. J Clin Nurs. 2019;28:351–61.
46. Poteat T, White J, van Griensven F. The HIV care continuum in black MSM in the USA. The Lancet HIV. 2014;1:e97–8.
47. Irvin R, Vallabhaneni S, Scott H, et al. Examining levels of risk behaviors among black men who have sex with men (MSM) and the association with HIV acquisition. PLoS One. 2015;10:e0118281.
48. Duncan DT, Hickson DA, Goedel WC, et al. The social context of HIV prevention and care among black men who have sex with men in three U.S. cities: the neighborhoods and networks (N2) cohort study. Int J Environ Res Public Health. 2019;16:E1922.
49. Duncan DT, Park SH, Hambrick HR, et al. Characterizing geosocial-networking app use among young black men who have sex with men: a multi-city cross-sectional survey in the southern United States. JMIR Mhealth Uhealth. 2018;6:e10316.
50. Franks J, Hirsch-Moverman Y, Loquere AS Jr, et al. Sex, PrEP, and stigma: experiences with HIV pre-exposure prophylaxis among New York City MSM participating in the HPTN 067/ADAPT study. AIDS Behav. 2018;22:1139–49.
51. Williams JK, Wilton L, Magnus M, et al. Relation of childhood sexual abuse, intimate partner violence, and depression to risk factors for HIV among black men who have sex with men in 6 US cities. Am J Public Health. 2015;105:2473–81.
52. Hotton A, Quinn K, Schneider J, Voisin D. Exposure to community violence and substance use among black men who have sex with men: examining the role of psychological distress and criminal justice involvement. AIDS Care. 2018;31:1–9.
53. Fields SD, Malebranche D, Feist-Price S. Childhood sexual abuse in black men who have sex with men: results from three qualitative studies. Cultur Divers Ethnic Minor Psychol. 2008;14:385–90.
54. Wilton L, Koblin B, Nandi V, et al. Correlates of Seroadaptation strategies among black men who have sex with men (MSM) in 4 US cities. AIDS Behav. 2015;19:2333–46.
55. Dyer TP, Regan R, Wilton L, et al. Differences in substance use, psychosocial characteristics and HIV-related sexual risk behavior between black men who have sex with men only (BMSMO) and black men who have sex with men and women (BMSMW) in six US cities. J Urban Health. 2013;90:1181–93.
56. Dyer TV, Khan MR, Regan R, et al. Differential patterns of risk and vulnerability suggest the need for novel prevention strategies for black bisexual men in the HPTN 061 study. J Acquir Immune Defic Syndr (1999). 2018;78:491–8.
57. Dyer TV, Khan MR, Sandoval M, et al. Drug use and sexual HIV transmission risk among men who have sex with men and women (MSMW), men who have sex with men only (MSMO), and men who have sex with women only (MSWO) and the female partners of MSMW and MSWO: a network perspective. AIDS Behav. 2017;21:3590–8.
58. Wilton L. Correlates of substance use in relation to sexual behavior in black gay and bisexual men: implications for HIV prevention. J Black Psychol. 2008;34:70–93.

59. Harris OO. Survival now versus survival later: immediate and delayed HIV risk assessment among young Jamaican men who have transactional sex with men. Cult Health Sex. 2018;21:1–15.
60. Ojikutu BO, Bogart LM, Mayer KH, Stopka TJ, Sullivan PS, Ransome Y. Spatial access and willingness to use pre-exposure prophylaxis among black/African American individuals in the United States: cross-sectional survey. JMIR Public Health Surveill. 2019;5:e12405.
61. Ojikutu BO, Mazzola E, Fullem A, et al. HIV testing among black and Hispanic immigrants in the United States. AIDS Patient Care STDs. 2016;30:307–14.
62. Rodriguez MM, Madera SR, Diaz NV. Stigma and homophobia: persistent challenges for HIV prevention among young MSM in Puerto Rico. Rev Let Cienc. 2013;26:50–9.
63. Malebranche DJ, Gvetadze R, Millett GA, Sutton MY. The relationship between gender role conflict and condom use among black MSM. AIDS Behav. 2012;16:2051–61.
64. Wilton L. Characteristics and correlates of lifetime suicidal thoughts and attempts among young black men who have sex with men (MSM) and transgender women. J Black Psychol. 2018;4:273–90.
65. Services USDoHaH. Mental health: culture, race, and ethnicity—a supplement to mental health: a report of the surgeon general. Rockville: US Department of Health and Human Services; 2001.
66. Sun CJ, Nall JL, Rhodes SD. Perceptions of needs, assets, and priorities among black men who have sex with men with HIV: community-driven actions and impacts of a participatory photovoice process. Am J Mens Health. 2019;13:1557988318804901.
67. Mays VM, Jones AL, Cochran SD, Taylor RJ, Rafferty J, Jackson JS. Chronicity and mental health service utilization for anxiety, mood, and substance use disorders among black men in the United States; ethnicity and nativity differences. Basel: Healthcare; 2018. p. 6.
68. Malebranche DJ, Peterson JL, Fullilove RE, Stackhouse RW. Race and sexual identity: perceptions about medical culture and healthcare among black men who have sex with men. J Natl Med Assoc. 2004;96:97–107.
69. Wheeler DP. Exploring HIV prevention needs for nongay-identified black and African American men who have sex with men: a qualitative exploration. Sex Transm Dis. 2006;33:S11–6.
70. Williams JK, Wyatt GE, Rivkin I, Ramamurthi HC, Li X, Liu H. Risk reduction for HIV-positive African American and Latino men with histories of childhood sexual abuse. Arch Sex Behav. 2008;37:763–72.
71. Meyer IH. Prejudice, social stress, and mental health in lesbian, gay, and bisexual populations: conceptual issues and research evidence. Psychol Bull. 2003;129:674–97.
72. la Roi C, Meyer IH, Frost DM. Differences in sexual identity dimensions between bisexual and other sexual minority individuals: implications for minority stress and mental health. Am J Orthopsychiatry. 2019;89:40–51.
73. Meyer IH. Identity, stress, and resilience in lesbians, gay men, and bisexuals of color. Couns Psychol. 2010;38:1–9.
74. Meyer IH. Does an improved social environment for sexual and gender minorities have implications for a new minority stress research agenda? Psychol Sex Rev. 2016;7:81–90.
75. Choi KH, Paul J, Ayala G, Boylan R, Gregorich SE. Experiences of discrimination and their impact on the mental health among African American, Asian and Pacific islander, and Latino men who have sex with men. Am J Public Health. 2013;103:868–74.
76. Sang JM, Matthews DD, Meanley SP, Eaton LA, Stall RD. Assessing HIV stigma on prevention strategies for black men who have sex with men in the United States. AIDS Behav. 2018;22(12):3879–86.
77. Wheeler DP. Working with positive men: HIV prevention with black men who have sex with men. AIDS Educ Prev. 2005;17:102–15.

Chapter 5
HIV/AIDS and the Latino Populations in the United States: Epidemiology, Prevention, and Barriers to Care and Treatment

Alex González

Introduction

In many ways, Latino (also referred to as Latinx, Hispanic, or Hispanic American) people in the United States are not a monolith. They vary by race, religion, socioeconomic and legal status, country of birth, English and Spanish language proficiency, and political affiliation. Yet almost all Latino subgroups are more likely than non-Hispanic whites to become HIV infected. This chapter presents a current snapshot of the HIV/AIDS epidemic among Latinos in the United States.

Latinos in the United States

With almost 60 million people in the United States, Latinos comprise 18.3% of the nation's population and form its largest ethnic or racial minority group. The Latino population in the United States has nearly doubled over the last two decades, and it is expected to account for almost 30% of the nation's total projected population in 2050 [1, 2]. Most Latinos – over 60% – are of Mexican origin, with the remainder comprised of people whose roots come from dozens of other countries and territories, including Puerto Rico (9.5%), El Salvador (3.9%), Cuba (3.9%), Dominican Republic (3.5%), Guatemala (2.5%), Colombia (2.1%), and Honduras (1.6%) [3]. Nineteen US states and territories reported Latino populations of at least 10% in the 2010 Census [4]. The predominant Latino-origin group in each area of the United States varies. Mexicans and Central Americans are more likely to reside in the Southwest United States, the Midwest, and Washington, D.C.; Puerto Ricans and

A. González (✉)
Fenway Health, Boston, MA, USA
e-mail: agonzalez@fenwayhealth.org

© Springer Nature Switzerland AG 2021
B. O. Ojikutu, V. E. Stone (eds.), *HIV in US Communities of Color*,
https://doi.org/10.1007/978-3-030-48744-7_5

Dominicans are more likely to reside in the Northeast United States; and Cubans and South Americans are more likely to be located in Florida [5, 6].

More than two-thirds of Latinos are US born. Compared to non US born or immigrant Latinos, US-born Latinos are on average younger (20 vs. 43 years old median age), wealthier ($53,000 vs. $45,200 median annual household income), more educated (53% vs. 29% attained some college or more), more likely to speak English proficiently (90% vs. 36%), and less likely to have ever married (49% vs. 25%). Despite these differences, US-born and immigrant Latinos have similar poverty rates (20% vs. 18%), fertility rates (6% vs. 8% cisgender women who have given birth in the past 12 months), unemployment rates (7% vs. 5%), and homeownership rates (49% vs. 46%) [1].

Compared to non-Hispanic whites, Latinos are on average younger (28 vs. 43 years old median age), less educated (37% vs. 64% some college or more), less wealthy ($50,486 vs. $68,145 median annual household income), and more likely to have children (2007 vs. 1666 births per 1000 women) [7–10]. Over 18% of Latinos (compared to 8% of whites) live in poverty, and Latinos account for a disproportionate share (27.2%) of the US population living in poverty [11].

The Latino population in the United States is racially diverse with 53% of Latinos identifying as white, 36.7% identifying as "some other race," 2.5% identifying as black or African American, and 6% identifying as multiracial according to the 2010 US Census [12]. A 2014 Pew Research Center survey of Latinos living in the United States noted that up to a third identify as *mestizo* (mix of white Latino and indigenous background), *mulatto* (mix of white Latino and black background), or some other mixed-race combination [13]. These terms demonstrate that US Census and other survey data routinely fail to capture the multiple dimensions of race and ethnicity with respect to Latino individuals.

Epidemiology of HIV/AIDS and Latino Populations

HIV Incidence and Prevalence

HIV affects Latinos in the United States disproportionately. While Latinos make up 18% of the US population, they were responsible in 2017 for 26% (9889 out of 38,739) of new HIV diagnoses in the United States and dependent areas. The majority (87%) of these new diagnoses among Latinos occurred in Latino men, with male-to-male sexual contact accounting for 86% of these. Only black/African-American male-to-male sexual contact accounted for more new infections. Equally concerning, the incidence of HIV among Latinos in this transmission category is continuing to rise, with roughly 18% more infections occurring in this group per year than a decade ago [14].

The HIV epidemic affects Latino men who have sex with men (MSM) of all ages. Latino MSM in the 25–34 year age group accounted for the greatest number of new HIV cases in 2017 (4100), followed by the 13–24 year age group (2100), the 35–44 year age group (1900), the 45–54 year age group (970), and the 55+ year age group (350). Overall, Latino MSM are estimated to have a 1 in 5 lifetime risk of becoming HIV infected [15].

Transgender Latinas are also at high risk of HIV infection, with some studies showing HIV prevalence rates of up to 50% and a recent meta-analysis estimating a prevalence of 25.8% (compared to an estimated HIV prevalence for US adults overall of less than 0.5%) [16, 17]. The Centers for Disease Control and Prevention reported that transgender Latinas represented 29% of all HIV infections among transgender women between the years 2009 and 2014 [18]. Too little is known about the epidemiology of HIV infection in this group, however, because HIV surveillance programs historically have not routinely collected and documented gender identity data in case report forms.

Despite the disturbing trends in HIV incidence among Latino MSM as well as transgender Latinas, new HIV diagnoses among Latinos in all other risk groups decreased between the years 2010 and 2016. Among men, this includes the transmission categories of injection drug use (down 39%), male-to-male sexual contact and injection drug use (down 21%), and heterosexual contact (down 17%). Among women, this includes the transmission categories of heterosexual contact (down 20%) and injection drug use (down 25%) [14]. Nevertheless, Latina women still have an HIV incidence rate that is four times the rate for white women, and Latino men still have an HIV incidence rate that is three times the rate for white men [19]. Moreover, Latina heterosexual women remain among the six most affected subpopulations experiencing new HIV infections, with 1058 women in this transmission category being newly infected in 2017 [14].

Perinatal HIV transmission from Latina mother to child accounted for only 10 cases in 2017, representing a 41% decrease over the previous 5 years [20].

At the end of 2016, an estimated 254,600 Latino people had HIV, representing 22% of all people living with HIV in the United States. Close to 80% of Latino people living with HIV are men, with about 75% of them having acquired HIV from male-to-male sexual contact. Of the over 40,000 Latina women living with HIV, roughly three quarters of them acquired HIV from heterosexual contact. Approximately 50% of all Latino people living with HIV are between the ages of 40 and 60 years old. Less than 300 Latinos living with HIV in 2016 were children under the age of 13, most (90%) of whom acquired the infection perinatally [21].

AIDS Incidence and Prevalence and HIV/AIDS Mortality

The incidence of AIDS (defined as the presence of an AIDS defining condition or a CD4 count less than 200 cells/mm^3 in a person with HIV) has decreased across all major race/ethnicity groups over the past decade. In 2017, 3857 Latinos – 3238 men and 619 women – were diagnosed with AIDS in the United States. While this represents a 24% decrease in new AIDS cases compared to 2012, Latinos still experience an AIDS incidence rate that is over three times the rate for whites. Male-to-male sexual contact accounted for 77% of all new AIDS cases in Latino men in 2017, whereas heterosexual contact accounted for 80% of all new AIDS cases in Latina women [21]. A 2014 Kaiser Family Foundation report revealed that 36% of Latinos (compared to 31% for black/African-American people and 32% for whites) are tested for HIV late in their illness and thus are diagnosed with AIDS within 1 year of testing positive for HIV [22]. Approximately 119,000 Latinos in the United States – about 23% of total AIDS cases in this country – are living with AIDS today [21].

Death rates for people living with HIV/AIDS have decreased across all major race/ethnicity groups over the past decade. In 2016, approximately 2500 Latinos – 1921 men and 576 women – with HIV/AIDS died, accounting for about 16% of all HIV/AIDS deaths. Latinos with HIV/AIDS still experience a mortality rate that is twice the rate for whites. The most common age group where these Latino deaths occurred was 50–54 years, compared to 65+ years among whites [20, 21]. Thus far, more than 125,000 US Latinos have died since the start of the HIV epidemic [15].

HIV/AIDS and Geography

Puerto Rico and seven states – California, Texas, Florida, New York, New Jersey, Arizona, and Illinois – account for roughly 80% of all new HIV diagnoses among Latinos [23]. In 2017, Latinos made up 30% (1803) of all new infections in the Northeastern United States, 12% (604) of all new infections in the Midwestern United States, 21% (4193) of all new infections in the Southeastern United States, 40% (2908) of all new infections in the Western United States, and 98% (449) of all new infections in US-dependent areas (of which Puerto Rico is a part) [24]. Together with Pennsylvania, the above seven states and Puerto Rico are also where roughly 80% of all people living with HIV/AIDS reside. Moreover, ten large metropolitan areas account for almost two-thirds of Latinos living with HIV, with New York City, Los Angeles, and Miami having the greatest numbers of these [22].

Among Latinos with new diagnoses of HIV infection, approximately half were born outside of the United States, with the highest percentages being from Mexico (19.4%) and Puerto Rico (15.8%). Although male-to-male sexual contact remains the predominant HIV transmission category for Latinos across all US regions and Latino-origin groups, more infections were attributed to injection drug use and heterosexual contact in the Northeast United States and in Puerto Rico (two areas where Latinos tend to be of Puerto Rican origin) than elsewhere [25].

Latinos and the HIV/AIDS Care Continuum

HIV Testing and Diagnosis

Among all Latino people living with HIV in the United States in 2015, 84% knew their diagnosis. This comes close to achieving the United Nations Programme on HIV/AIDS (UNAIDS) goal of 90% disease detection by 2020, but disparities exist across age groups and transmission categories, with some studies showing that half of young MSM Latinos are not aware of their HIV positive status [26]. Individuals who do not know they have HIV are much more likely to pass the infection to others. They may also be less likely to access screenings for sexually transmitted infections, such as gonorrhea, Chlamydia, syphilis, and herpes, all of which may increase a person's chance of acquiring or transmitting HIV. Cultural factors such as *machismo* (exaggerated masculinity rooted in the traditional expectation that a man is responsible for providing for, protecting, and defending his family) may contribute to risky behavior in the form of multiple sex partners, condomless sex, and unwillingness to seek testing [27]. Only 53% of Latinos ages 18–64 years old report ever having been tested for HIV [22].

Linkage to Care

In 2015, the linkage to care rate (defined as having one or more CD4 or viral load tests performed within a month of HIV diagnosis) was 75.4% for Latinos. This compares favorably with overall rates nationally, but falls short of the national goal of 85%. By transmission category and age group, males aged 55+ years with infection attributed to heterosexual contact accounted for the highest percentage of people linked to care (88%), whereas females aged 45–54 years with infection attributed to injection drug use accounted for the lowest percentage (61.4%). Prompt linkage to care after diagnosis is essential to the reduction of HIV transmission since it enables the initiation of HIV treatment [28].

Retention in Care

In 2015, the rate of retention among Latinos living with HIV (defined by the presence of at least two CD4 or HIV RNA tests at least 3 months apart during the calendar year) was only 58.3%. This again compares favorably with overall retention in care rates nationally, but falls short of the national goal of 90% [28]. Barriers to retention in HIV care for Latinos include stigma (negative attitudes and beliefs about HIV leading to the belief that having HIV is socially unacceptable), a perceived lack of social support upon disclosure of one's status to family members and friends, unaddressed trauma and substance use leading to interruption in care, failure to develop a trusting and motivating relationship between provider and patient, and the challenge of having to meet basic unmet needs that compete with the perceived value of HIV care [29].

Antiretroviral Use and Viral Suppression

In 2015, viral suppression rates (defined as the percentage of living people with HIV who had at least one viral load test during the calendar year and whose most recent HIV RNA level was less than 200 copies/mL) among Latinos with HIV reached almost 60% [28]. This rate is similar to that achieved by non-Hispanic whites, but falls short of the national 2020 goal of 80%. It is not believed that HIV treatment is less effective in Latinos. However, Latinos are at higher risk for other health problems such as cardiovascular disease, diabetes mellitus, and hepatitis C infection, which can make managing HIV more difficult. Latinos also have the highest uninsured (17.8%, three times the rate for non-Hispanic whites) rate of any racial or ethnic group within the United States, and immigrant Latinos – even those who entered the country lawfully – may be barred from receiving government benefits such as Medicaid. Without insurance coverage, Latinos with HIV may perceive antiretroviral medications as too expensive to afford. Lastly, they may deem too risky (because it may expose their or a family member's undocumented status), time consuming, or onerous to present for health care or pursue drug and care coverage through government programs for which they are eligible (such as the AIDS Drug Assistance Program) [30, 31].

Latinos aged 13–24 present an interesting paradox: Even though this group had the highest retention in care among all Latino age groups (60.5%), they had the lowest overall viral suppression (54.6%) [28]. Studies consistently show lower viral suppression rates for this age group compared to other age groups across all races. A recent Adolescent Medicine Trials Network for HIV/AIDS Interventions (ATN) cohort study failed to demonstrate an association between sustained viral suppression and adolescent age, race/ethnicity education, mental health indicators, illicit drug use, or geography; factors that did remain significantly associated with sustained viral suppression included living situation (living in one's own residence as opposed to foster housing, group home, halfway house, shelter, or on the street) and the absence of either heavy alcohol use or remote incarceration history [32].

Latinos and HIV Prevention

Prevention efforts have led to successful decreases in Latino HIV incidence among all transmission categories except male-to-male sexual contact (and, presumably, transgender female-to-male sexual contact). These efforts include increased HIV testing, the use of medications to prevent transmission (treatment of known HIV+ people, prevention of mother-to-child transmission, pre-exposure prophylaxis, post-exposure prophylaxis), syringe service programs for people who inject drugs, condom distribution programs, medication-assisted treatment for people with substance use disorders, and better STD diagnosis and treatment programs [33].

Why are current prevention efforts failing to curb new infections among Latino MSM and transgender Latinas? These individuals are not more likely to engage in HIV risk behavior than people in other racial/ethnic groups or transmission categories. Latinos are more likely to have sex with other Latinos; however, and since Latino MSM and transgender Latinas have relatively high prevalence rates of HIV and STDs, this makes an identical rate of HIV risk behavior significantly riskier for HIV transmission to occur.

Unlike their Latino counterparts in other transmission categories, Latino MSM and transgender Latinas are subject to additional minority stress in the form of homophobia and transphobia in everyday life, which in turn impact physical, mental, and financial health and may make it harder for them to seek HIV testing and care. Research shows that many Latinos experience discrimination, homophobia, and transphobia within health care settings, which can lead to mistrust of the health care system and delays in seeking care [14].

Lastly, one other important barrier to successful HIV prevention among Latino MSM and transgender Latinas is the underutilization of pre-exposure prophylaxis (PrEP). PrEP is known to reduce the risk for HIV transmission by approximately 99%, but in 2016, only 13% of PrEP users – one-fifth as many as non-Hispanic whites – were Latino [15]. Recent efforts have led to a 500% increase in PrEP use among MSM overall, but while 40% of non-Hispanic white MSM and 35% of MSM overall used PrEP in 2017, only 30% of Latino MSM had done so [34]. The CDC estimates that 300,000 Latinos – 25% of people who could potentially benefit from PrEP – across the nation could benefit from PrEP based on current clinical guidelines, but only 3% of those (7600) were prescribed PrEP [34]. Barriers to PrEP uptake by Latinos include drug costs, concerns about immigration status, a dearth of messaging about PrEP within the Latino community networks these Latinos trust, an undersupply of health care workers who speak Spanish and are competent in prescribing PrEP, and the isolating effects of discrimination and stigma [35].

Current and Future Efforts

"Ending the HIV Epidemic: A Plan for America" is a new initiative by the federal government that seeks to reduce the number of new HIV infections in the United States by 75% within 5 years and then by at least 90% within 10 years, for an estimated 250,000 total HIV infections averted. The effort will prioritize the 48 US counties with the highest number of new HIV diagnoses (most of which have large Latino populations); Washington, D.C.; San Juan, Puerto Rico; and 7 states with a substantial rural HIV burden (Alabama, Arkansas, Kentucky, Mississippi, Missouri,

Oklahoma, South Carolina). The initiative's four core strategies involve all of the following:

- Early diagnosis of HIV
- Early and effective treatment of HIV to achieve and sustain viral suppression
- Prevention of HIV, primarily through increased use of PrEP and syringe services programs
- Quick response to potential HIV outbreaks so that (a) additional infections can be prevented and (b) newly infected people can be linked to care

New HIV infections peaked at approximately 130,000 cases per year in the mid-1980s, dropped to approximately 50,000 cases per year in the 1990s, then dropped one last time in the early 2010s to a new plateau of approximately 39,000 cases per year [36]. A reduction in incidence of 75–90% will be unprecedented, if reached. Experts have expressed specific concerns about how the initiative will achieve its gains, specifically among sexual and racial/ethnic minority populations, and especially at a time when insurance coverage is shrinking and Spanish-speaking health care workforce shortages are increasing [37].

Started in 1990 by an act of Congress, the Ryan White HIV/AIDS Program (RWHAP) serves more than half of all people diagnosed with HIV in the United States – approximately 535,000 people in 2017. Latinos make up 23.1% of all RHWAP clients. RHWAP funding recipients include state and local agencies as well as local community-based organizations (such as AIDS service organizations, HIV clinics, and federally qualified health centers). Even though 65.8% of Latino RWHAP clients live at or below 100% of the federal poverty level, 87.9% of them have suppressed viral loads. Despite their unparalleled success with Latino patients, RWHAP clinics only serve half of all Latino people living with HIV/AIDS [38]. Continued and, likely, increased congressional appropriations in support of the program will be needed in order to reach the ambitious Ending the HIV Epidemic targets mentioned above.

Conclusion

Latinos in the United States are disproportionately affected by HIV. Recent prevention and treatment improvements evidenced by almost across-the-board reductions in HIV incidence among Latino transmission categories are countered by both (a) an unprecedented increase in new infections among Latino MSM and transgender Latinas and (b) an inability to meet that increase with concomitant improvements in the HIV continuum of care. Ending the epidemic will require culturally sensitive, swift, and effective interventions aimed at decreasing the number of undiagnosed HIV cases, increasing access to PrEP and syringe services programs to HIV negative people, and achieving greater rates of viral suppression more quickly among those who are diagnosed.

References

1. Noe-Bustamante L, Flores A. Facts on Latinos in the U.S. September 16 2019. https://www.pewresearch.org/hispanic/fact-sheet/latinos-in-the-u-s-fact-sheet/.
2. U.S. Census Bureau. 2017 National population projections tables. 2017. https://www.census.gov/data/tables/2017/demo/popproj/2017-summary-tables.html.
3. Krogstad JM, Noe-Bustamante L. 7 facts for national Hispanic heritage month. October 14 2019. https://www.pewresearch.org/fact-tank/2019/10/14/facts-for-national-hispanic-heritage-month/.
4. U.S. Census Bureau. Population by race and Hispanic or Latino origin for the United States, regions, divisions, states, Puerto Rico, and places of 100,000 or more population (PHC-T-6). April 2 2001. https://www.census.gov/population/www/cen2000/briefs/phc-t6/index.html.
5. Pew Research Center. Hispanic population and origin in select U.S. metropolitan areas, 2014. September 6 2016. https://www.pewresearch.org/hispanic/interactives/hispanic-population-in-select-u-s-metropolitan-areas/.
6. Lopez MH, Dockterman D. U.S. Hispanic country of origin counts for nation, top 30 metropolitan areas. May 26 2011. https://www.pewresearch.org/hispanic/2011/05/26/us-hispanic-country-of-origin-counts-for-nation-top-30-metropolitan-areas/
7. Flores A. How the U.S. Hispanic population is changing. September 18 2017. https://www.pewresearch.org/fact-tank/2017/09/18/how-the-u-s-hispanic-population-is-changing/.
8. Flores A. Hispanic population in the United States statistical portrait. 2015. September 18 2017. https://www.pewresearch.org/hispanic/2017/09/18/2015-statistical-information-on-hispanics-in-united-states/#hispanic-pop.
9. Ryan CL, Bauman K. Educational attainment in the United States: 2015. March 2016. https://www.census.gov/content/dam/Census/library/publications/2016/demo/p20-578.pdf.
10. Matthews TJ, Hamilton BE. Total fertility rates by state and race and Hispanic origin: United States, 2017. National Vital Statistics Reports; vol 68 no 1. Hyattsville: National Center for Health Statistics. p. 2018.
11. Edwards A. U.S. Hispanic poverty rate hit an all-time low in 2017. U.S. Census Bureau. February 27 2019. https://www.census.gov/library/stories/2019/02/hispanic-poverty-rate-hit-an-all-time-low-in-2017.html.
12. Humes KR, Jones NA, Ramirez R. Overview of race and Hispanic origin. 2010. 2010 Census Briefs; C2010BR-02. U.S. Census Bureau. March 2011.
13. Pew Research Center. Multiracial in America: proud, diverse, and growing in numbers. Washington, D.C.: June 2015.
14. Centers for Disease Control and Prevention. HIV and Hispanics/Latinos. October 15, 2019. https://www.cdc.gov/hiv/group/racialethnic/hispaniclatinos/index.html.
15. Centers for Disease Control and Prevention. HIV among Latinos. https://www.cdc.gov/nchhstp/newsroom/docs/factsheets/cdc-hiv-latinos-508.pdf.
16. Volpi C, Cahill S. Retaining transgender women in HIV care: best practices in the field. Boston: The Fenway Institute; 2018.
17. Centers for Disease Control and Prevention. HIV and transgender communities. April 2019. https://www.cdc.gov/hiv/pdf/policies/cdc-hiv-transgender-brief.pdf.
18. Centers for Disease Control and Prevention. HIV and transgender people. September 6, 2019. https://www.cdc.gov/hiv/group/gender/transgender/index.html.
19. U.S. Department of Health and Human Services Office of Minority Health. HIV/AIDS and Hispanic Americans. January 17, 2018. https://minorityhealth.hhs.gov/omh/browse.aspx?lvl=4&lvlid=66
20. Centers for Disease Control and Prevention. HIV and pregnant women, infants, and children. September 6, 2019. https://www.cdc.gov/hiv/group/gender/pregnantwomen/index.html.
21. Centers for Disease Control and Prevention. HIV surveillance report: diagnoses of HIV infection in the United States and dependent areas, 2017. Vol 29. November 2018. https://www.cdc.gov/hiv/pdf/library/reports/surveillance/cdc-hiv-surveillance-report-2017-vol-29.pdf.

22. Kaiser Family Foundation. Latinos and HIV/AIDS. April 15, 2014. https://www.kff.org/hivaids/fact-sheet/latinos-and-hivaids/.

23. Center for Latino Adolescent and Family Health. The invisible crisis: HIV among Hispanics/Latinos in the United States. 2019. https://drive.google.com/file/d/19c-vXMte97_RPMb4alcaiV1A2GMUuyHt/view.

24. Centers for Disease Control and Prevention. HIV in the United States by region. September 9 2019. https://www.cdc.gov/hiv/statistics/overview/geographicdistribution.html.

25. Centers for Disease Control and Prevention (CDC). Geographic differences in HIV infection among Hispanics or Latinos – 46 states and Puerto Rico, 2010. JAMA. 2012;308(23):2450–2.

26. Centers for Disease Control and Prevention. HIV and youth. September 9 2019. https://www.cdc.gov/hiv/group/age/youth/.

27. Diaz RM. Latino gay men and HIV: culture, sexuality, and risk behavior. New York: Routledge; 1998.

28. Gant Z, et al. HIV care outcomes among Hispanics or Latinos with diagnosed HIV infection – United States, 2015. MMWR. 2017;66(40):1065–72. https://www.cdc.gov/mmwr/volumes/66/wr/pdfs/mm6640a2.pdf.

29. Levison JH, et al. "Where it falls apart": barriers to retention in HIV care in Latino immigrants and migrants. AIDS Patient Care STDs. 2017;31(9):394–405.

30. HIV and Latinos. POZ Magazine. March 19, 2018. https://www.poz.com/basics/hiv-basics/hiv-latinos.

31. U.S. Department of Health and Human Services, Office of Minority Health. Profile: Hispanic/Latino Americans. August 22, 2019. https://minorityhealth.hhs.gov/omh/browse.aspx?lvl=3&lvlid=64.

32. Lally MA, et al. HIV continuum of care for youth in the United States. J Acquir Immune Defic Syndr. 2018;77(1):110–7.

33. U.S. Department of Health and Human Services. HIV prevention activities. May 20 2017. https://www.hiv.gov/federal-response/federal-activities-agencies/hiv-prevention-activities.

34. Centers for Disease Control and Prevention. HIV prevention pill not reaching most Americans who could benefit – especially people of color. March 6, 2018. https://www.cdc.gov/nchhstp/newsroom/2018/croi-2018-PrEP-press-release.html.

35. Page KR, et al. Promoting pre-exposure prophylaxis to prevent HIV infections among sexual and gender minority Hispanics/Latinxs. AIDS Educ Prevent. 2017;29(5):389–400.

36. U.S. Department of Health and Human Services. What is 'ending the epidemic: a plan for America'? September 3, 2019. https://www.hiv.gov/federal-response/ending-the-hiv-epidemic/overview.

37. League of United Latin American Citizens. Latino health disparities. 2014. https://lulac.org/programs/health/health_disparities/.

38. Health Resources and Services Administration. HRSA's Ryan White HIV/AIDS program population fact sheet. August 2019. https://hab.hrsa.gov/sites/default/files/hab/Publications/factsheets/population-factsheet-hispanic.pdf9.

Chapter 6
Women of Color and HIV

Charlene A. Flash, Syundai R. Johnson, and Valerie E. Stone

Epidemiology

Globally, it is estimated that 51% of those living with HIV are women [1]. In the United States, approximately 1 in 5 new HIV infections occur among women. Women of color comprise a disproportionate proportion of HIV infections among women in the United States, with African-American women accounting for 59% of new infections among women, Hispanic women comprising 19%, while only 17% of new infections among women are in white women. The prevalence of people living with HIV in African American and Hispanic/Latino communities and the fact that people tend to have sex with partners of the same race/ethnicity mean that women from these communities face a greater risk of HIV infection with each new sexual encounter [2].

Overall, the incidence of HIV among women in the United States is declining. In 2002, the HIV diagnosis rate among US women was 13 per 100,000. By 2011, that rate had decreased 49.2% to 6.6 per 100,000 [3]. Marked decreases in the rates of new HIV diagnosis occurred in nearly every demographic group and the US population of women experienced some of the largest decreases in HIV infection rates. Racial disparities in the rate of new HIV infections persist between African-Americans and white people in the United States; however, the disparities are

C. A. Flash
Legacy Community Health Center, Houston, TX, USA

Baylor College of Medicine, Houston, TX, USA

S. R. Johnson
Baylor College of Medicine, Houston, TX, USA

V. E. Stone (✉)
Divisions of General Internal Medicine, Division of Infectious Diseases, Department of Medicine, Brigham and Women's Hospital, Harvard Medical School, Boston, MA, USA
e-mail: vstone@bwh.harvard.edu

© Springer Nature Switzerland AG 2021
B. O. Ojikutu, V. E. Stone (eds.), *HIV in US Communities of Color*,
https://doi.org/10.1007/978-3-030-48744-7_6

narrowing among the population of women as evidenced by a 20% decrease between 2012 and 2016 in the annual number of new infections among African-American women between 2012 and 2016 while rates among white women remained stable during that timeframe [3]. Each year approximately 27,000 people in the United States are diagnosed with AIDS. The disparities in AIDS diagnoses between black women and white women steadily increased until 2002, and then the gap started to narrow slowly between 2006 and 2013. This is particularly notable as during that same period, 2006 and 2013 there was a marked increase in the black-white disparity in HIV infections and AIDS diagnoses among men [3].

In the United States, 10,292 Hispanics/Latinos were diagnosed with HIV in 2016. Twelve percent (1277) of Hispanics/Latinos who received an HIV diagnosis were women. The CDC estimates that 1 in 106 Hispanic/Latino women will be diagnosed with HIV at some point in their lifetime. Among Hispanic women/Latinas, 88% (1121) of diagnosed HIV infections were attributed to heterosexual contact [4]. In 2013, the estimated rate of HIV infections was almost four times greater among Hispanic/Latino females (7.0) than among white non-Hispanic females (1.8) [4]. From 2011 to 2015, Hispanic/Latina women diagnoses declined 14%. Of the total number of women living with diagnosed HIV at the end of 2015, 19% (43,086) were Hispanic/Latina. Given that Hispanics/Latinos are the largest and fastest growing minority group in the United States, with an estimated population of 55 million, addressing HIV/AIDS in their community is important to their health and the nation's health [5].

HIV Transmission

Heterosexual contact accounts for the majority of new HIV diagnoses among women in the United States. In 1988, early in the US HIV epidemic, 60% of new HIV infections among women were secondary to injection drug use (IDU). By 2002, a marked shift was apparent in transmission risk categories as the rates of new diagnoses attributed to IDU were 3892 per 100,000 while that due to heterosexual contact was 11,695 per 100,000. In the ensuing years, 2002 to 2011, a 68.7% decrease in the numbers of infections attributed to IDU occurred [3]. Over the years, the key transmission risks shifted and the 2017 data reveal that the majority of new infections (86%) among women are secondary to heterosexual sex [6]. However, the predominant routes of infection differ substantially by race: the most recent data show that 92% of African-American women and 80% of Latinas acquire HIV through heterosexual sex, while only 68% of white women acquire HIV through this route [6].

Various factors drive HIV risk for Black/African-American women in the United States. Sexual behaviors such as the number of sexual partners, the frequency of intercourse, and condom use trends impact the HIV risk. In addition, analysis of sexual networks informs transmission trends among women. Heterosexual partnerships in which partner concurrency occurs (i.e., having a sexual partner who has multiple sexual partners) is an independent risk factor for new HIV infection [7]. Risk factors for HIV infection among heterosexual African-American women who deny personal high-risk behavior (i.e., STD in prior year, sex trade, crack/cocaine use, binge alcohol use, IDU, or sexual contact with a man who had sex with men) included partner concurrency (i.e., a partner who had other sexual partners) as well as social determinants of health such as having less than a high school education, food insecurity [7], poverty, lack of employment, and resultant marital instability [8].

Focus groups among southern African-Americans detail the potential impact of social environment including the potential influence of lack of recreation, illicit substance use, experiences of adversity, gender inequity, and limited eligible male partners [8]. Additional focus group data reveal that women may not consistently demand condom use. In addition, low self-esteem was one of the key features driving condomless sex [9].

Both African-American and Latinas experience increased risk when they have a greater number of sexual partners, history of STIs, limited condom use even with primary sexual partner, and a belief that their primary sexual partner has low risk of being infected with HIV [10]. Socioeconomic factors such as high rates of poverty and unemployment, immigration and acculturation stress, and cultural values are among the many factors that increase HIV risk for Latinas. Negotiating safer sex practices becomes more difficult because of these risk factors. Additional risk factors that women may experience include being unaware of their partner's HIV status and/or risk, substance abuse, poor mental health, and history of violence victimization [11]. It appears that younger age may be associated with HIV transmission. This may, in part, be due to noncondom use and less education. Nonetheless, other factors that may or may not necessarily be limited to youth have also been identified such as having a known partner living with HIV, substance use during sex, and history of sexually transmitted infections [12, 13]. Some series reveal higher HIV incidence among young women in communities in which female adolescents have greater likelihood of partnership with older partners as compared to male adolescents [14].

HIV transmission risk varies by type of exposure. Blood transfusion has an estimated per-act risk of HIV transmission of 9250 per 100,000 exposures to an infected source. For mother to child transmission the per-act transmission risk is 2260 per 100,000, and for needle-sharing injection drug use it is 63 and for needle sticks 23 [15].

The most common route of HIV transmission among women in the United States is by heterosexual intercourse. Factors that facilitate male-to-female sexual HIV transmission include index partner with AIDS, sexual contact during menses, anal sex, and female partner age greater than 45 years [16]. Male-to-female transmission of HIV is two times more efficient than female-to-male transmission during vaginal intercourse [15]. During receptive vaginal intercourse, the exposed mucosal area for women is larger than that for men and includes the vagina, cervix, and uterus. By contrast, for men, the exposed mucosal area is limited to the head of the penis and the exposed urethra. In addition, women are exposed to a larger quantity and have a potentially longer time period of exposure to potentially infectious material from a man (ejaculate).

Heterosexual transmission of HIV includes transmission via anal sex. Receptive anal intercourse bears 34 times the per-act risk of HIV transmission of receptive vaginal intercourse. Approximately 30% of US women have engaged in anal sex at some point during their sexual lives, and only 16% report condom use during the last episode of anal sex. These results vary by age, race, and relationship factors. Women between 20 and 44 years of age were nearly twice as likely as adolescents to have ever had anal sex. White women were more like to report anal sex than black women or Hispanic women [17]. Cohabiting, having been previously (but not currently) married, and having more lifetime sex partners or having a nonmonogamous sex partner in the past year are all factors associated with being more likely to have had anal sex [17].

Oral sex bears a nominal but nonzero risk of HIV transmission. White women are more like to report engaging in oral sex than black or Hispanic women [17]. In addition, oral sex is more common among women who are married, have a higher number of lifetime partners, or have a nonmonogamous partners in the prior year [17].

Natural History

Our understanding of the natural history of HIV disease in women has evolved over the years. Initial studies suggested that there might be a difference in disease progression by gender. Subsequent studies have demonstrated no difference between men and women in progression to AIDS and death when matched by socioeconomic status, race, and HIV risk factor [44]. The previously noted gender disparities were most likely due to late presentation and poor access to care due to poverty, transportation difficulty, cultural and language barriers, and other issues.

Women have been noted to have lower viral loads than men at similar CD4 counts. In a study of the ALIVE (AIDS Linked to the Intravenous Experience) cohort, which is 95% African American, the initial median viral load was $0.5 \log_{10}$ (3.16 times) lower for women than it was for men. Multivariate proportional hazards models stratified by sex and controlling for initial CD4 cell count and age showed no significant difference between men and women in the risk of progression to AIDS in 5 years of follow-up, despite women starting with lower HIV RNA loads. Thus, although the relative viral load has a similar predictive value for progression to AIDS for men and women, the same absolute viral load seems to confer different risk of progression to AIDS between the sexes [18].

Women with CD4 counts >200, of comparable age and degree of clinical symptoms, have HIV-1 RNA levels that are 32–50% lower than men. HIV-1 RNA levels predict overall disease progression; however, men and women have comparable outcomes when access to resources is comparable. In addition, for women with CD4 counts <200, no differences in viral load persist when compared to men [18].

Availability of effective HIV treatment facilitates improved survival rates among women living with HIV [19]. In 2017, 16% of women with HIV were over 55 years of age [6]. For these patients, age-related comorbidities may complicate their HIV infection [19]. In fact, PLWH suffering immunologic and inflammatory changes that may lead to earlier onset of heart disease, cancer, and liver disease as well as neurocognitive impairment. The impaired liver and kidney function is more common in the elderly and may result in increased drug exposure by slowing down the metabolism of these agents [20]. Polypharmacy adds complexity to the management of the elderly and may lead to poor medication adherence or confusion about drug dosing [21]. It is recommended that elderly PLWH have lipids, glucose, bone health, and kidney function monitored closely to identify comorbidities and adverse impact of medications [22–26].

Gynecologic Issues and Clinical Manifestations in Women with HIV Infection

Early manifestations of HIV disease in women are often gynecological in nature. These are most commonly recurrent herpetic or candidal infections, pelvic inflammatory disease, and cervical cytologic abnormalities. Thus, it is imperative that women who present with or report a history of frequent recurrences of these problems, without other predisposing factors, be tested for HIV infection. In general, the treatment of STIs, pelvic inflammatory disease, and other genital infections among HIV-uninfected and HIV-infected women is the same; however, the clinical presentation may be more severe and/or more varied among women with HIV infection.

Menstrual abnormalities, particularly amenorrhea, are frequently seen in women living with HIV/AIDS. However, a prospective cohort analysis using the HERS and WIHS cohorts found no association between HIV infection alone and menstrual disorders. However, there was a correlation found between increasing likelihood of these disorders and lower CD4 counts and higher HIV viral loads. In addition, the higher frequency of menstrual disorders among the women with HIV was associated with other factors related to their health status, including weight loss, chronic disease, substance abuse, and the use of psychoactive medications. Studies have found that between 5 and 20% of women with HIV experience abnormalities in their menstrual cycles. For patients whose HIV has progressed to AIDS and experience high viral loads, low CD4 counts, and concomitant health challenges such as wasting syndrome, renal dysfunction, and liver dysfunction, this is often the setting in which amenorrhea occurs. The at-times concomitant substance use, poverty, multiple social stressors, and use of psychotropic drugs in setting of psychiatric comorbidity may also contribute to menstrual cycle abnormalities [27]. Some studies suggest that the decrease in testosterone levels associated with HIV may drive anovulatory cycles although additional studies are needed [28]. HIV may also cause elevated follicle-stimulating hormone (FSH), premature ovarian failure, and menopause, most notably among patients with low CD4 counts [29, 30]. Women with HIV infection, particularly those between 45 and 54 years of age, are more likely to experience psychological and vasomotor menopausal symptoms [31].

Human Papilloma Virus Infection and Cytologic Abnormalities

Human papillomavirus (HPV) infection, the most common sexually transmitted infection, has been identified as the most common causative agent in lower genital tract neoplasia such as cervical cancer and cancers of the vulva, vagina, and anus as well as oropharyngeal cancer. HPV may also cause genital warts. HPV has been strongly associated with HIV infection. HIV complicates the course of moderate and severe dysplasia and for this reason invasive cervical cancer is an AIDS defining condition. Women with HIV also experience higher prevalence of vulvar, vaginal, and perianal intraepithelial lesions [32]. The HIV virus itself has regulatory proteins that have been shown in vitro to increase expression of a regulatory gene for HPV-16 [33], one of the oncogenic strains of HPV. The immunosuppression that accompanies HIV also drives HPV reactivation, which in turn is associated with higher prevalence of squamous intraepithelial lesions for women with HIV infection (17–18%) as compared to matched controls without HIV infection (3–5%) [34, 35]. The more advanced the degree of immunosuppression, the more likely women are to have cervical, perianal, and/or vaginal squamous intraepithelial lesions. Although being infected with HIV has not been demonstrated to independently drive progression of cytological abnormalities, positive HPV serostatus and HIV RNA level > 4000 copies/ml do; nonetheless, the overall prevalence of high-grade lesions is low [36]. A cohort of HIV-infected adolescent girls had a 21.4% incidence of CIN as compared to age-matched HIV-negative controls. Confounding variables included the use of hormonal contraceptives, higher interleukin-12 concentrations that may indicate local immune dysregulation and HPV and low-grade squamous intraepithelial lesion (LSIL) persistence [37].

The influence of antiretroviral therapy (ART) on HPV persistence and the progression or regression of cytologic abnormalities has been difficult to ascertain. HIV treatment may improve immune function and potentially have an antiviral effect on HPV itself; however, not all women on ART experience regression of their cytologic lesions. Those without improvement in CD4 count to levels >200 are more likely to have persistence of HPV, increased progression, and decreased regression of cytologic lesions.

Cervical cancer screening recommendations for women with HIV differ by age. HIV-infected women under 30 years of age should undergo pap test within 1 year of onset of sexual activity or by age 21. Women between 21 and 29 years of age should have two pap tests during the year of HIV diagnosis at least 6 months apart. If three consecutive results show no cytologic abnormality, then follow-up pap test should be completed every 3 years. Abnormal cytologic results such as abnormal squamous cells of undetermined significance (ASCUS) with concomitant positive reflex HPV testing should be referred for colposcopy. If no HPV testing is done, then pap test should be repeated in 6–12 months. More advanced abnormalities than ASCUS, such as low-grade squamous intraepithelial lesion (LSIL) and high-grade squamous epithelial lesion (HSIL), should undergo evaluation with colposcopy. HIV-infected women aged 30 years or older should undergo pap test at the time of diagnosis (with HPV cotesting if available) and then annually even past age 65 when pap tests are no longer recommended for HIV-negative women. If three consecutive pap test results show no cytologic abnormality, then follow-up pap test should be completed every 3 years. During year 1, patients with abnormal cytology or positive HPV should be referred to colposcopy. Thereafter patients with HPV tests revealing high-risk genotypic strains 16 or 18 should undergo colposcopy and those with other strains should undergo repeat HPV test in 1 year. ASCUS-positive results warrant repeat pap test in 6–12 months with recurrent abnormalities referred for colposcopy. More severe lesions should be referred for colposcopy [38]. Treatment failure is associated with remaining HPV-positive and having a CD4 count <200. Treatment with 5-fluorouracil cream has been evaluated as an alternative to excisional therapy for cervical cytologic abnormalities [39].

HPV vaccination with the 9-valent vaccine has shown immunogenicity among HIV-infected women, though less so for women with low CD4 counts, and should be provided to women with HIV who are ages 13–26 years [38].

Trichomonas vaginalis Infections

Overall, the prevalence of genital Trichomonas vaginalis is higher among African-American women in the United States than among other races. In the United States, 13% of black women are affected compared with 1.8% of non-Hispanic white women. This infection is also quite common among women living with HIV, recent studies have shown that approximately 53% have trichomonas co-infection [40]. Trichomonas is associated with preterm delivery and low birth weight. There may be association with pelvic inflammatory disease among women with HIV. It is also associated with infertility [40]. Frequently asymptomatic women with HIV should undergo screening for trichomoniasis at the time of HIV diagnosis and then annually thereafter [41]. Women co-infected with HIV and with trichomonas also tend to have higher HIV viral loads. Usually, trichomoniasis can be effectively treated with single-dose therapy of an appropriate nitroimidazole antibiotic, but HIV-infected women should receive therapy for 7 days [42]. Three months after treatment, women with HIV should undergo repeat testing for trichomoniasis [41].

Bacterial Vaginosis

Bacterial vaginosis (BV) is a nonulcerative clinical vaginosis syndrome character-ized by shifts in the vaginal microbiota with decreases in vaginal lactobacilli and overgrowth of anaerobic and facultative aerobic bacteria such as *Gardnerella vagi-nalis* and *Mycoplasma hominis*, as well as *Atopobium, Mobiluncus, Bacteroides, Prevotella*, and *Peptostreptococcus* species [43]. It has been hypothesized that the pro-inflammatory nature of BV results in an increased risk of HIV acquisition [44]. Estimates of BV prevalence among black women (51.6%), Mexican American women (32.1%), and white, non-Hispanic women (23.2%) demonstrate substantial disparities in rates of infection [44]. These differences may well be contributing to the increased risk of HIV infection among women of color. The prevalence of BV has been associated with several demographic and behavioral factors, including race, age, country of origin, income status, number of sexual partners, hormonal contraceptive use, menopausal status, smoking, alcohol consumption, and douching [44, 45]. BV also is more likely to recur or persist among women with HIV and has increased clinical severity for women with CD4 counts less than 200 [46]. Diagnosis requires homogenous thin white discharge, vaginal fluid pH > 4.5; characteristic odor after application of 10% KOH and clue cells. BV treatment recommendations are the same as for women without HIV infection—oral metronidazole 500 mg twice daily for 7 days or metronidazole 0.75% gel daily for 5 days or clindamycin 2% cream intravaginally × 7 days [40].

Candidal Vaginal Infections

Women with HIV are more likely to have symptomatic vulvovaginal candidiasis than women without HIV. In addition, women with HIV have higher rates of colo-nization with candida and those rates increase with worsening degree of immuno-suppression. Unlike oropharyngeal candida, which is quite common among women living with HIV, is AIDS defining and can be quite refractory, vulvovaginal candi-diasis in women with HIV is rarely refractory to standard treatment with an azole [38]. Either topic or oral treatment with an azole is generally effective; although women with advanced immunosuppression may need longer courses. It is unclear if there is an association between treatment of candida and HIV transmission [40]. Fluconazole prophylaxis may promote resistant candida and nonalbicans strains and therefore should be avoided and discouraged [47].

Gonorrhea and Chlamydia

Both gonorrhea and chlamydia cause genital tract inflammation that can enhance the likelihood of HIV acquisition and yield a 1.8 greater odds of HIV infection [48]. Racial disparities exist in rates of gonorrheal and chlamydial infection, but appear to be related to other structural and demographic features such as poverty and access to health care. Rates of gonorrhea in the United States increased over the 2010–2014 time period. Of note, 25% of gonorrheal infections have antibiotic resistance mutations. In addition, asymptomatic infection is common [40]. Guidelines recommend annual screening for people living with HIV. However, only 60% of women at HIV clinic across the country undergo routine screening [49]. Standard methods of diagnosis and treatment of gonorrhea and chlamydia are recommended for women living with HIV [50, 51]. When screening women for these infections, it is important to screen extragenital sites such as rectum and pharynx for women as genital screening alone will miss a significant number of infections [50, 51].

Syphilis Infections in HIV-Infected Women

Syphilis facilitates the acquisition of HIV infection. Syphilis infection also is associated with increased HIV viral load and decreased CD4 count [52]. Syphilis and HIV co-infection are managed in the same way with a few special considerations. Patients with HIV are at an increased risk of developing neurosyphilis and should undergo careful clinical neurologic evaluation at the time of syphilis diagnosis. At times persons with HIV will have posttreatment syphilis serologic titers that either fluctuate or are higher than expected [40]. In addition, they may have a delay in serologic response after infection [53]. Despite fluctuations in syphilis rates among women over time, notable racial and ethnic disparities in syphilis diagnosis persist. The rate of diagnosis of primary and secondary syphilis among black women is 13.3 times that among white women (4.0 per 100,000 population versus 0.3) [54]. The rate among Hispanic women is 2.7 times that among white women (0.8 per 100,000 population versus 0.3) [54]. Given the potentially dire outcomes of neonatal syphilis, pregnant women should be screened for syphilis at the first prenatal visit [38]. In high prevalence populations, syphilis screening should be repeated during the third trimester and at delivery [38].

Herpes Simplex Virus Infections

Herpes simplex virus type 1 (HSV1) manifests most commonly with orolabial cold sores or fever blisters, but can also less commonly cause genital lesions. HSV1 is present in 60% of US adults and 90% of US adults with HIV infection. HSV2 usually manifests as genital lesions. HSV2 is present in 17% of US adults and up to 95% of those with HIV infection [55]. HSV2 has been found to increase the risk of HIV transmission [56]. For women, HSV2 is associated with a threefold increased risk of HIV acquisition [56]. HSV2 stimulates HIV1 replication in cervical tissues [57]. The recommended treatment for HSV is with 5–10 days of acyclovir 400 mg three times a day OR valacyclovir 1 g twice a day OR famciclovir 500 mg orally twice a day [58].

Patients with nonintact immune systems are also more likely to develop atypical lesions or resistant lesions [59, 60]. Although ART decreases the severity and frequency of outbreaks, asymptomatic subclinical shedding still persists for longer periods of time than for HIV-uninfected people. HSV shedding has been found to increase significantly during the first 90 days after ART initiation and then decreases steadily thereafter [61].

HSV type-specific serologic testing can be offered to persons with HIV infection during their initial evaluation if infection status is unknown, and suppressive antiviral therapy can be considered in those who have HSV-2 infection. Suppressive anti-HSV therapy in persons with HIV infection does not reduce the risk for either HIV transmission or HSV-2 transmission to susceptible sex partners [40].

An important consideration for women is the possible reactivation of HSV2 during the third trimester of pregnancy or at delivery and the potential for neonatal herpes infection [62]. Neonatal herpes most commonly occurs among women who acquire HSV2 during the second half of pregnancy or near term. Women with genital HSV2 lesions at the onset of labor should deliver via cesarean section. Prophylactic acyclovir may be used near term to prevent recurrences and decrease risk of neonatal herpes [62].

Contraception

More than half of the pregnancies that occur among women living with HIV are unplanned [63]. In the United States, 56.2% black women between ages 20 and 44 years who are at risk for unintended pregnancy use the most effective or moderately effective methods of FDA-approved contraception as compared to 59.1% of Hispanic/Latina women and 65.1% of white non-Hispanic women [64]. Unintended pregnancy is associated with delays in the initiation of prenatal care, poor maternal health, and preterm birth. When controlling for age, race and several other factors, having had a live-birth since time of diagnosis with HIV, having seen a clinician, and having had a patient-initiated discussion about pregnancy were all associated with having a lesser chance of unintended pregnancy [65].

Multiple observational studies have examined the impact of hormonal contraception on HIV acquisition. A meta-analysis found no evidence that combination oral contraceptives or norethisterone impacts HIV risk. However, the adjusted hazard ratio for HIV acquisition among women using depot medroxyprogesterone acetate (DMPA) for contraception was substantially increased at 1.5 [66]. The lack of randomized trials examining this question makes it difficult to determine if compounding behavioral factors such as decreased condom use, genital inflammation, or concomitant STIs may be influencing these results. Of possible importance, however, unlike other progestins, such as norethisterone and levonorgestrel, medroxyprogesterone acetate that is commonly used in the depot format as a 3-month injectable contraceptive, mimics cortisol in its effect on the human glucocorticoid receptor. This glucocorticoid-like activity may increase female mucosal permeability, facilitate HIV-1 uptake by increasing levels of the CCR5 coreceptor for HIV-1 entry [67]. Conversely, it has been found that when DMPA is used by HIV-infected women for contraception, it does not impact HIV shedding or impact risk of HIV transmission to sexual partner(s) [68].

HIV infection itself does not impact the effectiveness of contraception. However, there is an increasing body of literature on the interaction between antiretroviral therapy and contraceptive methods and how coadministration may impact the effectiveness of one or the other.

Sexually active women with HIV/AIDS not desiring a pregnancy should be counseled to always use one hormonal contraceptive method and one barrier method to prevent pregnancy as well as HIV transmission and to prevent the acquisition of sexually transmitted infections. The most effective forms of contraception are contraceptive implants with a less than 1% failure rate. Levonorgestrel-containing implants last 5 years, and etonogestrel-containing implants last 3 years. Even among patients taking efavirenz-based ART, which may slightly lessen implant effectiveness, implants are recommended as this incremental difference does not outweigh the benefits [69]. Depot medroxyprogesterone acetate (DMPA), a commonly used option, is a 3-month injectable contraceptive that has a 6% failure rate. Regimens containing the protease inhibitor combination lopinavir-ritonavir may cause a marginal nontoxic increase in DMPA levels that does not modify the contraceptive's effectiveness [69].

A variety of oral contraceptives with different types and concentrations of hormonal agents vary in their efficacy, with an average failure rate of 9% [69]. Drug-drug interactions with antiretroviral exist. There is potentially decreased progestin-based contraceptive efficacy for patients taking either of the nonnucleoside inhibitors (NNRTIs) efavirenz and nevirapine. There is increased progestin exposure with protease inhibitors. Ethinyl estradiol levels decrease when coadministered with protease inhibitors and recently have been found to increase by 25% with cobicistat-boosted elvitegravir. Cobicistat-boosted elvitegravir increases norethindrone exposure by 126% [69].

Intrauterine devices (IUDs) containing levonorgestrel have a 0.2% failure rate as compared to copper IUDs with a 0.8% failure rate. At minimum, screening for symptoms of sexually transmitted infection is recommended prior to placement of an IUD. No drug interactions with ART exist [69]. The World Health Organization recommends avoiding IUD placement for those with advanced AIDS; however, if one is already in place, however, removal is not necessary.

Vaginal rings and transdermal patches have, on average, a 9% failure rate. There is limited data on existence of drug interactions with antiretrovirals for these contraceptive methods [69]. Diaphragms have a 12% failure rate and no drug interactions [69]. Male condoms have an 18% failure rate and female condoms have a 21%, but both have the added benefit of preventing sexually transmitted infections.

Discourse on contraception among women living with HIV is incomplete without consideration that these women may experience community bias and even provider bias toward their pregnancy intentions and may feel unduly influenced to use contraception regardless of their personal pregnancy intention. Patient-centered unbiased preconception counseling is important.

Preconception Counseling

Despite the importance of discussing reproductive options and pregnancy intentions with HIV-infected women on an ongoing basis, it is estimated that only 31% of women have personalized discussions about preconception issues with a provider and most discussions are patient initiated. This is particularly important for US black women, as this group tends to have poorer pregnancy-related health outcomes. In addition, non-Hispanic black women in the United States have 1.8 times the chance of infertility as compared to Hispanic or non-Hispanic white or Asian women [70].

Approximately 60% of women with primary infertility problems intend to have a child in the future. Women with HIV have similar pregnancy desires as women without HIV. Those most likely to have pregnancy intentions are those who are younger and have fewer children and higher physical functioning and overall health. Black women are more likely to desire children in the future than other women living with HIV/AIDS. There is a difference between desire for children and expectation that they will have a child. This fact alone reflects the importance of and need for preconception counseling for all women [71].

Preconception counseling and care can identify and modify risks prior to pregnancy and help prevent unwanted pregnancy. These efforts improve maternal and fetal outcomes by helping HIV-infected women and their partners make informed reproductive decisions, optimize maternal and paternal health prior to pregnancy, and decrease the risk of HIV transmission to the partner or child [71].

Optimizing viral suppression prior to conception helps stabilize the women's health and decrease risk of transmission to her sexual partner and/or to the fetus. Attention to the possible teratogenicity of the antiretroviral treatment regimens such as those containing dolutegravir is extremely important [72]. The preconception period is the optimal time to consider this issue as well as potential ART side effect profile and drug interactions [72]. HIV negative sexual partners should be provided information about HIV preexposure prophylaxis (PrEP), which, with confirmed adherence, decreases the risk of HIV transmission by 90%. Condom use with timed condomless coitus at most fertile times of month for women with undetectable viral loads yields a less than 1% rate of mother-to-child HIV transmission risk [65]. Additional important topics to be covered in optimal preconception counseling include alcohol and tobacco cessation counseling and management and appropriate folic acid supplementation. At present, in the United States, it is recommended that women with HIV not breastfeed [72].

Nongynecologic Clinical Manifestations of HIV in Women

The nongynecologic manifestations of HIV disease differ little in women compared to men. The one exception is Kaposi's sarcoma, which occurs more frequently in men than in women, most likely due to a higher prevalence of co-infection with the etiologic agent of Kaposi's sarcoma, human herpesvirus 8, among men. Pneumocystis pneumonia (PCP) remains the most common opportunistic infection found in HIV-infected patients in the United States; men and women appear to have equivalent risk of infection. Older cohorts reported a higher incidence of esophageal candidiasis among women, but no recent cohorts have clarified whether this difference persists [73].

HIV and the Older Woman

Approximately 47% of those living with HIV in this country are over 50 years of age; this is a dramatic increase in the percent of people living with HIV who are "older" in just a decade [6, 12, 19]. Therefore, many women with HIV are or will be experiencing menopause. Unfortunately, there are few studies characterizing menopause in HIV-infected women. Those that have been published have noted an earlier mean age of menopausal onset (46 years vs. 49 years) [74]. Drug use may also contribute to this finding [75]. In addition, symptoms of menopause, hot flushes, and vaginal dryness may be more severe [76]. Whether older age and estrogen decline translate into differences in treatment response or clinical progression is unclear.

Both untreated HIV and HIV treated with antiretroviral therapy are associated with bone demineralization with increased prevalence of osteoporosis and osteopenia. Menopause may add to the predisposition for these disorders in women. In a study of 31 HIV-infected African-American and Hispanic women, a 43% prevalence of osteoporosis of the spine versus 23% in historical controls was noted [77]. Hormone replacement therapy is generally felt to be underutilized in women with HIV. We need additional studies to understand the risk and benefits and to further characterize the interactions with antiretroviral therapy.

Clinical Care of Women Living with HIV/AIDS

The care of women with living with HIV has two key components: (1) provision of medications to treat HIV disease (antiretroviral therapy) and (2) overall care—consisting of the care setting, organization of care, and the manner in which care is delivered. Related to the first of these, antiretroviral therapy—this aspect of care does not differ for women compared to men, because the efficacy of ART in women appears to be generally the same as in men [78]. However, the overall clinical care of women is much more complex and has many aspects that should be considered and optimized by clinical care sites. In 2011, Gardner et al. described the HIV care cascade, which details the percent of patients who are diagnosed, linked to care, retained in care, and virologically suppressed [79]. When initially described, this cascade documented clear-cut disparities in the linkage to care of women and black patients. These findings served to clarify the basis for the long-standing poorer outcomes seen among women and black patients. Fortunately, recent data seem to suggest that linkage to care among women overall has improved and now may be equal to that of men [80]. However, the rates of linkage to care is still far from optimal among all patients (57%) and remains lower among black patients [80, 81]. Moreover, recent studies have documented that black patients are more likely to miss clinic visits and more likely to have a detectable viral load [82, 83]. While all of these concerning findings can be extrapolated to black women, who comprise the majority of women with HIV/AIDS, one study recent study has clearly demonstrated higher mortality among black women with HIV/AIDS [84]. Therefore, it is extremely clear that efforts to optimize linkage to care, engagement in care, and retention in care among women of color are vitally important and can have important implications for their long-term outcomes.

To ideally engage women of color in care (and >80% of women living with HIV/AIDS are women of color), clinical care sites should demonstrate in multiple small ways that they are there to welcome and care for women living with HIV/AIDS. These approaches can include, but are not limited to, employing staff who are women and who are of the same culture as the patients being served, having magazines and educational materials of interest to women of color in the waiting room, and displaying art and flyers that are of interest to women, and making the environment appear more inviting and appealing. In addition, clinical care sites should host celebrations at special times of the year (such as holidays and World AIDS Day) that are fun and include foods from the cultures of the patients being served. Most importantly, clinical programs should be developed and offered that meet the special (and frequent) needs and concerns of women living with HIV/AIDS. These include ensuring on-site (or easy access to) social workers, mental health services, substance abuse services, gynecologic care especially colposcopy, dermatology, and nutritionists, as well as other weight-related care services. Finally, educational programs focused on the needs of the women who come to the clinical care site should be offered on a regular basis, and support groups should be available for women to decrease social isolation and to promote social support through contact with staff and with others living with HIV/AIDS.

Optimizing access to antiretroviral therapy should be a priority in the care of women living with HIV infection. Numerous studies over the years have found that women are less likely to receive antiretroviral therapy when indicated than are men with HIV infection [85, 86]. And, a series of more recent studies has found that minority women, particularly black women, are even less likely than other women to receive antiretroviral therapy when indicated [87, 88]. The reasons for this disparity in the receipt of antiretroviral therapy have not been clearly elucidated. Contributing factors to this disparity in the receipt of antiretroviral therapy may include (1) provider-patient encounter factors (e.g., miscommunications and misunderstandings in the clinical care setting), (2) medical comorbidities such as hepatitis C infection, depression, or substance abuse that cause the patient or her provider to delay prescribing antiretroviral therapy, and (3) competing life circumstances such as unstable living situation, personal relationship problems such as domestic violence, or needs of children, partners, parents, or others for which the patient serves as a caregiver. Finally, women appear to discontinue antiretroviral therapy due to side effects more often than men do [89]. While the causes are not entirely clear (and may be myriad), what is clear is that this disparity is one of the largest contributors to the disparity in death rates due to HIV/AIDS among minority women than among others [84].

Given this, providers should proactively encourage women who meet current US Department of Health and Human Services Guideline indications for HAART to start HAART and to stay on antiretroviral therapy. Strategies such as the use of peer counselors, treatments buddies, and frequent visits can be helpful in enhancing the patient's acceptance of antiretroviral therapy and engagement in treatment. The quality of the patient's relationship with her HIV primary provider has been found to be critically important for acceptance of treatment and adherence to treatment [90, 91]. Efforts to spend time with the patient, getting to know her, having relatively frequent visits, and spending some time during visits on nonclinical conversation can contribute to this goal. Having a second or third provider with whom the patient is consistently connected and can turn to in the primary provider's absence such as a primary nurse or case manager has also been shown to enhance engagement in care [92, 93].

Many women living with HIV/AIDS may have one or more of the documented barriers to adherence to antiretroviral therapy such as depression, substance abuse, alcohol abuse, low literacy, chaotic living situation, or nondisclosure of HIV status to family. Providers and care sites should therefore have a set of strategies and programmatic interventions that they consistently utilize to proactively optimize antiretroviral adherence and thereby optimize the outcomes of women of color on antiretroviral therapy [94, 95].

References

1. WHO. Number of women living with HIV: situation and trends. 2018. www.who.int/gho/hiv/epidemic_status/cases_adults_women_children_text/en/.
2. Centers for Disease Control. HIV among women. 2018. https://www.cdc.gov/hiv/group/gender/women/index.html.
3. Johnson AS, et al. Trends in diagnoses of HIV infection in the United States, 2002-2011. JAMA. 2014;312:432–4. https://doi.org/10.1001/jama.2014.8534.
4. Centers for Disease Control. HIV and Hispanics/Latinos. 2018. https://www.cdc.gov/hiv/group/racialethnic/hispaniclatinos/index.html.
5. Garcia D, Betancourt G, Scaccabarrozzi L, editors. The Latino Commission on AIDS. New York: Hispanic Health Network; 2015.

6. Centers for Disease Control and Prevention. HIV surveillance report, 2017; vol. 29. http://www.cdc.gov/hiv/library/reports/hiv-surveillance.html. Published November 2018. Accessed 13 July 2019.

7. Adimora AA, et al. Heterosexually transmitted HIV infection among African Americans in North Carolina. J Acquir Immune Defic Syndr. 2006;41:616–23.

8. Adimora AA, et al. Social context of sexual relationships among rural African Americans. Sex Transm Dis. 2001;28:69–76.

9. Forna FM, et al. A case-control study of factors associated with HIV infection among black women. J Natl Med Assoc. 2006;98:1798–804.

10. Moreno CL, El-Bassel N, Morrill AC. Heterosexual women of color and HIV risk: sexual risk factors for HIV among Latina and African American women. Women Health. 2007;45:1–15.

11. Peragallo N, Gonzalez-Guarda RM, McCabe BE, Cianelli R. The efficacy of an HIV risk reduction intervention for Hispanic women. AIDS Behav. 2012;16:1316–26. https://doi.org/10.1007/s10461-011-0052-6.

12. Clark RA, Kissinger P, Bedimo AL, Dunn P, Albertin H. Determination of factors associated with condom use among women infected with human immunodeficiency virus. Int J STD AIDS. 1997;8:229.

13. Sarkar K, et al. Young age is a risk factor for HIV among female sex workers- an experience from India. J Infect. 2006;53:255–9.

14. Heffernan R, Chiasson MA, Sackoff JE. HIV risk behaviors among adolescents at a sexually transmitted disease clinic in New York City. J Adolesc Health. 1996;18:429–34.

15. Patel P, et al. Estimating per-act HIV transmission risk: a systematic review. AIDS. 2014;28:1509–19. https://doi.org/10.1097/QAD.0000000000000298.

16. Duriux-Smith A, TW EC, Goodman JT. Comparison of female to male and male to female transmission of HIV in 563 stable couples. European Study Group on Heterosexual Transmission of HIV. BMJ. 1992;304:809–13.

17. Leichliter JS, Chandra A, Liddon N, Fenton KA, Aral SO. Prevalence and correlates of heterosexual anal and oral sex in adolescents and adults in the United States. J Infect Dis. 2007;196:1852–9. https://doi.org/10.1086/522867.

18. Sterling TR, Vlahav D, Astemborski J, et al. Initial plasma HIV-1 RNA levels and progression to AIDS in women and men. N Engl J Med. 2001;344:720–5.

19. Panel on Antiretroviral Guidelines for Adults and Adolescents. Guidelines for the use of antiretroviral agents in adults and adolescents with HIV. Department of Health and Human Services. Available at http://www.aidsinfo.nih.gov/ContentFiles/AdultandAdolescentGL.pdf. Accessed 13 July 2019.

20. Sitar DS. Aging issues in drug disposition and efficacy. Proc West Pharmacol Soc. 2007;50:16–20.

21. Steinman MA, Hanlon JT. Managing medications in clinically complex elders: "There's got to be a happy medium". JAMA. 2010;304:1592–601. https://doi.org/10.1001/jama.2010.1482.

22. Aberg JA, et al. Primary care guidelines for the management of persons infected with HIV: 2013 update by the HIV Medicine Association of the Infectious Diseases Society of America. Clin Infect Dis. 2014;58:1–10. https://doi.org/10.1093/cid/cit757.

23. Brown TT, et al. Recommendations for evaluation and management of bone disease in HIV. Clin Infect Dis. 2015;60:1242–51. https://doi.org/10.1093/cid/civ010.

24. Lucas GM, et al. Clinical practice guideline for the management of chronic kidney disease in patients infected with HIV: 2014 update by the HIV Medicine Association of the Infectious Diseases Society of America. Clin Infect Dis. 2014;59:e96–138. https://doi.org/10.1093/cid/ciu617.

25. Medicine, A. A. o. H. The HIV and aging consensus project: recommended treatment strategies for clinicians managing older patients with HIV. 2011. http://www.aahivm.org/Upload_Module/upload/HIV%20and%20Aging/Aging%20report%20working%20document%20FINAL.pdf.

26. Jacobson TA, et al. National lipid association recommendations for patient-centered management of dyslipidemia: part 1--full report. J Clin Lipidol. 2015;9:129–69. https://doi.org/10.1016/j.jacl.2015.02.003.
27. Cejtin HE. Gynecologic issues in the HIV-infected woman. Infect Dis Clin N Am. 2008;22:709–39. https://doi.org/10.1016/j.idc.2008.05.006.
28. Sinha-Hikim I, et al. The use of a sensitive equilibrium dialysis method for the measurement of free testosterone levels in healthy, cycling women and in HIV-infected women. J Clin Endocrinol Metab. 1998;83:1312–8.
29. Schoenbaum EE, et al. HIV infection, drug use, and onset of natural menopause. Clin Infect Dis. 2005;41:1517–24.
30. Seifer DB, et al. Biologic markers of ovarian reserve and reproductive aging: application in a cohort study of HIV infection in women. Fertil Steril. 2007;88:1645–52. https://doi.org/10.1016/j.fertnstert.2007.01.122.
31. Ferreira CE, et al. Menopause symptoms in women infected with HIV: prevalence and associated factors. Gynecol Endocrinol. 2007;23:198–205. https://doi.org/10.1080/09513590701253743.
32. Jamieson DJ, Paramsothy P, Cu-Uvin S, Duerr A, Group., H. E. R. S. Vulvar, vaginal, and perianal intraepithelial neoplasia in women with or at risk for human immunodeficiency virus. Obstet Gynecol. 2006;107:1023–8.
33. Vernon SD, Hart CE, Reeves WC, Icenogle JP. The HIV-1 tat protein enhances E2-dependent human papillomavirus transmission. Virus Res. 1993;27:133–45.
34. Massad LS, et al. Prevalence and predictors of squamous cell abnormalities in Papanicolaou smears from women infected with HIV-1. Women's Interagency HIV Study Group. J Acquir Immune Defic Syndr. 1999;21:33–41.
35. Duerr A, et al. Human papillomavirus-associated cervical cytologic abnormalities among women with or at risk of infection with human immunodeficiency virus. Am J Obstet Gynecol. 2001;184:584–90.
36. Massad LS, et al. Evolution of cervical abnormalities among women with HIV-1: evidence from surveillance cytology in the Women's Interagency HIV Study. JAIDS. 2001;27:432–42.
37. Moscicki AB, et al. Risk of high-grade squamous intraepithelial lesion in HIV-infected adolescents. J Infect Dis. 2004;190:1413–21. https://doi.org/10.1086/424466.
38. Panel on Opportunistic Infections in HIV-Infected Adults and Adolescents. Guidelines for prevention and treatment of opportunistic infections in HIV-infected adults and adolescents. https://aidsinfo.nih.gov/contentfiles/lvguidelines/adult_oi.pdf. Accessed 20 May 2019.
39. Maiman M, et al. Vaginal 5-fluorouracil for high-grade cervical dysplasia in human immunodeficiency virus infection: a randomized trial. Obstet Gynecol. 1999;94:954–61.
40. Workowski KA, Bolan GA, Prevention., C. f. D. C. a. Sexually transmitted diseases treatment guidelines, 2015. MMWR Recomm Rep. 2015;64:1–137.
41. Meites E, et al. A review of evidence-based Care of Symptomatic Trichomoniasis and Asymptomatic Trichomonas vaginalis infections. Clin Infect Dis. 2015;61(Suppl 8):S837–48. https://doi.org/10.1093/cid/civ738.
42. Kissinger P, et al. A randomized treatment trial: single versus 7-day dose of metronidazole for the treatment of Trichomonas vaginalis among HIV-infected women. J Acquir Immune Defic Syndr. 2010;55:565–71.
43. Chehoud C, et al. Associations of the vaginal microbiota with HIV infection, bacterial vaginosis, and demographic factors. AIDS. 2017;31:895–904. https://doi.org/10.1097/QAD.0000000000001421.
44. Alcendor DJ. Evaluation of health disparity in bacterial Vaginosis and the implications for HIV-1 Acquisition in African American Women. Am J Reprod Immunol. 2016;76:99–107. https://doi.org/10.1111/aji.12497.
45. Koumans EH, et al. The prevalence of bacterial vaginosis in the United States, 2001-2004; associations with symptoms, sexual behaviors, and reproductive health. Sex Transm Dis. 2007;34:864–9. https://doi.org/10.1097/OLQ.0b013e318074e565.

46. Jamieson DJ, et al. Longitudinal analysis of bacterial vaginosis: findings from the HIV epidemiology research study. Obstet Gynecol. 2001;98:656–63.
47. Vazquez JA, et al. Evolution of antifungal susceptibility among Candida species isolates recovered from human immunodeficiency virus-infected women receiving fluconazole prophylaxis. Clin Infect Dis. 2001;33:1069–75.
48. Johnson LF, Lewis DA. The effect of genital tract infections on HIV-1 shedding in the genital tract: a systematic review and meta-analysis. Sex Transm Dis. 2008;35:946–59. https://doi.org/10.1097/OLQ.0b013e3181812d15.
49. Berry SA, et al. Brief report: gonorrhea and chlamydia testing increasing but still lagging in HIV clinics in the United States. J Acquir Immune Defic Syndr. 2015;70:275–9. https://doi.org/10.1097/QAI.0000000000000711.
50. Travassos AG, et al. Anogenital infection by chlamydia trachomatis and Neisseria gonorrhoeae in HIV-infected men and women in Salvador, Brazil. Braz J Infect Dis. 2016;20:569–75. https://doi.org/10.1016/j.bjid.2016.09.004.
51. Tao G, et al. Infrequent testing of women for rectal chlamydia and Gonorrhea in the United States. Clin Infect Dis. 2018;66:570–5. https://doi.org/10.1093/cid/cix857.
52. Kofoed K, Gerstoft J, Mathiesen LR, Benfield T. Syphilis and human immunodeficiency virus (HIV)-1 coinfection: influence on CD4 T-cell count, HIV-1 viral load, and treatment response. Sex Transm Dis. 2006;33:143–8. https://doi.org/10.1097/01.olq.0000187262.56820.c0.
53. Kingston AA, et al. Seronegative secondary syphilis in 2 patients coinfected with human immunodeficiency virus. Arch Dermatol. 2005;141:431–3. https://doi.org/10.1001/archderm.141.4.431.
54. Patton ME, Su JR, Nelson R, Weinstock H. Primary and secondary syphilis--United States, 2005-2013. MMWR Morb Mortal Wkly Rep. 2014;63:402–6.
55. Xu F, et al. Trends in herpes simplex virus type 1 and type 2 seroprevalence in the United States. JAMA. 2006;296:964–73. https://doi.org/10.1001/jama.296.8.964.
56. Freeman EE, et al. Herpes simplex virus 2 infection increases HIV acquisition in men and women: systematic review and meta-analysis of longitudinal studies. AIDS. 2006;20:73–83.
57. Rollenhagen C, Lathrop MJ, Macura SL, Doncel GF, Asin SN. Herpes simplex virus type-2 stimulates HIV-1 replication in cervical tissues: implications for HIV-1 transmission and efficacy of anti-HIV-1 microbicides. Mucosal Immunol. 2014;7:1165–74. https://doi.org/10.1038/mi.2014.3.
58. Warren T, Harris J, Brennan CA. Efficacy and safety of valacyclovir for the suppression and episodic treatment of herpes simplex virus in patients with HIV. Clin Infect Dis. 2004;39(Suppl 5):S258–66. https://doi.org/10.1086/422362.
59. Levin MJ, Bacon TH, Leary JJ. Resistance of herpes simplex virus infections to nucleoside analogues in HIV-infected patients. Clin Infect Dis. 2004;39(Suppl 5):S248–57. https://doi.org/10.1086/422364.
60. Safrin S, et al. Correlation between response to acyclovir and foscarnet therapy and in vitro susceptibility result for isolates of herpes simplex virus from human immunodeficiency virus-infected patients. Antimicrob Agents Chemother. 1994;38:1246–50.
61. Ford ES, et al. Increase in HSV shedding at initiation of antiretroviral therapy and decrease in shedding over time on antiretroviral therapy in HIV and HSV-2 infected persons. AIDS. 2018;32:2525–31.
62. Sheffield JS, Hollier LM, Hill JB, Stuart GS, Wendel GD. Acyclovir prophylaxis to prevent herpes simplex virus recurrence at delivery: a systematic review. Obstet Gynecol. 2003;102:1396–403.
63. Halperin DT, Stover J, Reynolds HW. Benefits and costs of expanding access to family planning programs to women living with HIV. AIDS. 2009;23(Suppl 1):S123–30. https://doi.org/10.1097/01.aids.0000363785.73450.5a.
64. Department of Health and Human Services, Office of Disease Prevention and Health Promotion. National survey of family growth. https://www.healthypeople.gov/2020/datasource/national-survey-of-family-growth. Accessed 20 May 2019.

65. Rahangdale L, et al. Pregnancy intentions among women living with HIV in the United States. J Acquir Immune Defic Syndr. 2014;65:306–11.
66. Morrison CS, et al. Hormonal contraception and the risk of HIV acquisition: an individual participant data meta-analysis. PLoS Med. 2015;12:e1001778. https://doi.org/10.1371/journal.pmed.1001778.
67. Hapgood JP, Kaushic C, Hel Z. Hormonal contraception and HIV-1 acquisition: biological mechanisms. Endocr Rev. 2018;39:36–78.
68. Chinula L, et al. Effect of the depot medroxyprogesterone acetate injectable and levonorgestrel implant on HIV genital shedding: a randomized trial. Contraception. 2018;98:193–8. https://doi.org/10.1016/j.contraception.2018.05.001.
69. Patel RC, Bukusi EA, Baeten JM. Current and future contraceptive options for women living with HIV. Expert Opin Pharmacother. 2018;19:1–12. https://doi.org/10.1080/14656566.2017.1378345.
70. Chandra A, Copen CE, Stephen EH. Infertility and impaired fecundity in the United States, 1982-2010: data from the National Survey of Family Growth. Natl Health Stat Report. 2013:1–18, 11 p following 19.
71. Chen JL, Philips KA, Kanouse DE, Collins RL, Miu A. Fertility desires and intentions of HIV-positive men and women. Fam Plann Perspect. 2001;33:144–52, 165.
72. Panel on Treatment of Pregnant Women with HIV Infection and Prevention of Perinatal Transmission. Recommendations for use of antiretroviral drugs in transmission in the United States. Available at http://aidsinfo.nih.gov/contentfiles/lvguidelines/PerinatalGL.pdf. Accessed 13 July 2019.
73. Clark RA, Brandon W, Dumestre J, Pindaro C. Clinical manifestations of infection with the human immunodeficiency virus in women in Louisiana. Clin Infect Dis. 1993;17:165–70.
74. Cejtin HE. Gynecologic issues in the HIV-infected woman. Obstet Gynecol Clin N Am. 2003;30(4):711–29.
75. Santoro N, Arsten JH, Buono D, et al. Impact of street drug use, HIV infection, and highly active antiretroviral therapy on reproductive hormones in middle-aged women. J Women's Health. 2005;14:898–905.
76. Fantry LE, Zhan M, Taylor GH, et al. Age of menopause and menopausal symptoms in HIV-infected women. AIDS Patient Care STDs. 2005;19:703–11.
77. Yin M, Dobkin J, Brudney K, et al. Bone mass and mineral metabolism in HIV+ postmenopausal women. Osteoporos Int. 2005;16:1345–52.
78. Soon GG, Min M, Struble KA, et al. Meta-analysis of gender differences in efficacy outcomes for HIV-positive subjects in randomized controlled clinical trials of antiretroviral therapy (2000-2008). AIDS Patient Care STDs. 2012;26:444–9.
79. Gardner EM, McLees MP, Steiner JF, del Rio C, Burman WJ. The spectrum of engagement in HIV care and its relevance to "test and treat" strategies for prevention of HIV infection. Clin Infect Dis. 2011;52:793–800.
80. Horberg MA, Hurley LB, Klein DB, et al. The HIV care cascade measured over time and by age, sex, and race in a large integrated care system. AIDS Patient Care and STDs. 2015;29:582–8.
81. Center for Disease Control and Prevention. Selected national HIV prevention and care outcomes in the United States. https://www.cdc.gov/hiv/pdf/library/slidesets/cdc-hiv-prevention-and-care-outcomes.pdf. June 2018. Accessed 14 July 2019.
82. Mugavero MJ, Westfall AO, Cole SR, et al. Beyond core indicators of retention in HIV care: missed clinic visits are independently associated with all cause mortality. Clin Infet Dis. 2014;59:1471–9.
83. Nance RM, Delaney JAC, Simoni JM, et al. HIV viral suppression trends over time among HIV-infected patients receiving care in the U.S. 1997-2015. Ann Intern Med. 2018;169:376–84.
84. Lesko CR, Cole SR, Miller WC, et al. Ten year survival by race/ethnicity and sex among treated, HIV-infected adults in the U.S. Clin Infect Dis. 2015;60:1700–7.
85. Shapiro MF, Morton SC, DF MC, et al. Variations in the care of HIV-infected adults in the United States. JAMA. 1999;281:2305–15.

86. Gebo KA, Fleishman JA, Conviser R, et al. Racial and gender disparities in receipt of highly active antiretroviral therapy persist in a multistate sample of HIV patients in 2001. J Acquir Immune Defic Syndr. 2005;38(1):96–103.

87. Cohen MH, Cook JA, Grey D, et al. Medically eligible women who do not use HAART: the importance of abuse, drug use, and race. AM J Pub Health. 2004;94(7):1147–51.

88. Lillie-Blanton M, Stone VE, Snow Jones A, et al. Association of race, substance use and health insurance coverage with use of highly active antiretroviral therapy in HIV-infected women. Am J Public Health. 2010;100(8):1493–9.

89. Lucas GM, Chaisson RE, Moore RD. Highly active antiretroviral therapy in a large urban clinic: risk factors for virologic failure and adverse drug reactions. Ann Intern Med. 1999;131:81–9.

90. Malcolm SE, Ng JJ, Rosen RK, Stone VE. An examination of HIV/AIDS patients who have excellent adherence to HAART. AIDS Care. 2003;15:251–61.

91. Stone VE, Clarke J, Lovell J, et al. HIV/AIDS patients' perspectives on adhering to regimens containing protease inhibitors. J Gen Intern Med. 1998;13(9):586–93.

92. Stone VE, Weissman JS, Cleary P. Satisfaction with ambulatory care of persons with AIDS: predictors of patient ratings of quality. J Gen Intern Med. 1995;10:239–45.

93. Stein MD, Fleishman J, Mor V, Dresser M. Factors associated with patient satisfaction among symptomatic HIV-infected persons. Med Care. 1993;31:182–8.

94. Stone VE, Smith KY. Improving adherence to highly active antiretroviral therapy. J Natl Med Assoc. 2004;96(2):27S–9S.

95. Berg KM, Demas PA, Howard AA, et al. Gender differences in factors associated with antiretroviral therapy. J Gen Intern Med. 2004;11:1111–7.

Chapter 7
HIV and Immigrants from Sub-Saharan Africa and the Caribbean Living in the United States

Bisola O. Ojikutu, Chioma Nnaji, and Jessy G. Dévieux

Introduction

Significant racial disparities exist within the HIV epidemic in the United States (US) with Black or African-American individuals bearing a disproportionate burden of new infections and the highest mortality rate compared to other racial groups [1]. Though progress has been made to reduce these disparities, little attention has focused on non-US-born (immigrant, foreign-born) Black individuals, most of whom are from sub-Saharan Africa (African-born) and the Caribbean (Caribbean-born) and comprise an increasing proportion of the Black population throughout the United States [2]. Non-US-born Black individuals are categorized within most nationally representative databases as Black or African-American. Therefore, their unique characteristics and needs are often unrecognized and underreported [3]. However, important differences regarding HIV infection by nativity exist within the Black population in the United States. Nationally, non-US-born Black individuals have a new HIV diagnosis rate that is higher than US-born Black individuals [4]. Most notably, in 2014, African-born women had an annual HIV diagnosis rate that was more than five times higher than US-born Black women (100.5 versus 19.1 per 100,000 population) [5].

It is important to note that these data may be an underrepresentation of the actual burden of infection. Country of origin is not a required component of HIV surveillance data collection. Therefore, it is often incompletely collected or may be

B. O. Ojikutu (✉)
Divisions of Global Health Equity, Division of Infectious Diseases, Department of Medicine, Brigham and Women's Hospital, Harvard Medical School, Boston, MA, USA
e-mail: bojikutu@mgh.harvard.edu

C. Nnaji
Multicultural AIDS Coalition, Boston, MA, USA

J. G. Dévieux
Department of Health Promotion and Disease Prevention, Florida International University, Miami, FL, USA

© Springer Nature Switzerland AG 2021
B. O. Ojikutu, V. E. Stone (eds.), *HIV in US Communities of Color*,
https://doi.org/10.1007/978-3-030-48744-7_7

inaccurately assigned [6]. In an analysis describing the epidemiology of HIV infection among non-US-born individuals conducted by the Center for Disease Control and Prevention (CDC) using the National HIV Surveillance System, 18.7% or 35,806 records were missing country of origin data [7].

In addition to these epidemiologic disparities, cultural and structural factors among Black individuals differ by nativity and may impact HIV risk and access to services. Studies comparing US- and non-US-born Black individuals across regions of origin have identified divergent HIV-related cultural norms and beliefs, as well as differences in HIV knowledge, HIV-related stigma, and self-perceived behavioral risk [8–10]. Furthermore, diverse norms and beliefs regarding HIV exist by specific country of origin and have received little attention in the medical literature [11, 12].

Immigration, as a social determinant of health, also poses unique challenges for African- and Caribbean-born individuals [13]. Migratory populations face numerous structural barriers secondary to immigration status, including limited access to health insurance, health care, and employment [13]. These structural impediments are compounded by individual-level barriers, such as language discordance with health care providers, lack of familiarity with a foreign health care system, and poverty, all of which may impact use of HIV prevention, care, and treatment services and behavioral risk [14–16].

For non-US-born Black individuals, the intersectionality of race and migratory experience must also be acknowledged. Newly acquired minority status, racism, discrimination, and mistrust of institutions led and staffed by non-Black individuals serve as important barriers to health care access [17]. Non-US-born Black individuals may also be transnational and maintain strong, multi-stranded social relationships within their home countries which may impact HIV risk, norms, and beliefs [18]. Moreover, the complex interplay of displacement, acculturative stress, and mental health disorders has been described as a unique challenge to the provision of health care services, including HIV prevention, care, and treatment [19, 20]. Given these important differences between US- and non-US-born Black individuals, disaggregation by country (or region) of origin is critical to eliminating persistent racial disparities and achieving health equity [6].

This chapter focuses on describing challenges and barriers to HIV prevention, care, and treatment among non-US-born Black individuals living in the United States from sub-Saharan Africa (African-born) and the Caribbean (Caribbean-born). Salient gaps in knowledge and unmet needs regarding HIV within these diverse and often marginalized populations are highlighted. Strategies and interventions that have proven successful in overcoming the barriers noted are also described. In addition, the authors provide recommendations regarding the collection of HIV surveillance data, service delivery, community engagement, and future research.

Immigration from Africa and the Caribbean

Over the course of the last four decades, a steady growth in the number of immigrants to the United States from sub-Saharan Africa and the Caribbean has been noted. From 1980 to 2017, the number of non-US-born Black individuals living in the United States rose from approximately 800,000 to 4.2 million. In 2017, approximately 10% of the Black population in the United States was non-US born [21, 22]. The primary drivers of migration from Africa and the Caribbean to the United States are rooted in historical and contemporary oppression, imperialism, political upheaval, and socioeconomic deprivation. For example, beginning in the mid-1950s in sub-Saharan Africa, the struggle for independence from colonial powers heralded a phase of state formation during which internal tensions and violence led to increased migration both within the continent and to Europe and North America [23]. Further highlighting the impact of Western countries on migration, in Haiti, from the mid-1950s through the 1980s, the rise of brutal, violent dictatorships supported and maintained by certain US political and economic interests drove thousands of Haitians to migrate to the United States [24, 25].

More recently, changes to US immigration policy allowing the entry of a wider variety of migrants, including the Immigration Act of 1990 which created the Diversity Immigrant Visa Program, have contributed to increased immigration from sub-Saharan Africa and the Caribbean [26]. Though more restrictive immigration policies have subsequently been sought and enacted [27], voluntary migration to access economic and educational opportunities, as well as flight from war, natural disasters, adverse social events, and political instability will continue to drive immigration to the United States from sub-Saharan Africa and the Caribbean. According to the US Census Bureau, by 2060, 16.5% of Black individuals living in the United States will be African- or Caribbean-born [28]. These newcomers will continue to be a heterogeneous group, differentiated by their cultural, linguistic, religious, social, socioeconomic backgrounds, and immigration status [22, 29].

Much of the rise in Black immigrant population has been due to increased migration from sub-Saharan Africa. The population of African-born individuals in the United States has doubled every decade since 1970. In 2016, there were 1.6 million African-born individuals in the United States, and immigrants from sub-Saharan Africa comprised 39% of the overall non-US-born Black population [22, 29]. Most are from Western (e.g., Nigeria, Ghana, and Liberia) and Eastern (e.g., Ethiopia, Kenya, and Somalia) sub-Saharan Africa. In regard to post-migration residence, African-born individuals tend to be diffusely spread throughout the United States with the largest number living within the greater New York City and Washington, DC, metropolitan areas [30]. Only 27% report limited English proficiency, compared to 48% of the overall immigrant population [31]. Approximately 40% of African-born individuals hold a bachelor's degree or higher compared to 31% and 32% of all non-US-born and US-born individuals, respectively. However, educational attainment is not an accurate predictor of socioeconomic status among African-born individuals who experience poverty at a higher rate than the non-US-born population overall [31].

In 2016, 49% of the non-US-born Black population living in the United States were from the Caribbean with Jamaica and Haiti being the largest source countries [22]. In recent decades, the United States has experienced a significant increase in the number of immigrants from Haiti secondary to political instability, poverty, and natural disasters. Following the 2010 earthquake, the number of Haitian immigrants in the United States rose from 587,000 to 676,000 [32]. Approximately 51% of

Haitian Immigrants report limited English proficiency [33]. Overall, non-US-born Black individuals from the Caribbean (including Haiti) are more geographically concentrated than non-US-born individuals from sub-Saharan Africa. More than 60% of Caribbean immigrants reside in greater New York City or the Miami metropolitan area [32, 33]. A lower percentage of non-US-born individuals from the Caribbean have bachelor's degrees or higher (20%) compared to other non-US-born individuals (31%). Approximately 17% of Caribbean immigrants live in poverty versus 15% of immigrants overall [32, 33].

HIV Epidemiology

More than one in every six individuals newly diagnosed with HIV is non-US born [4, 7]. Among immigrants, African- and Caribbean-born individuals are disproportionately affected. From 2010–2014, African and Caribbean-born individuals accounted for 13.9% of the US-foreign-born population, but combined represented 38.8% of HIV cases with known country of origin data among immigrants [4]. Gender differences by region of origin have also been noted. Most non-US-born women recently diagnosed with HIV are from Africa (39.5%) or the Caribbean (27%). Among non-US-born males, most are from Mexico and Central America (combined: 42.4%) and the Caribbean (18.9%) [4]. Geographic disparities by nativity have also been noted with disproportionate rates of new HIV diagnoses among non-US-born Black individuals reported within specific cities, states, and jurisdictions (e.g., New York City; Massachusetts; King County, Washington State; Washington D.C.; Minnesota; Miami-Dade County, Florida, Utah) [34–41]. For example, in King County, Washington State, non-US-born individuals comprised 34% of the newly diagnosed population in 2015; 34% of the newly diagnosed non-US-born population were African-born [34]. In Massachusetts, non-US-born individuals comprise 36% of recently diagnosed HIV infections; 29% are from sub-Saharan Africa, 28% from the Caribbean, and 27% from Central and South America [35].

Comparing non-US-born to US-born Black individuals diagnosed with HIV reveals a number of important differences. Among Black individuals in the United States, African-born women have the highest rate of new HIV diagnoses. In 2014, the HIV diagnosis rate among African-born Black women was 1.4 times the rate of US-born Black men, 2.0 times the rate of African-born men, and 5.3 times the rate of US-born Black women [5]. More than half of newly diagnosed African-born individuals are women (60.7%) versus 27.0% among US-born Black individuals [7]. Among Caribbean-born women, the diagnosis rate is 1.6 times the rate in US-born Black women [5] (See Table 7.1). While a decrease in annual HIV diagnoses rate has been noted among Black women, the decrease among African-born women is the smallest of all subgroups by region [42].

Differences in transmission risk category by region of origin have also been noted. The most common transmission risk factor for African- and Caribbean-born

Table 7.1 Annual HIV diagnoses rates, 2014 per 100,000 population

African-born women	100.5
US-born Black men[a]	72.8
African-born men	51.3
Caribbean-born men	40.6
Caribbean-born women	31.8
US-born Black women	19.1

Reference: Demeke et al. [6]
[a]Data include US-born Black MSM

newly diagnosed individuals is heterosexual sex versus male-to-male sexual contact for individuals born in other regions of the world [5].

Additionally, late diagnosis which is defined as presenting with an AIDS diagnosis (CD4 count <200 cells/ml^3) ≤3 months post a positive HIV test is more common among non-US Black individuals (36.6%) compared to US-born Black individuals (25.8%) [5]. However, survival is higher among non-US-born Black individuals compared to their US-born counterparts [5].

Location of HIV Acquisition

As mentioned earlier, late presentation is more common among non-US-born compared to US-born Black individuals living with HIV [5]. Most non-US-born Black individuals emigrate from countries (e.g., Nigeria, Ethiopia, Jamaica, and Haiti) where the prevalence of HIV is higher than in the United States [21, 43–46]. Therefore, the predominant assumption has been that they acquired HIV pre-immigration in their home countries, and the delay in presentation is a result of the prolonged timeline of migration, not HIV acquisition post-migration in the United States [47]. However, African- and Caribbean-born individuals may be at risk in the United States and require increased HIV testing and prevention strategies. Determining the location of HIV acquisition may help promote the development of HIV prevention services that specifically address the needs of non-US-born Black individuals.

Evidence has emerged that a significant proportion of non-US-born Black individuals acquired HIV infection post-immigration [48–52]. Patient life histories, rate of CD4 decline, surveillance data, and phylogenetic analysis provide evidence to support this theory. Harawa et al. compared age at HIV diagnosis, number of years in the United States, and age at immigration among HIV positive, non-US-born individuals at public health clinics in Los Angeles County and concluded that the relatively young age at arrival and long time since arrival suggested that many were infected post-migration [48]. In a similar study, Wiewel et al. utilized data on length of time in United States, HIV testing, and life history and concluded that approximately 65% of HIV-infected Caribbean-born and 34% of HIV-infected African-born individuals were most likely infected in the United States [49]. Lin et al. reported that the North American subtype B genotype was detected among most newly diagnosed non-US-born individuals, including individuals from the Caribbean and Africa, indicating probable transmission in the United States [51]. In order to better understand transmission risk post-migration, the Centers for Disease Control of Prevention (CDC) constructed a genetic distance–based transmission network using HIV-1 polymerase nucleotide sequences reported to the US National HIV Surveillance System for persons with diagnosed HIV infection during 2001–2013. Among African-born and Caribbean-born individuals, 48% and 65% of transmission partners were born in the United States, respectively, indicating probable post-migration transmission [52]. Additional research is needed to confirm these findings at the local (city or state) level. These data could be used to advocate for funding to increase HIV testing and to design of culturally appropriate HIV prevention interventions.

Behavioral HIV Risk

The Behavioral Risk Factor Surveillance System (BRFSS), the nationally representative database that captures HIV/STI behavioral risk does not collect data by country or region of origin [53]. Therefore, we do not have a comprehensive understanding of behavioral risk among non-US-born Black individuals. In lieu of these data, a number of smaller studies have explored the contextual nature of HIV risk among African- and Caribbean-born individuals [8, 54–65]. These studies have noted a complex array of behavioral, cultural, psychosocial, and structural issues that predict HIV risk among this diverse population. Though these factors may differ by gender, similar themes have been noted across countries and regions of origin.

Among non-US-born Black women, heterosexual transmission accounts for the majority of new HIV diagnoses [5, 7]. Culturally based gender inequality, which contributes to inability to negotiate condom use, low condom use self-efficacy, engagement in sexual relationships with high-risk male partners, and lack of open communication regarding sex, has been described as a predictor of HIV risk [54–57]. Consistent condom use may be further comprised by cultural expectations regarding procreation, the importance of childbearing within the context of a heterosexual relationship, and religious beliefs that do not support the use of contraception [58, 59]. Several studies have also described community acceptance of forced sex and intimate partner violence (IPV) which increase women's HIV risk [60–62]. Low HIV knowledge (and low general health literacy), inaccurate risk perception, and high levels of HIV-related stigma leading to non-disclosure of HIV status among sexual partners serve as barriers to HIV services and promoters of HIV risk [8, 9, 16, 63–66]. Across diverse populations of non-US-born Black women, conditions of poverty, undocumented immigration status, and survival needs have also been associated with the increased HIV risk behavior (e.g., condomless and transactional sex) [9, 56, 63, 64]. While some of these factors may be similar to the experience of US-born Black women who are also disproportionately affected by HIV, others are unique to the experience of non-US-born Black women and should be reflected in the development of novel, culturally appropriate interventions.

Among non-US-born Black men, the percentage of new diagnoses attributed to heterosexual sex is significantly higher than among US-born Black men (49% versus 14%, respectively). Male-to-male sexual contact is the second highest HIV transmission risk factor among non-US-born Black men [5]. Limited data are available exploring HIV risk behavior among African- or Caribbean-born men who have sex with men (MSM). Available studies suggest that increasing risk behavior with greater acculturation and length of time in the United States, selecting partners from high risk sexual networks, chem sex (engaging in sexual activity while using stimulants), and low rates of HIV testing are drivers of HIV risk among non-US-born Black MSM [67, 68]. Obasanjo et al. noted that a number of pre- and post-migration factors are associated with substance use among African-born MSM, including forced sex and transactional sex pre-migration in their home country, internalized homophobia, and housing instability [69]. Sandfort et al. also noted that structural factors, such as housing instability, were strongly associated with sexual risk among African-born MSM. Additional research exploring HIV risk and barriers to uptake of HIV prevention strategies among this vulnerable population are needed [70].

HIV Testing

Suboptimal uptake of HIV testing may compromise clinical outcomes and promote HIV transmission risk with African- and Caribbean-born communities in the United States. Therefore, strategies to overcome the barriers to testing and to improve HIV testing uptake are warranted. Ojikutu et al. determined the rate of HIV testing among non-US-born Black individuals using data collected by the National Health Interview Survey. Of non-Hispanic, non-US-born Black participants ($n = 1368$), 49.2% were from the Caribbean and 39.2% were from Africa. Among participants, only 69% of individuals with known HIV risk factors reported ever having obtained an HIV test in their lifetime. Low self-perceived risk was the most common reason for not testing. Younger (≤ 25 years of age) and older participants (≥ 45 years of age), US citizens, and individuals who had not talked to a health care provider in the prior 12 months were less likely to have obtained an HIV test [71].

Research conducted in partnership with African- and Caribbean-born community partners has determined numerous barriers to HIV testing. In a cross-sectional study conducted in Massachusetts, Ojikutu et al. found that non-US-born Black individuals were significantly less likely to report recent testing than US-born Black individuals (41.9% versus 55.6%, $p < 0.0001$). Lower educational attainment, not having a primary care provider, and recent immigration were associated with non-testing. HIV-related stigma, low HIV knowledge, and fear of deportation were also noted among participants and may serve as barriers to uptake of HIV testing [8, 72]. Similar findings have been noted by other researchers. Bova et al. noted suboptimal rates of HIV testing among African-born men participating in a community-based soccer tournament to raise HIV awareness. HIV testing stigma, HIV-related stigma, mistrust (test result confidentiality), and respondents not wanting to know their status were noted barriers to HIV testing uptake [73].

Qualitative data provides important insight into cultural and community-level barriers to HIV testing. De Jesus et al. explored HIV testing among East African-born women living in the United States. Barrier to testing themes included the negative implications of HIV testing, fear of partner reactions, fear that their community would judge them negatively for testing, and that the results would not be confidential [74]. In a second study, De Jesus et al. noted the centrality of cultural and religious beliefs in HIV testing uptake among African-born women. Participants expressed that HIV testing may imply immoral behavior and should not be discussed with male partners [75].

Biomedical HIV Prevention (Pre-exposure Prophylaxis)

Pre-exposure prophylaxis (PrEP) has been one of the most important recent biomedical advances in HIV prevention. Treatment with a combination tablet containing tenofovir and emtricitabine has been shown to be safe and effective, among MSM, heterosexual men and women, injection drug–using populations, and transgender individuals and should be offered to all who are at risk [76–78]. Yet, uptake has been low among Black individuals, and little is known about its use among non-US-born populations [79]. In a subset analysis of data from the 2016 National Survey on HIV in the Black Community (NSHBC) conducted by Ojikutu et al. which included 101 non-US-born individuals, only 19% were aware of PrEP and only 22% were willing to use it [80]. In a qualitative study which included African-born women, PrEP use during timed intercourse for conception was perceived to enhance intimacy and overcome stigma [81]. In a needs assessment for African-born women, health care providers suggested that PrEP should be included in comprehensive sexual health programming [82]. At the 2018 Empowering Women's Health Summit in Miami, Florida, 279 participants, including Haitian-born women, were convened to discuss barriers and facilitators to PrEP uptake. Cultural gender norms, religiosity and religious stigma, economic dependence on sexual partners, and "sexual silence" or lack of discussion regarding sex and sexual behaviors were identified barriers (J. Dévieux, personal communication, January 25, 2020). Additionally, HIV-related stigma and challenges identifying those at risk using current guideline criteria will pose significant challenges to increasing uptake of PrEP among non-US-born Black individuals [83]. To address this critical need, African- and Caribbean-born community members and stakeholders should be engaged to develop a research agenda focused on biomedical HIV prevention. Failure to create the evidence base for providing PrEP, and other biomedical interventions in the pipeline, to at-risk non-US-born Black individuals will further exacerbate existing racial and ethnic disparities.

HIV Care and Treatment

Few studies describing care and treatment outcomes among non-US-born Black individuals living with HIV have been published. What is known from the data that are available is that though late presentation is common, clinical outcomes are largely favorable once care is established. The Medical Monitoring Project (MMP) is a surveillance system that provides national estimates of behavioral and clinical characteristics of people living with HIV (PLWH) receiving medical care in the United States [84]. In an analysis that included 1721 people living with HIV (16% Caribbean/10% African), a higher percentage of PLWH achieved viral suppression compared with US-born individuals. No major disparities in receipt of ART prescription or viral suppression were noted by nativity despite higher rates of poverty and uninsurance among the non-US-born population [85].

Studies focused on non-US-born Black populations living with HIV within specific states and jurisdictions have revealed mixed findings regarding clinical outcomes. In an analysis of Florida HIV surveillance data from 2000 to 2014 ($N = 7675$), Sheehan et al. noted higher rates of non-retention and virologic failure among non-US-born Black individuals compared to their US-born Black counterparts in Florida [86]. Also in Florida, Cyrus et al. sought to determine retention and viral suppression among non-US-born Black individuals from the Caribbean. Caribbean-born Black individuals were less likely to be retained in care or be virally suppressed than US-born Black individuals, non-Hispanic White, and Hispanic individuals. Specifically, Bahamians, Haitians, and Trinidadians and Tobagonians had increased odds of non-retention and virologic failure compared to non-Hispanic White individuals [87].

Several studies have described clinical outcomes among Haitian-born individuals living with HIV. In a retrospective chart review of patients living with HIV receiving care at two clinics in Florida, Colasanti et al. noted that fewer Haitian-born individuals (58.5%) achieved viral suppression than US-born Black individuals (74.1%) or Latino (82.8%) patients. Linguistic and cultural factors were suggested barriers to treatment adherence [88]. Saint-Jean G et al. sought to determine barriers to routine use of HIV primary care among Haitian-born individuals living with HIV in Florida. Twenty-one percent of patients ($N = 96$) did not complete four or more visits in the past year. Patients without formal education or those with high levels of psychological distress were significantly less likely to have used HIV primary care regularly [89].

A small cohort study focused on African-born individuals living with HIV noted that rates of progression to AIDS once initiated in care were similar and no worse compared to US-born individuals. However, African-born individuals initiated care with more advanced HIV disease [90]. Additional research is needed to better elucidate differences in clinical outcomes by nativity, particularly in regions of the country with a high proportion of non-US-born Black individuals.

HIV-Related Stigma

As mentioned, many structural, cultural, community, and individual-level factors serve as barriers to utilizing HIV services for non-US-born Black individuals. Among these, HIV-related stigma deserves dedicated attention. Numerous studies have noted the persistence of HIV-related stigma across diverse non-US-born Black communities living in the United States [8, 63, 91–95]. Therefore, there is a critical need to improve our understanding of HIV-stigma within African- and Caribbean-born communities and to develop novel strategies to overcome its pervasive impact on access to HIV prevention, care, and treatment services.

Conceptualizing HIV-related stigma among non-US-born Black individuals requires an understanding of early work defining stigma. Goffman described stigma as an attribute that leads to "social devaluation and profound discrediting of the individual possessing the attribute or characteristic" [96]. HIV-related stigma involves negative attitudes and beliefs about people living with HIV and often results in avoidant or maladaptive coping, marginalization, and discrimination [97]. Further, HIV-related stigma undermines access to resources, social interactions, and intimate relationships and leads to adverse health outcomes for individuals living with or at risk for HIV [98–100]. When HIV-related stigma intersects with other forms of stigma and marginalization, it can be deadly, particularly for women [101–104]. High rates of HIV, stigma, and violence against women (and sexual minorities) converge in the countries of origin for non-US-born Black individuals where gender-based barriers are prevalent and few legal protections exist [105–112]. Once in the United States, these individuals transition into more complex webs of stigma and trauma as they become an ethnic cultural minority [113].

HIV-related stigma directed toward, perceived, and internalized by both African- and Caribbean-born individuals has been fueled by racism and xenophobic fear of contagion [95, 114]. Though all non-US-born Black populations have been impacted, Haitian immigrants have inarguably borne the brunt of HIV-related stigma throughout the history of the HIV epidemic in the United States. In 1982, the CDC identified Haitians as the only ethnic group among four high-risk groups (in addition to heroin-users, hemophiliacs, homosexuals) for HIV infection [115]. The ramifications of this stigmatizing pronouncement were far-reaching. In 1984, the Food and Drug Administration (FDA) informed all registered blood establishments that Haitian-born individuals who came to this country after 1977 should be disallowed from donating blood [116]. In the ensuing years, many Haitian-born individuals suffered loss of employment and housing due to HIV-related stigma [114]. By 1987, the "HIV Travel Ban" which barred the entrance of immigrants living with HIV into the United States was enacted further demonstrating the extent of the xenophobic fear of contagion [117]. Though data supporting the inclusion of Haitian-born individuals in the "high risk" category have proved erroneous, and the travel ban has been lifted [118], HIV-related stigma has persisted within Haitian-born communities in the United States and continues to contribute to late HIV testing, status non-disclosure, and delays in accessing care [119–121].

Among all individuals, HIV-related stigma may serve as a barrier to the uptake of HIV testing, lead to delays in accessing care for those who test positive, and contribute to non-adherence to antiretroviral therapy [122–124]. Among non-US-born Black individuals, high levels of HIV-related stigma may exacerbate these challenges. Ojikutu et al. conducted a study to determine barriers to HIV testing, including HIV-related stigma, among a venue-based, convenience sample ($N = 1060$) of Caribbean-, African-, and US-born Black individuals and found Caribbean-born individuals (majority Haitian) had the highest levels of HIV-related stigma (65% with high scores using a validated HIV stigma index), followed by African-born individuals (52%), and US-born Black individuals (44%) [8]. Additional research should be conducted to confirm these findings on a national level.

There are numerous challenges to overcoming HIV-related stigma among non-US-born Black individuals. Stigmatized attitudes regarding HIV should be understood and addressed within the context of the norms and values of diverse cultures. HIV-related stigma is often manifested within African- and Caribbean-born communities through communal fear, avoidance of persons with HIV, and the belief that HIV infection occurs due to moral failure and is a divine punishment or "curse" [95]. Within this setting of communal fear, communication between intimate partners and within families regarding HIV status, sexual preferences, and condom use is often avoided [58, 125, 126]. Among non-US-born Black individuals living with HIV, HIV-related stigma has led to social isolation, status non-disclosure, and lack of integration into the larger US community [16, 63]. To combat the devastating impact of HIV-related stigma on African- and Caribbean-born individuals, community-based solutions to reduce stigma, increase HIV testing, enhance HIV education, and improve access to HIV treatment must be developed.

Promising Strategies and Interventions

There is a critical need for interventions to address barriers to HIV services among non-US-Black individuals. The development of new interventions or cultural adaptation of evidence-based practices in partnership with stakeholders from diverse African- and Caribbean-born communities enhances commitment to implementation and program sustainability [127]. Few evidence-based practices have been described in the literature. However, there are limited data on promising strategies and innovative programming.

Much of the published literature has focused on community-based HIV testing. An overarching strategy to increase uptake of HIV testing is the establishment of meaningful, equitable partnerships with diverse stakeholders (e.g., civic associations, faith communities, hair salons, and businesses) [128]. In Washington State, a community-based health fair held within apartment complexes where large numbers of African-born residents reside was successful in increasing uptake of HIV testing, as well as other health screenings [129]. The partnership leading the initiative consisted of a local AIDS serving organization with a history of serving African-born individuals, the managerial staff of the apartment complexes, and an academic institution. A second HIV testing intervention example is led by the Africans For Improved Access (AFIA) program located in Massachusetts. AFIA has partnered with local African-born stakeholders for over 10 years to host the African Health Cup, an annual soccer tournament to increase HIV testing among African-born men and increase HIV awareness. Increasing HIV testing among African-born men may be particularly challenging given cultural norms and gender dynamics [130, 131]; hence, convening members of the African-born community to play soccer, celebrate their respective cultures, and simultaneously engage in HIV education has been a successful strategy for increasing testing uptake and destigmatizing HIV [132].

An additional strategy to overcome barriers to HIV testing is the integration of HIV testing with other diagnostic and preventative health screenings in community-based settings. Integration of health services supports the need to address other prevention gaps within populations with limited health access and increases willingness to engage in HIV testing as a component of a comprehensive prevention effort [133]. Over a 3-year period, the African Diaspora Health Initiative located in Philadelphia convened 352 "Clinics Without Walls" in collaboration with African- and Caribbean-born stakeholders and community members to provide services in community-based settings. "Clinics without Walls" has provided HIV testing, blood pressure assessment, and diabetes screening to more than 4000 African- and Caribbean-born individuals [134].

Providing HIV education and HIV testing within established social networks has also been successful. The Safety Net Party (SNP) is a group-level intervention which encourages African-born women to recruit other women in their social network to participate in HIV prevention. Using interactive activities, social network members are engaged in discussions focused on female body anatomy, HIV and other STDs, condom use, and health resources. HIV testing was provided onsite. In an evaluation of 14 SNPs in Greater Boston reaching 144 women, this intervention resulted in increased knowledge and awareness regarding HIV, reproductive health, and sexual health. A majority of participants ($n = 75$; 63%) received onsite HIV testing [135].

Community-wide engagement is important to understanding barriers, determining promising strategies, and developing successful culturally relevant interventions [136]. The Tulumbe! Partnership ("Let's engage!" in Luganda, a Ugandan language) was developed to address the need for culturally appropriate HIV prevention strategies designed for African-born individuals living in the United States. The project is comprised of a multidisciplinary group of stakeholders, including community members, health care providers, government officials, and researchers and is housed within the AFIA Program at the Multicultural AIDS Coalition in Massachusetts. Throughout 2017 and 2018, Tulumbe! conducted comprehensive community outreach throughout the state and convened a series of community-based forums to determine topics applicable to research and service delivery that are critical to addressing HIV within African-born communities. Reducing HIV stigma was determined to be a priority area, and intervention development is underway [137].

Few HIV prevention interventions have been adapted for use among Caribbean-born individuals. Malow et al. culturally adapted Becoming a Responsible Teen (BART), an HIV intervention that has been shown to be effective in other ethnically diverse, at-risk adolescent populations, for use among Haitian-born adolescents. In a randomized controlled trial [general health education ($N = 101$) compared to the BART intervention ($N = 145$) at 1 month following the 8-week intervention, the BART intervention group demonstrated greater HIV knowledge, greater intentions to use condoms, higher safer sex self-efficacy, improved condom use attitudes, and an enhanced ability to use condoms [126].

Interventions that focus on the multifaceted needs of non-US-born individuals living with HIV are also needed. The authors are aware of only one such intervention that has been developed and piloted. In Washington State, a multimedia, culturally appropriate behavioral intervention to address HIV-related stigma and depression among African-born individuals, the Positive Living Program, was developed and piloted in a small sample of African immigrant PLWH. At 1-week post-intervention, participants reported reduced symptoms of depression [138].

Recommendations

In order to overcome the multifaceted barriers to HIV testing, prevention, care, and treatment experienced by non-US-born Black individuals living in the United States, we suggest the following:

1. *Disaggregate race and ethnicity data by country of origin in all federally funded nationally representative databases.* The unique health needs of this diverse population are often missed because non-US-born Black individuals are subsumed under the umbrella of Black/African-Americans. Disaggregation of nationally representative datasets will provide a more comprehensive understanding of HIV risk behaviors, and potentially lead to more equitable allocation of funding and services.

2. *Develop or culturally adapt behavioral HIV prevention interventions for use among African- and Caribbean-born individuals in both clinical and community settings.* As mentioned, few behavioral interventions have been developed to address needs in this population. Engagement of key stakeholders and community members from African- and Caribbean-born communities is necessary to ensure that any interventions that are developed are sustainably integrated into outreach and clinical practice.

3. *Design and conduct research specifically dedicated to determining biomedical HIV prevention preferences, needs, and challenges to uptake.* Few data are available describing the use of PrEP among non-US-born Black individuals. This is a critical gap that must be filled. Research should include determining the best ways of informing non-US-born Black individuals about PrEP and innovative solutions to increase knowledge, acceptance, and adherence. This

research will require investment in community engagement and academic-community partnerships.

4. *Measure and track immigration as a social determinant of health.* Immigration is "both socially determined and a social determinant of health" [13]. Immigration policy places significant barriers to accessing critical services, including health care and employment. Irrespective of immigration status, these policies promote fear of institutions, reinforce mistrust that immigrants have in the health care system, and deter immigrants from accessing needed prevention, care, and treatment. Recognizing immigration as a social determinant of health will lead to increased awareness of the impact of immigration policy on health care outcomes.

5. *Integrate the assessment of social determinants of health as a routine component of primary care.* Social determinants of health contribute significantly to clinical outcomes of care among all patients, including African- and Caribbean-born individuals. Therefore, social determinants should be assessed in clinical practice. Clinical-community linkages should be developed to connect patients to available resources. In regards to immigration as a social determinant, innovative practice models have integrated legal navigators into primary care practice [139, 140].

6. *Develop community-clinical partnerships that support culturally appropriate outreach.* For marginalized communities experiencing stigma, mistrust in the health care system, anti-immigrant pressures, and other social issues, the development of community-clinical partnerships is helpful to increase uptake of HIV services. Employing culturally competent staff who are African- and Caribbean-born builds trust and promotes the formation of long-term, sustainable relationships with communities. In addition, providing services (e.g., HIV testing and prevention education) outside of business hours and offering patient navigation to clinical sites have been identified as successful strategies to promote engagement in care.

7. *Provide quality and culturally appropriate language access.* In order to ensure that non-English proficient individuals are able to understand and act on public health information and fully engage in clinical services, access to language-appropriate services must be ensured. Federal law and executive orders mandate compliance with language access requirements for any agency receiving federal funds [141]. Culturally and linguistically appropriate patient education materials have been developed, such as MedlinePlus and EthnoMed [142, 143]. However, language access and interpreter services for many common languages spoken by non-US-born Black individuals are not widely available (e.g., Somali, Haitian Creole, Amharic) [144]. Without expanded language access within communities where disproportionately high numbers of African- and Caribbean-born individuals live, disparities noted within the HIV epidemic will deepen.

8. *Establish coalitions dedicated to advocating for the HIV-related needs of non-US-born Black immigrants within all jurisdictions where disparities have been noted.* These coalitions would shed light on emerging issues, create pathways

to civic engagement for PLWH, and make recommendations on how to improve the quality of life of the growing population of non-US-born Black individuals. This strategy has proven effective in metropolitan areas, such as in Washington DC (Mayor's Office on African Affairs) and the Bronx, New York City (African Advisory Council) where these bodies focus on overall health needs.

9. *Recognize the intersection of race and migration.* Immigrants in the United States are policed, detained, and deported at increasing rates. Non-US-born Black communities are disproportionately vulnerable to these acts of structural violence due to the intersection of racism and xenophobia. These practices negatively affect health outcomes by creating barriers to seeking, accessing, and utilizing HIV services [145, 146]. The intersection of racism and health is a growing area of research [147]. Increased awareness and additional research should be conducted to understand and address racism in the context of the Black immigrant experience.

10. *Continue to support the establishment of national HIV awareness days.* Awareness days have been established by community-led mobilization campaigns to increase national attention and galvanize communities to address challenges facing highly impacted, at-risk populations. Caribbean-American HIV/AIDS Awareness Day has historically been celebrated on June 8. Though not federally recognized, National African Immigrant and Refugee HIV/AIDS and Hepatitis Awareness (NAIRHHA) Day has been observed annually on September 9 since 2014. If NAIRHHA Day were federally recognized, resources to support culturally and linguistically appropriate programming and to ensure African-born individuals are represented in local and national policy discussions might increase [148].

Acknowledgment We would like to acknowledge Joel Piton MD for his contribution to this chapter.

References

1. Centers for Disease Control and Prevention. HIV surveillance report, 2018 (Preliminary); vol. 30. http://www.cdc.gov/hiv/library/reports/hiv-surveillance.html. Published November 2019. Accessed 5 Dec 2019.
2. Pew Research Center. Key facts about black immigrants in the U.S. Available at: http://www.pewresearch.org/fact-tank/2018/01/24/key-facts-about-black-immigrants-in-the-u-s/. Accessed on: 5 Dec 2019.
3. Singh GK, Rodriguez-Lainz A, Kogan MD. Immigrant health inequalities in the United States: use of eight major national data systems. Sci World J. 2013;2013:512313. Published online 27 Oct 2013.
4. Kerani RP, Satcher Johnson A, Buskin SE, Rao DK, Golden MR, Hu X, Hall HI. The epidemiology of HIV in people born outside the United States, 2010–2014. In: Conference on Retroviruses and Opportunistic Infections (CROI). Boston; March 4–7, 2018, Abstract 851.
5. Demeke HB, Johnson AS, Wu B, Nwangwu-Ike N, King H, Dean HD. Differences between U.S.-born and non-U.S.-born black adults reported with diagnosed HIV infection: United States, 2008–2014. J Immigr Minor Health. 2018;1007(10):699–4.

6. Koku EF, Rajab-Gyagenda WM, Korto MD, Morrison SD, Beyene Y, Mbajah J, Ashton C. HIV/AIDS among African Immigrants in the US: the need for disaggregating HIV surveillance data by country of birth. J Health Care Poor Underserved. 2016;27(3):1316–29.
7. Prosser AT, Tang T, Hall HI. HIV in persons born outside the United States, 2007-2010. JAMA. 2012;308(6):601–7.
8. Ojikutu B, Nnaji C, Sithole J, Schneider KL, Higgins-Biddle M, Cranston K, Earls F. All black people are not alike: differences in HIV testing patterns, knowledge, and experience of stigma between U.S.-born and non-U.S.-born blacks in Massachusetts. AIDS Patient Care STDS. 2013;27(1):45–54.
9. De Jesus M, Taylor J, Maine C, Nalls P. A one-size-fits-all HIV prevention and education approach?: interpreting divergent HIV risk perceptions between African American and East African immigrant women in Washington, DC using the proximate-determinants conceptual framework. Sex Transm Dis. 2016;43(2):78–83.
10. Hoffman S, Beckford Jarrett ST, Kelvin EA, Wallace SA, Augenbraun M, Hogben M, Liddon N, McCormack WM, Rubin S, Wilson TE. HIV and sexually transmitted infection risk behaviors and beliefs among black west Indian immigrants and US-Born Blacks. Am J Public Health. 2008;98(11):2042–50.
11. De Jesus M. HIV/AIDS and immigrant Cape Verdean women: contextualized perspectives of Cape Verdean community advocates. Am J Community Psychol. 2007;39(1–2):121–31. PMID:17340187.
12. Ebrahim NB, Davis S, Tomaka J. Psychosocial determinants of intention to use condoms among Somali and Ethiopian immigrants in the U.S. Psychol Health Med. 2017;22(5):611–7.
13. Castañeda H, Holmes SM, Madrigal DS, Young ME, Beyeler N, Quesada J. Immigration as a social determinant of health. Annu Rev Public Health. 2015;36:375–92.
14. Simbiri KO, Hausman A, Wadenya RO, Lidicker J. Access impediments to health care and social services between Anglophone and Francophone African immigrants living in Philadelphia with respect to HIV/AIDS. J Immigr Minor Health. 2010;12(4):569–79.
15. Ahad FB, Zick CD, Simonsen SE, Mukundente V, Davis FA, Digre K. Assessing the likelihood of having a regular health care provider among African American and African Immigrant women. Ethn Dis. 2019;29(2):253–60.
16. Foley EE. HIV/AIDS and African immigrant women in Philadelphia: structural and cultural barriers to care. AIDS Care. 2005;17:1030–43.
17. Wafula EG, Snipes SA. Barriers to health care access faced by black immigrants in the US: theoretical considerations and recommendations. J Immigr Minor Health. 2014;16(4):689–98.
18. Zhou YR, Coleman WD, Huang Y, Sinding C, Wei W, Gahagan J, Micollier E, Su HH. Exploring the intersections of transnationalism, sexuality and HIV risk. Cult Health Sex. 2017;19(6):645–52.
19. Williams DR, Haile R, González HM, Neighbors H, Baser R, Jackson JS. The mental health of Black Caribbean immigrants: results from the National Survey of American Life. Am J Public Health. 2007;97(1):52–9.
20. Alegría M, Álvarez K, DiMarzio K. Immigration and mental health. Curr Epidemiol Rep. 2017;4(2):145–55.
21. U.S. Census Bureau; American Community Survey. 2017 American Community survey 1-year estimates, table B06004B; generated by Bisola Ojikutu; using American FactFinder. http://factfinder.census.gov. December 6, 2019.
22. Pew Research Center. Key facts about Black immigrants in the U.S. Available at: http://www.pewresearch.org/fact-tank/2018/01/24/key-facts-about-black-immigrants-in-the-u-s/. Accessed on: 6 Dec 2019.
23. Flahaux M, De Haas H. African migration: trends, patterns, drivers. Comp Migr Stud. 2016;4:1.
24. Plummer G. Haitian migrants and backyard imperialism. Race Class. 1985;26(4):35–43.
25. Glick-Schiller N, Fournon G. "Everywhere we go, we are in danger": Ti manno and the emergence of a Haitian transnational identity. Am Ethnol. 1990;17:329–47.

26. Lobo AP. US diversity visas are attracting Africa's best and brightest. Popul Today. 2001;29:1–2.
27. Migration Policy Institute. Immigration-related policy changes in the first two years of the Trump Administration. May 2019. Available at: www.migrationpolicy.org/research/immigration-policy-changes-two-years-trump-administration. Accessed on: 10 Jan 2020.
28. The U.S. Census Bureau projections for 2060 include only non-Hispanic foreign-born blacks. See "U.S. immigrant population projected to rise, even as share falls among Hispanics, Asians," by Anna Brown, Pew Research Center. 2015. https://www.pewresearch.org/fact-tank/2015/03/09/u-s-immigrant-population-projected-to-rise-even-as-share-falls-among-hispanics-asians/.
29. Pew Research Center. Statistical portrait of the U.S. black immigrant population. Available at: http://www.pewsocialtrends.org/2015/04/09/chapter-1-statistical-portrait-of-the-u-s-black-immigrant-population/. Accessed on: 19 Dec 2018.
30. Pew Research Center. African immigrant population in U.S. steadily climbs. Available at: http://www.pewresearch.org/fact-tank/2017/02/14/african-immigrant-population-in-u-s-steadily-climbs/. Accessed on: 6 Dec 2019.
31. Migration Policy Institute. Sub-Saharan African immigrants in the United States. https://www.migrationpolicy.org/article/sub-saharan-african-immigrants-united-states. Accessed on: 6 Dec 2019.
32. Migration Policy Institute. Caribbean immigrants in the United States. https://www.migrationpolicy.org/article/caribbean-immigrants-united-states. Accessed on: 6 Dec 2019.
33. Migration Policy Institute. Haitian immigrants in the United States. https://www.migrationpolicy.org/article/haitian-immigrants-united-states. Accessed on: 6 Dec 2019.
34. Kerani R, Bennett AB, Golden M, Castillo J, Buskin SE. Foreign-born individuals with HIV in King County, WA: a glimpse of the future of HIV? AIDS Behav. 2018;22(7):2181–8.
35. Massachusetts Department of Public Health, Bureau of Infectious Disease and Laboratory Sciences. 2018 Massachusetts HIV/AIDS epidemiologic profile: individuals born outside the United States. Available at: https://www.mass.gov/lists/hivaids-epidemiologic-profiles. Accessed on: 22 Dec 2019.
36. Kerani RP, Kent JB, Sides T, Dennis G, Ibrahim AR, Cross H, Wiewel EW, Wood RW, Golden MR. HIV among African-born persons in the United States: a hidden epidemic? J Acquir Immune Defic Syndr. 2008;49(1):102–6.
37. HIV among foreign born individuals in New York City. 2018. Available at: https://www1.nyc.gov/assets/doh/downloads/pdf/dires/hiv-aids-in-foreign-born.pdf. Accessed on: 6 Dec 2019.
38. Hoffman S, Ransome Y, Adams-Skinner J, Leu CS, Terzian A. HIV/AIDS surveillance data for New York City West Indian–born blacks: comparisons with other immigrant and US-born groups. Am J Public Health. 2012;102(11):2129–34.
39. Willis LA, Opoku J, Murray A, West T, Johnson AS, Pappas G, Sutton MY. Diagnoses of human immunodeficiency virus (HIV) infection among foreign-born people living in the District of Columbia. J Immigr Minor Health. 2015;17(1):37–46.
40. Minnesota Department of Health (MDH). HIV prevalence and mortality report. 2015. Available from: http://www.health.state.mn.us/divs/idepc/diseases/hiv/stats/2015/pm2015.pdf. Accessed on: 12 Nov 2018.
41. Ashton C, Lowe M, Barnhardt S. Comparison of HIV/ AIDS incidence rates between U.S.-born Blacks and African- born Blacks in Utah, 2000– 2009. Open AIDS J. 2012;6:156–62. Epub 7 Sep 2012
42. Demeke HB, Johnson AS, Wu B, Moonesinghe R, Dean HD. Unequal declines in absolute and relative disparities in HIV diagnoses among Black women, United States, 2008 to 2016. Am J Public Health. 2018;108(S4):S299–303. PMCID: PMC6215380.
43. UNAIDS. Nigeria. Available at: https://www.unaids.org/en/regionscountries/countries/nigeria. Accessed on: 22 Dec 2019.
44. UNAIDS. Ethiopia. Available at: https://www.unaids.org/en/regionscountries/countries/ethiopia. Accessed on: 22 Dec 2019.

45. UNAIDS. Jamaica. Available at: https://www.unaids.org/en/regionscountries/countries/jamaica. Accessed on: 22 Dec 2019.
46. UNAIDS. Haiti. Available at: https://www.unaids.org/en/regionscountries/countries/haiti. Accessed on: 22 Dec 2019.
47. Winston SE, Beckwith CG. The impact of removing the immigration ban on HIV-infected persons. AIDS Patient Care STDs. 2011;25:709.
48. Harawa NT, Bingham TA, Cochran SD, Greenland S, Cunningham WE. HIV prevalence among foreign- and US-born clients of public STD clinics. Am J Public Health. 2002;92(12):1958–63.
49. Wiewel EW, Torian LV, Hanna DB, Bocour A, Shepard CW. Foreign-born persons diagnosed with HIV: where are they from and where were they infected? AIDS Behav. 2015;19(5):890–8. PMID:25524308.
50. Rice BD, Elford J, Yin Z, Delpech VC. A new method to assign country of HIV infection among heterosexuals born abroad and diagnosed with HIV. AIDS. 2012;26(15):1961–6.
51. Lin HH, Gaschen BK, Collie M. Genetic characterization of diverse HIV-1 strains in a foreign-born population living in New York City. J Acquir Immune Defic Syndr. 2006;41(4):399–404. PMID:16652046.
52. Valverde EE, Oster AM, Xu S, Wertheim JO, Hernandez AL. HIV transmission dynamics among foreign-born persons in the United States. J Acquir Immune Defic Syndr. 2017;76(5):445–52. PMCID:PMC5680123.
53. Chowdhury P, Balluz L, Town M. Surveillance of certain health behaviors and conditions among states and selected local areas-behavioral risk factor surveillance system, United States. Morb Mortal Wkly Rep. 2010;59(supplement 1):1–220. PMID:20134401.
54. Okoro ON, Whitson SO. HIV risk and barriers to care for African-born immigrant women: a sociocultural outlook. Int J Womens Health. 2017;9:421–9. PMCID:PMC5476631.
55. Worthington C, Este D, Strain KL, Huffey N. African immigrant views of HIV service needs: gendered perspectives. AIDS Care. 2013;25(1):103–8. PMID:22672154.
56. Hoffman S, Higgins JA, Beckford-Jarrett ST, Augenbraun M, Bylander KE, Mantell JE, Wilson TE. Contexts of risk and networks of protection: NYC West Indian immigrants' perceptions of migration and vulnerability to sexually transmitted diseases. Cult Health Sex. 2011;13(5):513–28.
57. Ebrahim NB, Davis S, Tomaka J. Correlates of condom use among Somali and Ethiopian immigrants in the U.S. J Immigr Minor Health. 2016;18(5):1139–47.
58. Cyrus E, Gollub EL, Jean-Gilles M, Neptune S, Pelletier V, Dévieux J. An exploratory study of acculturation and reproductive health among Haitian and Haitian-American Women in Little Haiti, South Florida. J Immigr Minor Health. 2016;18(3):666–72.
59. Fordyce L. Responsible choices: situating pregnancy intention among Haitians in South Florida. Med Anthropol Q. 2012;26(1):116–35.
60. Sabri B. Perspectives on factors related to HIV risk and preventative interventions at multiple levels: a study of African immigrant women survivors of cumulative trauma. AIDS Educ Prev. 2018;30(5):419–33.
61. Akinsulure-Smith AM, Chu T, Keatley E, Rasmussen A. Intimate partner violence among West African immigrants. J Aggress Maltreat Trauma. 2013;22(1):109–29.
62. Lacey KK, Mouzon DM. Severe physical intimate partner violence and the mental and physical health of U.S. Caribbean Black women. J Womens Health (Larchmt). 2016;25(9):920–9.
63. Ojikutu BO, Nnaji C, Sithole-Berk J, Masongo D, Nichols K, Weeks N, Ngminebayihi M, Bishop E, Bogart LM. African born women living with HIV in the United States: unmet needs and opportunities for intervention. AIDS Car. 2018;30(12):1542–50.
64. Akinsulure-Smith AM. Exploring HIV knowledge, risk and protective factors among west African forced migrants in New York City. J Immigr Minor Health. 2014;16(3):481–91.
65. Marcelin LH, McCoy HV, Diclemente RJ. HIV/AIDS knowledge and beliefs among Haitian adolescents in Miami-Dade County, Florida. J HIV AIDS Prev Child Youth. 2006;7(1):121–38.

66. Dévieux JG, Rosenberg R, Saint-Jean G, Bryant VE, Malow RM. The continuing challenge of reducing HIV risk among Haitian youth: the need for intervention. J Int Assoc Provid AIDS Care. 2015;14(3):217–23.
67. Lewis NM, Wilson K. HIV risk behaviours among immigrant and ethnic minority gay and bisexual men in North America and Europe: a systematic review. Soc Sci Med. 2017;179:115–28.
68. Akin M, Fernández MI, Bowen GS, Warren JC. HIV risk behaviors of Latin American and Caribbean men who have sex with men in Miami, Florida, USA. Rev Panam Salud Publica. 2008;23(5):341–8.
69. Ogunbajo A, Anyamele C, Restar AJ, Dolezal C, Sandfort TGM. Substance use and depression among recently migrated African gay and bisexual men living in the United States. J Immigr Minor Health. 2019;21(6):1224–32.
70. Sandfort T, Anyamele C, Dolezal C. Correlates of sexual risk among recent gay and bisexual immigrants from Western and Eastern Africa to the USA. J Urban Health. 2017;94(3):330–8.
71. Ojikutu BO, Mazzola E, Fullem A, Vega R, Landers S, Gelman RS, Bogart LM. HIV testing among black and Hispanic Immigrants in the United States. AIDS Patient Care STDs. 2016;30(7):307–14.
72. Ojikutu B, Nnaji C, Sithole-Berk J, Bogart LM, Gona P. Barriers to HIV testing in Black immigrants to the U.S. J Health Care Poor Underserved. 2014;25(3):1052–66. PMCID:PMC4442684.
73. Bova C, Nnaji C, Woyah A, Duah A. HIV stigma, testing attitudes and health care access among African-born men living in the United States. J Imm Minority Health. 2014;18:187.
74. De Jesus M, Carrete C, Maine C, Nalls P. Attitudes, perceptions and behaviours towards HIV testing among African-American and East African immigrant women in Washington, DC: implications for targeted HIV testing promotion and communication strategies. Sex Transm Infect. 2015;91(8):569–75.
75. De Jesus M, Carrete C, Maine C, Nalls P. "Getting tested is almost like going to the Salem witch trials": discordant discourses between Western public health messages and sociocultural expectations surrounding HIV testing among East African immigrant women. AIDS Care. 2015;27(5):604–11.
76. US Public Health Service. Pre-exposure prophylaxis for the prevention of HIV infection in the United States. A clinical practice guideline 2014. Available at: http://www.cdc.gov/hiv/pdf/prepguidelines2014.pdf. Accessed on: 29 Nov 2018.
77. Baeten JM, Donnell D, Ndase P. Antiretroviral prophylaxis for HIV prevention in heterosexual men and women. N Engl J Med. 2012;367:399–410. PMID:22784037.
78. Marrazzo JM, Ramjee G, Richardson BA. Tenofovir-based pre-exposure prophylaxis for HIV infection among African women. N Engl J Med. 2015;372:509–18. PMCID:PMC4341965.
79. Huang YA, Zhu W, Smith DK, Harris N, Hoover KW. HIV pre-exposure prophylaxis, by race and ethnicity - United States, 2014-2016. MMWR Morb Mortal Wkly Rep. 2018;67(41):1147–50. PMCID:PMC6193685.
80. Ojikutu BO, Bogart LM, Higgins-Biddle M, Dale SK, Allen W, Dominique T, Mayer KH. Facilitators and barriers to pre-exposure prophylaxis (PrEP) use among Black individuals in the United States: results from the National Survey on HIV in the Black Community (NSCHBC). AIDS Behav. 2018;22(11):3576–87. PMCID:PMC6103919.
81. Bazzi AR, Leech AA, Biancarelli DL, Sullivan M, Drainoni ML. Experiences using preexposure prophylaxis for safer conception among HIV serodiscordant heterosexual couples in the United States. AIDS Patient Care STDs. 2017;31(8):348–55.
82. Okoro ON, Whitson SO. Sexual health, HIV care and pre-exposure prophylaxis in the African immigrant population: a needs assessment. J Immigr Minor Health. 2019;22:134.
83. Ojikutu BO, Mayer KH. Hidden in plain sight: identifying women living in the United States who could benefit from HIV preexposure prophylaxis. J Infect Dis. 2019;24:jiz416.
84. Centers for Disease Control and Prevention. The medical monitoring project. Available at: https://www.cdc.gov/hiv/statistics/systems/mmp/index.html. Accessed on: 23 Dec 2019.

85. Myers TR, Lin X, Skarbinski J. Antiretroviral therapy and viral suppression among foreign-born HIV-Infected persons receiving medical care in the United States. A complex sample, cross-sectional survey. Medicine (Baltimore). 2016;95(11):e3051.
86. Sheehan DM, Fennie KP, Mauck DE, Maddox LM, Lieb S, Trepka MJ. Retention in HIV care and viral suppression: individual- and neighborhood-level predictors of racial/ethnic differences, Florida, 2015. AIDS Patient Care STDs. 2017;31(4):167–75.
87. Cyrus E, Dawson C, Fennie KP, Sheehan DM, Mauck DE, Sanchez M, Maddox LM, Trepka MJ. Disparity in retention in care and viral suppression for Black Caribbean-born immigrants living with HIV in Florida. Int J Environ Res Public Health. 2017;14:E285.
88. Colasanti J, Nguyen L, Kiem JT, Deeb K, Jayaweera D. Disparities in HIV-treatment responses between Haitians, African-Americans, and Hispanics living in Miami-Dade County, Florida. J Health Care Poor Underserved. 2012;23(1):179–90.
89. Saint-Jean G, Metsch L, Gomez-Marin O, Pierre C, Jeanty Y, Rodriguez A, Malow R. Use of HIV primary care by HIV-positive Haitian immigrants in Miami, Florida. AIDS Care. 2011;23(4):486–93.
90. Page LC, Goldbaum G, Kent JB, Buskin SE. Access to regular HIV care and disease progression among black African immigrants. J Natl Med Assoc. 2009;101(12):1230–6.
91. Rosenthal L, Scott DP, Kelleta Z, Zikarge A, Momoh M, Lahai-Momoh J, Ross MW, Baker A. Assessing the HIV/AIDS health services needs of African immigrants to Houston. AIDS Educ Prev. 2003;15(6):570–80.
92. Othieno J. Understanding how contextual realities affect African born immigrants and refugees living with HIV in accessing care in the Twin Cities. J Health Care Poor Underserved. 2007;18(3):170–88.
93. Airhihenbuwa CO, Webster JD. Culture and African contexts of HIV/AIDS prevention, care and support. SAHARA J. 2004;1(1):4–13.
94. Nnaji C, Metzger N. Black is decidedly not just Black: a case study on HIV among African-born populations living in Massachusetts. Trotter Rev. 2014;22(1):120–50.
95. Koku EF. HIV-related stigma among African immigrants living with HIV/AIDS in USA. Sociol Res Online. 2010;15(3):5.
96. Goffman E. Notes on the management of spoiled identity. New York: Simon & Schuster; 1963.
97. Earnshaw VA, Bogart LM, Laurenceau JP, Chan BT, Maughan-Brown BG, Dietrich JJ, Courtney I, Tshabalala G, Orrell C, Gray GE, Bangsberg DR, Katz IT. Internalized HIV stigma, ART initiation and HIV-1 RNA suppression in South Africa: exploring avoidant coping as a longitudinal mediator. J Int AIDS Soc. 2018;21(10):e25198.
98. Mahajan AP, Sayles JN, Patel VA, Remien RH, Sawires SR, Ortiz DJ, Szekeres G, Coates TJ. Stigma in the HIV/AIDS epidemic: a review of the literature and recommendations for the way forward. AIDS. 2008;22(Suppl 2):S67–79.
99. Hatzenbuehler ML, Phelan JC, Link BG. Stigma as a fundamental cause of population health inequalities. Am J Public Health. 2013;103(5):813–21.
100. Earnshaw VA, Bogart LM, Dovidio JF, Williams DR. Stigma and racial/ethnic HIV disparities: moving toward resilience. Am Psychol. 2013;68(4):225–36.
101. Ammon N, Mason S, Corkery JM. Factors impacting antiretroviral therapy adherence among human immunodeficiency virus-positive adolescents in Sub-Saharan Africa: a systematic review. Public Health. 2018;157:20–31.
102. Mugoya GC, Ernst K. Gender differences in HIV-related stigma in Kenya. AIDS Care. 2014;26(2):206–13.
103. Gómez-Suárez M, Mello MB, Gonzalez MA, Ghidinelli M, Pérez F. Access to sexual and reproductive health services for women living with HIV in Latin America and the Caribbean: systematic review of the literature. J Int AIDS Soc. 2019;22(4):e25273.
104. Pantelic M, Boyes M, Cluver L, Meinck F. HIV, violence, blame and shame: pathways of risk to internalized HIV stigma among South African adolescents living with HIV. J Int AIDS Soc. 2017;20(1):21771.

105. Hamilton A, Shin S, Taggart T, Whembolua GL, Martin I, Budhwani H, Conserve D. HIV testing barriers and intervention strategies among men, transgender women, female sex workers and incarcerated persons in the Caribbean: a systematic review. Sex Transm Infect. 2020 May;96(3):189–196. https://doi.org/10.1136/sextrans-2018-053932. Epub 2019 Sep 10. PMID: 31506346; PMCID: PMC7062576.
106. Ross J, Cunningham CO, Hanna DB. HIV outcomes among migrants from low-income and middle-income countries living in high-income countries: a review of recent evidence. Curr Opin Infect Dis. 2018;31(1):25–32.
107. Thapa S, Hannes K, Cargo M, et al. Stigma reduction in relation to HIV test uptake in low- and middle-income countries: a realist review. BMC Public Health. 2018;18(1):1277. Published 20 Nov 2018.
108. Egbe TO, Nge CA, Ngouekam H, Asonganyi E, Nsagha DS. Stigmatization among people living with HIV/AIDS at the Kumba Health District, Cameroon. J Int Assoc Provid AIDS Care. 2020;19:2325958219899305.
109. Peltzer K, Pengpid S. Prevalence and associated factors of enacted, internalized and anticipated stigma among people living with HIV in South Africa: Results of the First National Survey. HIV AIDS (Auckl). 2019;11:275–85. Published 7 Nov 2019.
110. Rubens M, Saxena A, Ramamoorthy V, McCoy HV, Beck-Sagué C, Jean-Gilles M, George F, Shehadeh N, Dévieux JG. HIV-related stigma, quality of care, and coping skills: exploring factors affecting treatment adherence among PLWH in Haiti. J Assoc Nurses AIDS Care. 2018;29(4):570–9.
111. Hintzen P, Vertovec J, Cyrus E, Padilla M, Varas-Díaz N. Introduction to the special issue: applying a Caribbean perspective to an analysis of HIV/AIDS. Glob Public Health. 2019;14(11):1547–56.
112. Kane JC, Elafros MA, Murray SM, Mitchell EMH, Augustinavicius JL, Causevic S, Baral SD. A scoping review of health-related stigma outcomes for high-burden diseases in low- and middle-income countries. BMC Med. 2019;17(1):17. Published 15 Feb 2019.
113. Saint-Jean G, Dévieux J, Malow R, Tammara H, Carney K. Substance abuse, acculturation, and HIV risk among Caribbean-Born Immigrants in the United States. J Int Assoc Physicians AIDS Care (Chic). 2011;10(5):326–32.
114. Farmer P. AIDS and accusation: Haiti and the geography of blame. 2nd ed. Berkeley: University of California Press; 2006.
115. Centers for Disease Control and Prevention. Opportunistic infections and Kaposi's sarcoma among Haitians in the United States. MMWR Morb Mortal Wkly Rep. 1982;31(26):353–4.
116. Leveton LB, Sox HC Jr, Stoto MA, editors. Institute of Medicine (US) Committee to Study HIV Transmission Through Blood and Blood Products. Washington, D.C.: National Academies Press (US); 1995. Office of Biologics, National Center for Drugs and Biologics, Memorandum to All Establishments Collecting Blood for Transfusions, March 24, 1983.
117. Fairchild AL, Tynan EA. The politics of containment: immigration in the era of AIDS. Am J Public Health. 1994;84(12):2011–22.
118. Center for Disease Control and Prevention. Final rule removing HIV infection from U.S. immigration screening. Available at: https://www.cdc.gov/immigrantrefugeehealth/laws-regs/hiv-ban-removal/final-rule.html. Accessed on: 20 Jan 2020.
119. Conserve DF, King G. An examination of the HIV serostatus disclosure process among Haitian immigrants in New York City. AIDS Care. 2014;26(10):1270–4.
120. Marc LG, Patel-Larson A, Hall HI, Hughes D, Alegría M, Jeanty G, Eveillard YS, Jean-Louis E, National Haitian-American Health Alliance. HIV among Haitian-born persons in the United States, 1985–2007. AIDS. 2010;24(13):2089–97.
121. Cyrus E, Sheehan DM, Fennie K, Sanchez M, Dawson CT, Cameron M, Maddox L, Jo TM. Delayed diagnosis of HIV among Non-Latino Black Caribbean immigrants in Florida 2000–2014. J Health Care Poor Underserved. 2018;29(1):266–83.
122. Valdiserri RO. HIV/AIDS stigma: an impediment to public health. Am J Public Health. 2002;92(3):341–2.

123. Shubber Z, Mills EJ, Nachega JB, Vreeman R, Freitas M, Bock P, et al. Patient-reported barriers to adherence to antiretroviral therapy: a systematic review and meta-analysis. PLoS Med. 2016;13(11):e1002183.
124. Grossman CI, Stangl AL. Global action to reduce HIV stigma and discrimination. J Int AIDS Soc. 2013;16(3 Suppl 2):18881.
125. Dévieux JG, Jean-Gilles M, Frankel A, Attonito J, Saxena A, Rosenberg R. Predictors of sexual activity in Haitian-American adolescents. J Immigr Minor Health. 2016;18(1):161–72.
126. Malow RM, Stein JA, McMahon RC, Dévieux JG, Rosenberg R, Jean-Gilles M. Effects of a culturally adapted HIV prevention intervention in Haitian youth. J Assoc Nurses AIDS Care. 2009;20(2):110–21.
127. Marsiglia FF, Booth JM. Cultural adaptation of interventions in real practice settings. Res Soc Work Pract. 2015;25(4):423–32.
128. Kingori C, Esquivel CL, Hassan Q, Elmi A, Mukasa B, Reece M. Recommendations for developing contextually relevant HIV/AIDS prevention strategies targeting African-Born immigrants and refugees in the United States. AIDS Patient Care STDs. 2016;30(10):476–83.
129. Roberts DA, Kerani R, Tsegaselassie S, Abera S, Lynes A, Scott E, Chung K, Yohannes E, Basualdo G, Stekler JD, Barnabas R, James J, Cooper-Ashford S, Patel R. Harambee!: a pilot mixed methods study of integrated residential HIV testing among African-born individuals in the Seattle area. PLoS One. 2019;14(5):e0216502.
130. Mane P, Aggleton P. Gender and HIV/AIDS: what do men have to do with it? Curr Sociol. 2001;49:23–37.
131. Johannessen A. Are men the losers of the antiretroviral treatment scale-up? AIDS. 2011;25:1225–6.
132. Woyah A, Nnaji C, Bova C. Planning and implementing a statewide soccer HIV awareness and health promotion intervention for African-born men. J Assoc Nurses AIDS Care. 2014;25(6):675–81.
133. Bassett IV, Walensky RP. Integrating HIV screening into routine health care in resource-limited settings. Clin Infect Dis. 2010;50(Suppl 3):S77–84.
134. Kwakwa HA, Wahome R, Goines DS, Jabateh V, Green A, Bessias S, Flanigan TP. Engaging African and Caribbean immigrants in HIV Testing and Care in a large US City: lessons learned from the African Diaspora Health Initiative. J Immigr Minor Health. 2017;19(4):818–24.
135. Nnaji C, Slopadoe S, Rao T, Babirye J, Pwamang A. Safety Net Party: a group-based program to prevent HIV/STDs in African-born women in the United States. J Assoc Nurses AIDS Care. 2016;27(5):731–9.
136. Vaughn LM, Jacquez F, Lindquist-Grantz R, Parsons A, Melink K. Immigrants as Research Partners: a Review of Immigrants in Community-Based Participatory Research (CBPR). J Immigr Minor Health. 2017;19(6):1457–68.
137. Patient Centered Outcomes Research. The Tulumbe project (PI Nnaji). Available at: https://www.pcori.org/research-results/2017/tulumbe-project-tier-ii. Accessed on: 30 Oct 2018.
138. Lipira L, Nevin PE, Frey S, Velonjara J, Endeshaw M, Kumar S, Mohanraj R, Kerani RP, Simoni JM, Rao D. The positive living program: development and pilot evaluation of a multimedia behavioral intervention to address HIV-related stigma and depression among African-Immigrant people living with HIV in a large, Northwestern U.S. Metropolitan Area. J Assoc Nurses AIDS Care. 2019;30(2):224–31.
139. Nuruzzaman N, Broadman M, Kourouma K, Olson D. Making the social determinants of health a routine part of medical care. J Health Care Poor Underserved. 2015;26:321–7.
140. Tobin TE. Medical-legal partnership in primary care: moving upstream in the clinic. Am J Lifestyle Med. 2017;13(3):282–91. Published 2017 Mar 23.
141. U.S. Department of Justice. Enforcement of title VI of the Civil Rights Act of 1964- National Origin Discrimination against persons with limited english proficiency; notice. Washington, D.C.: National Archives and Records Administration: Federal Register; 2000. Available at: http://www.justice.gov/crt/about/cor/Pubs/eolep.pdf. Accessed on: 3 Jan 2020.

142. EthnoMed. Patient education. Available at: https://ethnomed.org/patient-education. Accessed on: 26 Jan 2020.
143. MedlinePlus. Available at: https://medlineplus.gov/languages/languages.html. Accessed on: 26 Jan 2020.
144. Shippee ND, Pintor JK, McAlpine DD, Beebe TJ. Need, availability, and quality of interpreter services among publicly insured Latino, Hmong, and Somali individuals in Minnesota. J Health Care Poor Underserved. 2012;23(3):1073–81.
145. Martinez O, Wu E, Sandfort T, Dodge B, Carballo-Dieguez A, Pinto R, Rhodes SD, Moya E, Chavez-Baray S. Evaluating the impact of immigration policies on health status among undocumented immigrants: a systematic review. J Immigr Minor Health. 2015;17(3):947–70.
146. Kerani RP, Kwakwa HA. Scaring undocumented immigrants is detrimental to public health. Am J Public Health. 2018;108(9):1165–6.
147. Bailey ZD, Krieger N, Agénor M, Graves J, Linos N, Bassett MT. Structural racism and health inequities in the USA: evidence and interventions. Lancet. 2017;389(10077):1453–63.
148. National African Immigrant and Refugee HIV/AIDS and Hepatitis Awareness Day. Available at: https://www.facebook.com/NAIRHHA. Accessed on: 26 Jan 2020.

Chapter 8
HIV in the South

M. Keith Rawlings and Deborah Parham-Hopson

Demographics, Data, and Disparities

Geography matters! The impact of the HIV/AIDS epidemic is not uniformly distributed in the USA. The epicenter of HIV management long ago shifted from the Northeast and West Coast to the 16 states and District of Columbia that make up the South.[1] The South, in which 38% of the US population resides,[2] vastly outnumbers new HIV diagnoses in every other region.[3] It accounts for about 45% of all people living with an HIV diagnosis in the USA and half the new diagnoses in 2017.[4] Ten jurisdictions[5] accounted for about three-quarters (72%) of HIV diagnoses among adults and adolescents in 2017. Of the ten jurisdictions with the highest rate of newly diagnosed HIV infections, eight were in the South[6] (Table 8.1).

Though 86% of estimated PLWH were aware of their HIV infection at the end of 2015, in 12 out of 16 Southern states, the percentage of people aware of their

---

[1] According to the CDC, 16 states and the District of Columbia make up the South – AL, AR, DC, DE, FL, GA, KY, LA, MS, NC, OK, MD, TN, TX, SC, VA, WV

[2] US Census Data, 2018. https://www.census.gov/popclock/data_tables.php?component=growth

[3] AIDSVu. Ending the HIV Epidemic: A Plan for America. https://aidsvu.org/ending-the-epidemic

[4] Centers for Disease Control and Prevention. HIV in the United States by Region. https://www.cdc.gov/hiv/statistics/overview/geographicdistribution.html. Published November 27, 2018.

[5] Jurisdictions include states, US territories, Washington DC and San Juan, Puerto Rico.

[6] Centers for Disease Control and Prevention. HIV Surveillance Report, Diagnoses of HIV Infection in the United States and Dependent Areas, 2017, Vol. 29, November 2018.

M. K. Rawlings (✉)
ViiV Healthcare, Research Triangle Park, Durham, NC, USA
e-mail: Keith.m.rawlings@viivhealthcare.com

D. Parham-Hopson
MayaTech Corporation, Silver Spring, MD, USA

© Springer Nature Switzerland AG 2021
B. O. Ojikutu, V. E. Stone (eds.), *HIV in US Communities of Color*,
https://doi.org/10.1007/978-3-030-48744-7_8

Table 8.1 Number and rate of new HIV diagnoses (adults and adolescents), 2017

Top ten states/areas by number	
State	New HIV diagnoses, # (%)
Florida	4800 (12%)
California	4500 (12%)
Texas	4364 (11%)
New York	2772 (7%)
Georgia	2595 (7%)
North Carolina	1315 (3%)
Illinois	1265 (3%)
New Jersey	1109 (3%)
Pennsylvania	1094 (3%)
Louisiana	1033 (3%)
Subtotal	*27,847 (72%)*
US Total	*38,739 (100%)*

Top ten states/areas by rate	
State/area	New HIV diagnoses, per 100,000
District of Columbia	46.3
Georgia	24.9
Florida	22.9
Louisiana	22.1
Maryland	17.0
Nevada	16.5
Texas	15.4
Mississippi	14.3
South Carolina	14.3
New York	14.0
–	–
US rate	*11.8*

CDC HIV Surveillance Report: Diagnoses of HIV Infection in the United States and Dependent Areas, 2017; vol. 29. https://www.cdc.gov/hiv/statistics/overview/index.html

infection was lower than the national estimate.[7] In 2016, a closer assessment of states in the *Deep South*[8] revealed a higher AIDS diagnosis rate (10.3 per 100,000) than the USA overall (6.7 per 100,000) and the highest number of individuals diagnosed with AIDS compared to the other US regions.[9] The HIV epidemic in the South is also more suburban and rural focused than in other regions. According to

---

[7] Centers for Disease Control and Prevention. HIV in the United States by Region. https://www.cdc.gov/hiv/statistics/overview/geographicdistribution.html. Published November 27, 2018.

[8] Alabama, Florida, Georgia, Louisiana Mississippi, North Carolina, South Carolina, Tennessee and Texas

[9] https://www.cdc.gov/nchhstp/atlas/index.htm

analyses by the Southern HIV/AIDS Strategy Initiative (SASI), 29% of PLWH in the Deep South live in rural areas and smaller cities.[10] In some Deep South states, there is a heavier HIV burden outside the large urban areas than within them.[11] For example, more than 60% of PLWH in Alabama and Mississippi live outside a large urban area.

This shift in demographics and geography can also be seen among persons who inject drugs (PWID). In 2017, of the 2389 newly diagnosed HIV infections among people who inject drugs, the greatest number were in the South (954), followed by PWID in the Northeast (620).[12] The distribution of the current opioid epidemic further highlights the potential significances of demographic and geographic changes for individuals living with or at risk for both diseases.

Following the US President's 2019 State of the Union address, the Secretary of the federal Department of Health and Human Services (HHS) announced a plan (Plan) to end the HIV epidemic in 10 years.[13] To achieve the goals set forth in the Plan (75% reduction in new case in 5 years, 90% in 10 years), it is necessary to assess how and where HIV transmission is occurring in the USA. Federal data highlighted that more than 50% of the new HIV diagnoses in 2016 and 2017 occurred in just 48 counties, Washington, DC, and San Juan, Puerto Rico.[14] Half of those counties are in southern states, and six of the seven states with a disproportionate occurrence of HIV in rural areas are also in the South[15] (Fig. 8.1). The Plan also calls for a significant uptake of the use of pre-exposure prophylaxis (PrEP) by the nearly 1.2 million people in the USA believed to be a substantial risk of acquiring HIV.

Though there have been significant improvements in HIV incidence in recent years, racial disparities in HIV demographics persist. Black Americans made up approximately 13% of the US population but accounted for 42% of HIV infections[16]

---

[10] Deep South Continues to Have Significant HIV Burden Outside the Large Urban Areas Demonstrating a Need for Increased Federal Resources; https://southernaids.files.wordpress.com/2018/06/deep-south-hiv-burden-outside-large-urban-areas2.pdf

[11] The Office of Management and Budget (OMB) subdivides Metropolitan Statistical Areas (MSAs) as follows: (1) ≥ 500,000 population; (2) 50,000–499,999 population, (3) nonmetropolitan (<50,000 population). For purposes of this policy brief, we define "large urban area" or "large MSA" as having ≥500,000 population.

[12] Centers for Disease Control and Prevention. https://www.cdc.gov/hiv/pdf/library/slidesets/cdc-hiv-surveillance-persons-who-inject-drugs-2017.pdf

[13] Azar A. https://www.hhs.gov/blog/2019/02/05/ending-the-hiv-epidemic-a-plan-for-america.html. Published February 5, 2019.

[14] Azar A. https://www.hhs.gov/blog/2019/02/05/ending-the-hiv-epidemic-a-plan-for-america.html. Published February 5, 2019.

[15] Centers for Disease Control and Prevention. http://www.cdc.gov/hiv/library/reports/hiv-surveillance.html

[16] Centers for Disease Control and Prevention. HIV Supplemental Surveillance Report "Estimated HIV Incidence and Prevalence in the United States 2010–2016". Retrieved from: https://www.cdc.gov/hiv/library/reports/hiv-surveillance.html

Of the 48 counties targeted by the "Ending the HIV Epidemic" initiative, almost half of the counties with highest HIV burden are in southern states[1]

State	Counties	State	Counties	State	Counties
AZ	Maricopa County	NJ	Essex County	TX	Bexar County
			Hudson County		Dallas County
CA	Alameda County				Harris County
	Los Angeles County	NY	Bronx County		Tarrant County
	Orange County		Kings County		Travis County
	Riverside County		New York County	WA	King County
	Sacramento County		Queens County		Washington, DC
	San Bernardino County	NC	Mecklenburg County	PR	San Juan Municipio
	San Diego County	OH	Cuyahoga County		
	San Francisco County		Franklin County		**States with substantial rural HIV burden**
GA	Cobb County		Hamilton County		AL AR KY MO MS OK SC
	DeKalb County	PA	Philadelphia County		
	Fulton County	TN	Shelby County		
	Gwinnett County				
IL	Cook County				
IN	Marion County				
LA	East Baton Rouge Parish				
	Orleans Parish				
MD	Baltimore City				
	Montgomery County				
	Prince George's County				
MA	Suffolk County				
MI	Wayne County				
NV	Clark County				
FL	Broward County				
	Duval County				
	Hillsborough County				
	Miami-Dade County				
	Orange County				
	Palm Beach County				
	Pinellas County				

Fig. 8.1 Forty-eight highest burdened counties, Washington, DC, San Juan, Puerto Rico, and seven states with substantial rural HIV burden. AL Alabama, AR Arkansas, AZ Arizona, CA California, DC District of Columbia, FL Florida, GA Georgia, IN Indiana, IL Illinois, KY Kentucky, LA Louisiana, MA Massachusetts, MD Maryland, MI Michigan, MO Missouri, MS Mississippi, NC North Carolina, NJ New Jersey, NV Nevada, NY New York, OH Ohio, OK Oklahoma, PA Pennsylvania, PR Puerto Rico, SC South Carolina, TN Tennessee, TX Texas, WA Washington. (Centers for Disease Control and Prevention. http://www.cdc.gov/hiv/library/reports/hiv-surveillance.html. Accessed April 24, 2019. AIDSVu.org. https://aidsvu.org/resources/deeper-look-south/. Accessed April 25, 2019)

Table 8.2 HIV Transmissions in 2016

People with HIV (%)	Status of care	Transmissions (%)
15	Unaware that they have HIV	38
23	Aware of infection, but not connected to care	43
11	In care, not virally suppressed	20
51	Taking ART and adherent	0

and 50% of new HIV diagnosis in the South.[17] Gay and bisexual black men make up a disproportionate share of people with HIV in the South and black women account for 69% of all HIV diagnoses among women in the South.[18,19] Southern black people living with HIV are less likely to be tested, receive and *be* retained in care, and less likely to be virally suppressed than their black counterparts living in other parts of the country.[20]

Viral Suppression

A significant underpinning of the Plan is predicated on the diagnosis and treatment of those who are living with HIV. This approach is supported by research showing that PLWH who are adherent on HAART and virally suppressed pose effectively no risk of HIV transmission to their sexual partners.[21] Approximately 80% of new US HIV transmissions are from persons who are unaware they are HIV positive or are not receiving regular care (Table 8.2). This continuum of diagnosis to treatment to viral suppression has had variable success. In 2016, overall only 51% of PLWH in the USA had achieved viral suppression. To put this *in a* global context, a comparison of overall rates of VS with 10 African countries found the US ranked 7th (Fig. 8.2). Viral suppression rates differ by region. In 2015, the South had the greatest concentration of states with low rates of viral suppression in PLWH ≥13 years of age[22] (Fig. 8.3). That same year, the rate of viral suppression among black PLWH nationally was among the lowest of any racial or ethnic group. When low viral suppression rates are coupled with the low proportion of people being prescribed

[17] Centers for Disease Control and Prevention. Estimated HIV incidence and prevalence in the United States, 2010–2016. HIV Surveillance Supplemental Report 2018;24(No. 1). Published February 2019.

[18] Centers for Disease Control and Prevention (CDC). HIV Surveillance Report, 2014; vol. 26. Available at http://www.cdc.gov/hiv/library/reports/surveillance/. Published December 2015.

[19] Maulsby, C., Millett, G., Lindsey, K., Kelley, R., Johnson, K., Montoya, D., & Holtgrave, D. R. (2014). HIV among black men who have sex with men (MSM) in the United States: A review of the literature. AIDS and Behavior, 18(1), 10–25. https://doi.org/10.1007/s10461-013-0476-2

[20] https://www.cdc.gov/hiv/group/racialethnic/africanamericans/index.html

[21] Li Z, et al. MMWR Morb Mortal Wkly Rep. 2019; 68:267–272

[22] Centers for Disease Control and Prevention. https://www.cdc.gov/hiv/pdf/library/slidesets/cdc-hiv-prevention-and-care-outcomes.pdf

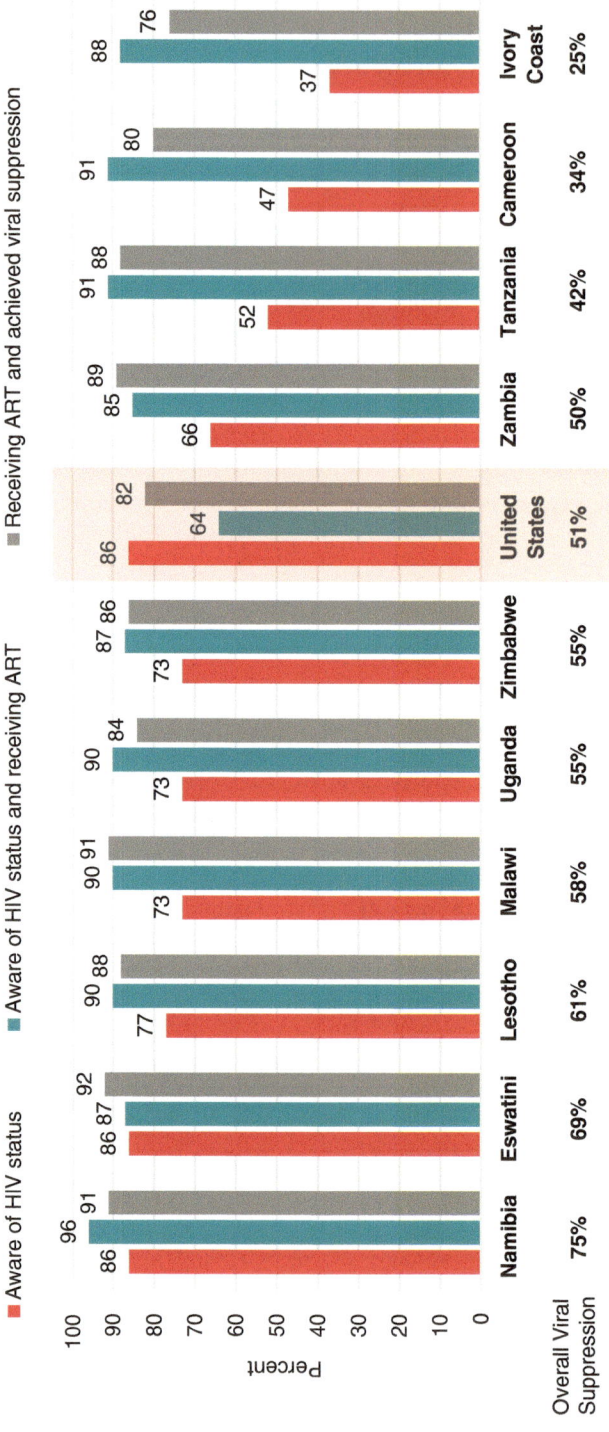

Fig. 8.2 Diagnosis and treatment status of PLWH in 10 African countries and the USA. ART antiretroviral treatment, PLWH people living with HIV. (El-Sadr W et al. *N Engl J Med.* 2019; doi: https://doi.org/10.1056/NEJMp1904113)

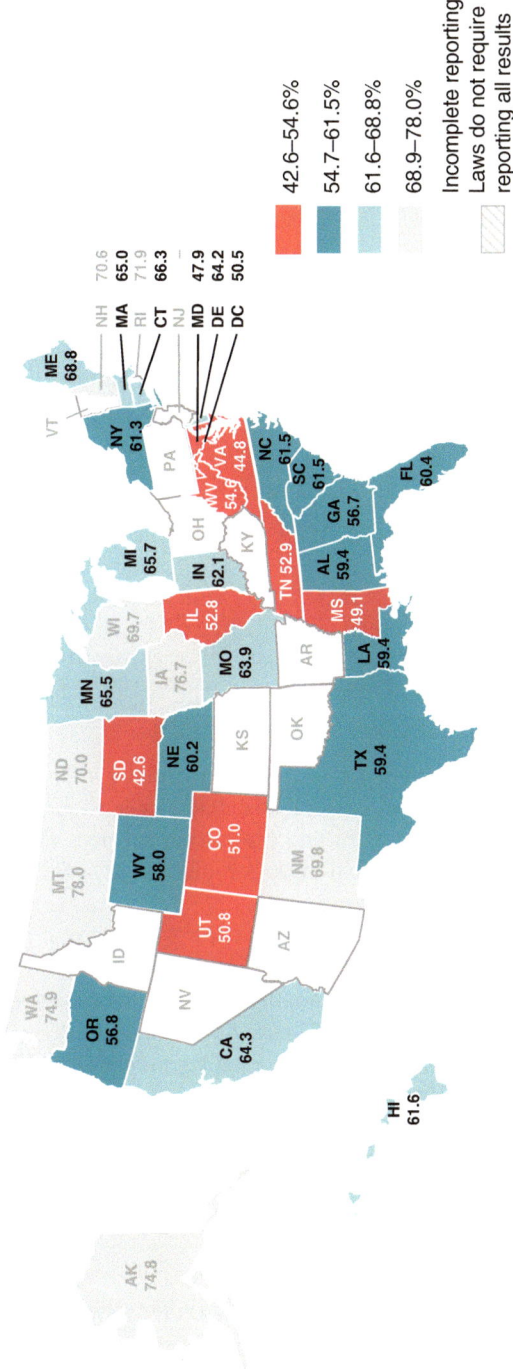

Fig. 8.3 Viral suppression among persons aged ≥ 13 years living with diagnosed HIV infection, 2015, 39 states, and the District of Columbia. AK Alaska, AL Alabama, AR Arkansas, AZ Arizona, CA California, CO Colorado, CT Connecticut, DC District of Columbia, DE Delaware, FL Florida, GA Georgia, HI Hawaii, IA Iowa, ID Idaho, IL Illinois, IN Indiana, KS Kansas, KY Kentucky, LA Louisiana, MA Massachusetts, MD Maryland, ME Maine, MI Michigan, MN Minnesota, MO Missouri, MS Mississippi, MT Montana, NC North Carolina, ND North Dakota, NE Nebraska, NH New Hampshire, NJ New Jersey, NM New Mexico, NV Nevada, NY New York, OH Ohio, OK Oklahoma, OR Oregon, PA Pennsylvania, RI Rhode Island, SC South Carolina, SD South Dakota, TN Tennessee, TX Texas, UT Utah, VA Virginia, VT Vermont, WA Washington, WI Wisconsin, WV West Virginia, WY Wyoming. (Centers for Disease Control and Prevention. https://www.cdc.gov/hiv/pdf/library/slidesets/cdc-hiv-prevention-and-care-outcomes.pdf. Accessed April 12, 2019)

Table 8.3 HIV prevention profiles for selected southern states

State	Virally suppressed (%)	Number of people who could potentially benefit from PrEP	Number of people who prescribed PrEP in 2017
Alabama	59%	11,840	899
Arkansas	60%	4610	391
Delaware	a	a	a
District of Columbia	51%	13,820	1869
Florida	60%	115,200	7594
Georgia	57%	35,700	2656
Kentucky	60%	a	a
Louisiana	59%	13,390	1078
Maryland	48%	27,390	2015
Mississippi	49%	5010	363
North Carolina	62%	29,820	1798
Oklahoma	60%	9140	481
South Carolina	62%	9040	590
Tennessee	53%	a	a
Texas	59%	117,180	6436
Virginia	a	a	a
West Virginia	a	a	a

aData not reported. Division of HIV/AIDS Prevention, National Center for HIV/AIDS, Viral Hepatitis, STD, and TB Prevention, Centers for Disease Control and Prevention. Retrieved from https://www.cdc.gov/hiv/policies/index.html#HIV%20Prevention%20Profiles

pre-exposure prophylaxis (PrEP), compared with state estimates of people who could potentially benefit, it paints a disturbing picture that people living with HIV in the South are not receiving adequate care and prevention services (Table 8.3). Thus, to have any chance of reaching the goal of 90% reduction in new HIV infections by 2029, we must get it right in the South.

Racial/ethnic differences in sustained viral suppression were present across all sex, age, and transmission categories. This is worth noting because though blacks make up approximately 13% of the total US population, they account for almost 60% of the population in the South.[23,24] In a 2014 assessment, only 40.8% of blacks living with diagnosed HIV infection had sustained viral suppression vs 50.1% for Hispanics and 56.3% for whites. Blacks experienced longer periods of time with viral loads >1500 copies/mL, a circumstance which can adversely affect health outcomes and pose a risk for further transmission. The mean number of days with a viral load >1500 copies/mL was also higher among blacks (190 days, 52.1% of the

---

[23] US Census Bureau. https://www.census.gov/quickfacts/fact/table/US/PST045218

[24] Office of Minority Health (HHS). https://www.minorityhealth.hhs.gov/omh/browse.aspx?lvl=3&lvlid=61

12-month period) than among Hispanics (172 days, 47.2%) or whites (149 days, 40.8%).[25]

Drivers of the Southern HIV Epidemic

In addition to geography, people with HIV who live in the South face many social, economic, cultural, and health system challenges that affect their overall health status. These factor also impact the ability of people living in the South to access healthcare *more broadly*. As a result, the mortality rate of people with AIDS is higher in the South. In 2016, of the 15,807 deaths among people with diagnosed HIV in the USA, nearly half (47%) were in the South.[26]

Poverty Poverty is associated with poorer health outcomes for everyone. In 2013, it was reported that 40% of people living with HIV in the South have an annual household income at or below $10,000 per year. Many are homeless or unstably housed while others live in houses with no electricity or running water. Others in geographically isolated communities lack adequate food and transportation.[27] The poverty rate is higher among African Americans than other racial/ethnic groups.[28] And, according to the CDC, "the socioeconomic issues associated with poverty—including limited access to high-quality health care, housing, and HIV prevention education—directly and indirectly increase the risk for HIV infection and affect the health of people living with and at risk for HIV. These factors may explain why African Americans have worse outcomes on the HIV continuum of care, including lower rates of linkage to care and viral suppression particularly in the South."[29]

Stigma and Criminalization The stigma of HIV is persistent and may be more prevalent in the South.[30] Stigma prevents people from getting tested for HIV and disclosing their status. It also inhibits people at high risk of acquiring HIV from using PrEP consistently. Stigma associated with HIV leads to fear of being judged and ostracized by family and friends and within communities. The number of people acquiring HIV through injection drug use is increasing in the South. Limited

---

[25] Crepaz N, Dong X, Wang X, Hernandez AL, Hall HI. Racial and ethnic disparities in sustained viral suppression and transmission risk potential among persons receiving HIV care — United States, 2014. MMWR Morb Mortal Wkly Rep. 2018; 67:113–118

[26] CDC. Diagnoses of HIV infection in the United States and dependent areas, 2017. HIV Surveillance Report 2018;29.

[27] https://www.centerforhealthjournalism.org/2013/07/10/hivaids-hotspots-america

[28] US Census Bureau. Income and poverty in the United States, Table 3. 2017.

[29] https://www.cdc.gov/hiv/group/racialethnic/africanamericans/index.html

[30] CDC Issue brief, HIV in the Southern United States. https://www.cdc.gov/hiv/pdf/policies/cdc-hiv-in-the-south-issue-brief.pdf September 2019

public support for a proven HIV prevention intervention such as syringe services programs in the region is a potential barrier.

HIV criminalization is the wrongful use of one's HIV status in a criminal prosecution and includes alleged, perceived, or potential HIV exposure; alleged nondisclosure of a known HIV-positive status prior to sexual contact; or non-intentional HIV transmission.[31] These laws were enacted early in the HIV/AIDS epidemic when legislators thought such laws would reduce transmission of HIV. Currently, 34 states and 2 US territories have laws which criminalize behavior of HIV-positive people. Many of these laws are quite harsh and carry significant penalties. For example, in Louisiana, a person with HIV who knows their status and intentionally exposes another through sexual contact can face 10 years in prison.

HIV criminal laws lead to stigma and discourage people at risk from getting tested or treated – especially young black gay and bisexual men and other people of color living in the South.

Patient/Client Factors   Lack of basic information about HIV prevention, abstinence-based sex education in schools, lack of trust in the health care system, increased rates of substance abuse and incarceration, and anti-gay attitudes all contribute to higher rates of HIV in the South. For example, 1 in 7 blacks/African Americans with HIV are unaware they have it.[27] This lack of knowledge inhibits one's ability to access HIV care and treatment and may lead to unknowingly pass HIV to others.

Providers   The maldistribution of health care providers in the USA has been a long-standing challenge. As a result, there are not enough health care professionals practicing in rural areas and many rural hospitals are closing. Providers in rural areas often have limited experience with HIV and are less likely to provide testing or PrEP to people at risk for contracting HIV. In a recent article it was noted: "One in 8 PrEP-eligible MSM (108 758/844 574; 13%) lived in 30-minute-drive deserts, and a sizable minority lived in 60-minute-drive deserts (38 804/844 574; 5%). Location in the South and lower urbanicity were strongly associated with increased odds of PrEP desert status."[32]

According to the CDC, providers in southern states have yet to widely adopt HIV prevention advances such as antigen/antibody combination HIV test that can detect HIV in early acute stages when it is most easily transmitted.[33] In addition, there is a lack of dental and specialty care for uninsured patients or those with Medicaid as their only insurance. Earlier this year, "the Trump administration finalized a health care regulation to protect the statutory conscience rights of health care providers and staff who have religious objections to certain procedures can refuse to provide

---

[31] https://elizabethtayloraidsfoundation.org/what-is-hiv-criminalization/

[32] Siegler AJ, Bratcher A, Weiss KM. Geographic Access to Preexposure Prophylaxis Clinics Among Men Who Have Sex with Men in the United States. Am J Public Health. Published online ahead of print July 18, 2019: e1–e8. doi:https://doi.org/10.2105/AJPH.2019.305172

[33] CDC Issue Brief, HIV in the Southern United States

them to patients. While the final rule focuses on abortion, assisted suicide, and sterilization, the language mirrors that of religious refusal laws in 12 states that authorize the denial of services, including health care, based on religious or moral belief. Potential conduct protected by the final rule could include a refusal to provide care to LGBT people, same-sex couples, and their children."[34] Such regulations may further reduce availability to high-quality HIV treatment and prevention.

Health Status Inadequate access to high-quality health care and lack of health care providers contribute to poor health outcomes. People living in the South suffer from higher rates of obesity, diabetes, sexually transmitted infections, cancer, and higher rates of HIV when compared to those that live in other regions of the country.[35] Support services such as case management are proven strategies to help people with HIV to find services and remain in clinical care. Too often, these services are lacking in the South.

Health Insurance The highest proportion of people without any health insurance live in the South. Of the HIV and AIDS patients with insurance, most rely on Medicaid. States in the South have the least expansive Medicaid programs and the strictest eligibility requirements to qualify for assistance. For example, in South Carolina, people with HIV must be disabled before qualifying for Medicaid. Alabama, Georgia, Florida, Louisiana, Mississippi, North Carolina, South Carolina, Tennessee, and Texas have never expanded Medicaid under the Affordable Care Act. These are the very same states that have the highest fatality rates from HIV in the country. Without Medicaid or other health care insurance, people with HIV rarely visit primary care doctors and often cannot afford their medications.

Federal HIV Funding Federal spending policies contribute to the challenge of addressing the HIV epidemic in the South. Because there are higher HIV diagnosis rates in suburban and rural areas in the South when compared to other regions of the country, there is a need for increased federal funding to community-based healthcare organizations located outside the large urban areas in the Deep South. Despite this, in recent years, the CDC has provided direct HIV prevention funding only to community-based organizations located in the large urban areas.[36] Most federal money to care for people with HIV distributed through the Ryan White HIV/AIDS Program (RWHAP) go to states and cities heavily impacted by the HIV epidemic. As a result, most rural areas and smaller cities have limited access to RWHAP funding. The Trump administration proposed significant cuts to the Medicaid and Medicare programs and changes to the Affordable Care Act which also impacts people with HIV.

---

[34] Sean Cahill, Trump Shreds LGBT Health Protections. https://www.publichealthpost.org/research/trump-shreds-lgbt-health-protections/
[35] HIV in the Southern United States. CDC Issue Brief. Updated May 2016
[36] SASI Analysis of Funds Distributed in the United States by the Centers for Disease Control and prevention Pursuant to PS15–2502 and PS17–1704

Clinical Research New and better tolerated methods of anti-retroviral delivery are showing exciting potential. However, the composition of HIV clinical trials remains mostly white, cis-gender, and males who have access to health care. The failure to prioritize representation in clinical trials that reflects the demographics of the epidemic, or at levels that allows statistical analysis between groups of participants, means that "we have products that have not been tested in all types of people, even though they are going to be used in all types of people."[37] This often translates into the inconsistent implementation of new interventions across all populations.

The disconnect between those who are included in clinical trials and those frequently seen in clinical practices in the USA shifts the burden to health care providers to determine how these innovations work for the various groups of people living with HIV in their practices. The lack of appropriate representation in clinical trials can also translate into a reluctance to make the implementation available or acceptable to different populations, often meaning that they will not garner the benefit at all.

Conclusion

Since the beginning of the AIDS epidemic in the USA, there have been different responses to the PLWH and those individuals at risk for acquiring it. Early discussions of the origin of the infection; policies related to willful transmission, moralization, and criminalization of sexual behavior and substance use; and conspiracies related to access or denial of care have punctuated the conversation. As a result, the implementation of effective interventions has often been hindered or delayed. The codification of discrimination and stigma have been both causes and manifestations of the health care systems and social norms in which PLWH and those providing services for them work.

While social and structural disparities have been embedded in the framework of our country from its inception, the near 40-year epidemic of HIV in this country has been, and continues to be, a microcosm of what can be achieved and what must be understood for all people to be treated equally. To truly "leave no one behind," as we strive to end the epidemic, will require us to look beyond our biases and assumptions and to explore new approaches. We must redirect our efforts toward what faces us now and test the preconceived limitations of what we can do. As the US epidemic has concentrated in the South, we must focus our efforts on the South in order to end this HIV epidemic. We have reached the inflection point where demographic shifts, new technologies, and evolving social priorities are redefining America, and we must redefine our actions as individuals, organizations, corporations, and governments as, together, we strive to end this epidemic.

---

[37] Heather Boerner. The New Face of HIV and Treating the 'Hardly Reached'. Medscape July 17, 2019. Quote by Dr. Linda-Gail Bekker of the Desmond Tutu Center, the University of Cape Town, South Africa, former president of the International AIDS Society

Chapter 9
Neighborhood-Level Structural Factors, HIV, and Communities of Color

Dustin T. Duncan, Byoungjun Kim, Yazan A. Al-Ajlouni, and Denton Callander

> *Like real estate, health is location, location, location …*
> --George Kaplan, PhD

Overview: Why Focus on Neighborhoods and HIV?

Neighborhoods matter. As George Kaplan highlights, neighborhoods (considered geographical places that can have social and cultural meaning to residents and non-residents alike and as sub-divisions of larger places) can have an enduring impact on various health outcomes and health behaviors [1]. To date, neighborhoods and health studies have focused on a wide range of health outcomes, including HIV outcomes such as condomless sex and HIV acquisition. This growing body of research connecting neighborhoods to sexual behaviors [e.g., condomless anal intercourse], HIV prevention behaviors [e.g., pre-exposure prophylaxis (PrEP) use], and HIV care behaviors [e.g., antiretroviral therapy (ART) use] has been conducted in different populations across geographic regions. For example, a review by Bauermeister and colleagues focused on neighborhoods in relation to HIV prevention and care outcomes in young gay, bisexual, and other men who have sex with men (MSM) in the United States [2], a high risk group for HIV acquisition [3]. The literature search discovered 126 peer-reviewed articles, of which 17 were eligible for inclusion based on the review criteria. This review found that neighborhood characteristics were associated with HIV-related prevention and care outcomes in MSM, especially HIV prevention outcomes. In addition, a systematic review was conducted to examine the relationship between neighborhood environments and HIV sexual risk behaviors among adult US women [4]. Seven articles identified

D. T. Duncan (✉) · B. Kim · Y. A. Al-Ajlouni · D. Callander
Columbia Spatial Epidemiology Lab, Department of Epidemiology, Mailman School of
Public Health, Columbia University, New York, NY, USA
e-mail: dd3018@cumc.columbia.edu; bk2767@cumc.columbia.edu; ya295@cam.ac.uk;
dc3480@cumc.columbia.edu

© Springer Nature Switzerland AG 2021   147
B. O. Ojikutu, V. E. Stone (eds.), *HIV in US Communities of Color*,
https://doi.org/10.1007/978-3-030-48744-7_9

from three databases or additional hand searches met inclusion criteria and were summarized. Findings were mixed with several studies indicating associations between neighborhood environments and HIV sexual risk behaviors. Another review identified studies that leveraged geographic information systems (GIS) methods (discussed later in the chapter) to examine the barriers to ART initiation, adherence, and viral suppression of people living with HIV (PLWH) [5]. Overall, 33 relevant studies were identified, excluding those not utilizing explicit GIS methodology or not examining Treatment as Prevention (TasP)-related outcomes. Findings from the study highlight geospatial variation in ART success and inequitable distribution of HIV care in racially segregated, economically disadvantaged, and, by some accounts, increasingly rural areas, particularly in the United States.

In this chapter, we overview studies focused on neighborhood factors and HIV outcomes, with special attention to relevant research focused on communities of color in the United States (defined in earlier chapters in this book and briefly includes Black and Hispanic/Latinx individuals in the United States). In this chapter, as appropriate, we highlight key populations of color for HIV such as Black gay, bisexual, and other MSM, recognizing the importance of intersectionality. Intersectionality is defined as a theoretical framework, which posits that multiple social categories (e.g., race, ethnicity, gender, sexual orientation, socioeconomic status, nativity) *intersect* to produce unique experiences and expressions of privilege and oppression (e.g., racism, sexism, heterosexism) [6]. Given that other chapters in the book describe (in detail) the epidemiology of HIV among communities of color (such as Chap. 6 which focuses on Black women and HIV and Chap. 8 which focuses on HIV in the South), we intentionally do not focus on HIV epidemiology in this chapter.

Neighborhoods and Overall Health

Early neighborhoods and health research focused on mortality as the health outcome of interest [1]. For example, Louis-René Villermé, an economist and physician, conducted a neighborhoods and health study in 1826. Villermé connected mortality rates with wealth and based on neighborhoods (arrondissements) in Paris, France [7]. The next generation of neighborhoods and health research largely focused on chronic diseases, especially obesity and obesogenic behaviors, likely given the rise of the obesity epidemic that received significant public health and media attention in the 1990s and 2000s. However, neighborhoods have been associated with a range of mental and physical health outcomes in a variety of populations across a range of geographic contexts [8–13]. With strong consistency and potency, neighborhood disadvantage impacts various health outcomes, including chronic diseases such as cardiovascular disease [14–17]. Overall, in the field of neighborhoods and health, the assessment of neighborhoods (discussed below) varies from study to study, making it difficult to compare findings and therefore difficult to summarize the accumulating literature.

Assessment of Neighborhoods

Across social science disciplines (sociology, geography, demography, psychology, etc.), neighborhoods research is typically defined into two buckets—"social environment" characteristics and "built environmental" characteristics. Examples of social environment characteristics include residential segregation, neighborhood disadvantage, and neighborhood disorder. Examples of built environmental characteristics include walkability and access to neighborhood services. In neighborhood health research, it is common to study the social and built environmental characteristics in isolation and to treat them as two separate categories. Put differently, studies often focus on either on the social environment or the built environment; however, neighborhoods coexist with both social and built environments [18]. For instance, one study found that parks were independently and positively associated with neighborhood collective efficacy (an aspect of neighborhood social capital), while alcohol outlets were negatively associated with neighborhood collective efficacy [19]. Neighborhood walkability can influence neighborhood crime: for example, one study found that neighborhoods with more retail space, restaurants, and public transit service had higher robbery rates [20].

Measuring Neighborhood Characteristics

There are several methods for measuring the neighborhood environment. These methods often include three categories. Traditional methods are the first category and include self-report surveys and systematic field observation. The second method includes current methods—in particular, geographic information systems (GIS) and web-based geospatial tools. The final class of methods includes emerging methods (e.g., wearable geospatial monitors, crowdsourcing and social media platforms).

A self-report measure relies on the participant self-reported responses to items of a survey or a questionnaire. The items in the survey can either have response options from which the participant chooses, or a free-text answer that can be later coded and grouped. Traditionally, surveys have been administered using simple methods (e.g., pen-and-paper surveys). However, more novel platforms emerged in recent years, including telephone questionnaires, tablets, face-to-face computer-assisted interview (CAPI), and audio computer-assisted self-interview (ACASI) delivered via a desktop computer. Furthermore, another example of traditional methods is systematic field observation (SFO), which can take the form of either sending trained auditors into neighborhoods with a pen and clipboard or capturing data from video-mounted vehicles. The latter has been utilized more often recently, and it involves photographic assessments from vehicle-mounted cameras traveling through neighborhoods (e.g., Google Street View).

On the other hand, current methods for characterizing neighborhoods include GIS, which is a framework that allows for organizing layers of geographic information into visualizations, using maps and 3D scenes, and for spatial location analyses. Examples of GIS layers include those with locations of park or local supermarkets and fast-food restaurants. This can allow for the measurement of proximity to specific services and/or density in a given neighborhood, as variables processed from GIS data can include both distances metrics and density metrics [21]. Furthermore, another example of current methods includes web-based geospatial tools such as Walk Score, which is a platform that allows users to receive numerical score assigned to any address they enter on their website (www.walkscore.com) that measures walkability [22].

Finally, emerging methods include utilizing the latest technology to measure specific neighborhood characteristics. An example includes wearable geospatial monitors, which allow for the logging of real-time geospatial data. It is also important to note that while wearable devices are used to measure specific characteristics, they can also play an important role in defining neighborhood boundaries in neighborhood research (discussed in the next section of the chapter). Social media platforms (e.g., Instagram, a mobile application for photo and video capturing and sharing) was used to provide empirical quantitative evidence in the neighborhood environment including food environments of specific neighborhoods) [23], and crowdsourcing geospatial data (e.g., Yelp, a free-for-all website with the purpose of helping people finding services in a neighborhood and reviewing them) was also utilized [24]. In this next section of the chapter, we discuss measurement of neighborhood boundaries.

Measuring Neighborhood Boundaries

It should be noted that there is no consensus definition of neighborhood in the field of health research. Hundreds of neighborhood definitions have been employed to define the neighborhood boundaries, and those various definitions are based on different assumptions of neighborhood in terms of geographical extend, types of experience in, and cognition and perception. The diverse methods of defining neighborhoods include perceived neighborhood boundaries, administrative units (e.g., census tract and Zone Improvement Plan [ZIP] code), GIS-based buffers, and global positioning system (GPS)-based activity space buffers [25]. Each method has benefits and caveats.

Early neighborhoods research mostly employed perceived neighborhood boundaries and administrative units. Perceived neighborhood boundaries are often assessed via survey measures. The perceived neighborhood would be more helpful to understand participants' behaviors in their own neighborhood boundaries; however, such measured response is commonly not consistent among survey participants [25]. And, responses are highly individualized based on characteristics of participants. Such individualized neighborhood definition may not closely be related to policy implications of research. Geographically defined administrative neighborhood boundaries are the most common method of operationalizing neighborhood via objective means, and the first strength of this definition is relatively easy translation to policy intervention. In addition, a plethora of data availability by such administrative units is another benefit of using such definition. Nevertheless, there is an issue of "spatial misclassification" with the administrative unit boundaries. Spatial misclassification refers to the incorrect characterization of a neighborhood-level exposure based on the definition used [26]. To illustrate, a neighborhood boundary may not reflect the actual daily experiences of people who live within.

With the wide use of GIS technologies, health research uses GIS-based buffer neighborhood definitions, for instance, 400-meter radius of an individual's residential address. This type of neighborhood definition is egocentric (i.e., individualized) so it varies from person to person, which can reduce the spatial misclassification to some degree. However, it is still a static boundary and cannot fully capture mobility patterns of individual. Thus, spatial misclassification remains as an issue with the GIS-based buffer neighborhood. In order to overcome such limitations of GIS-based buffer, recent research employs "activity space" neighborhood boundaries, including GPS-based "activity space" neighborhood definitions. An activity space refers to a set of spatial locations visited by an individual during a given period, and a GPS device enables identifying latitude and longitude coordinates using satellite and ground-based system. The GPS-based activity space definition can capture various neighborhood experiences and mobility patterns beyond participants' static residential area. This unfixed neighborhood definition can overcome the spatial misclassification by measuring actual travel patterns without assumptions about neighborhoods [27, 28]. However, lack of standardized GPS data collection methods remains as the first limitation of the GPS-based activity space. It is also worth noting that researchers proposed different methods in terms of the period of data collection (e.g., 1-week vs. 2-week) as well as time interval of each data point (e.g., 10-second vs. 30-second). There are also varied data processing metrics for defining activity space from collected data, such as daily path area, convex hall, and standard deviation ellipse [25, 29, 30]. In addition, GPS-based method has technical errors in data collection [31], privacy issues, and several biases due to GPS tracking [32], thus regarded as one of the most challenging methods to implement.

At the time of publication, we are not aware of any studies connecting GPS-based neighborhoods and HIV outcomes, although studies have examined connections between GPS-based neighborhoods and chronic disease such as obesity [33] and obesity risk behaviors [34]. We do note that we have several studies recently completed and in the field using GPS methods to connect with HIV outcomes. Preliminary analyses of The P18 Neighborhood Study show that a larger GPS activity space is associated with increased condomless sex among young MSM in New York City.

Research on Neighborhoods and HIV in Communities of Color

Various social and built neighborhood environments influence HIV prevalence. For example, high concentrations of racial/ethnic minorities, low educational attainment, unemployment, and crime, as well as prevailing abandoned lots/buildings and

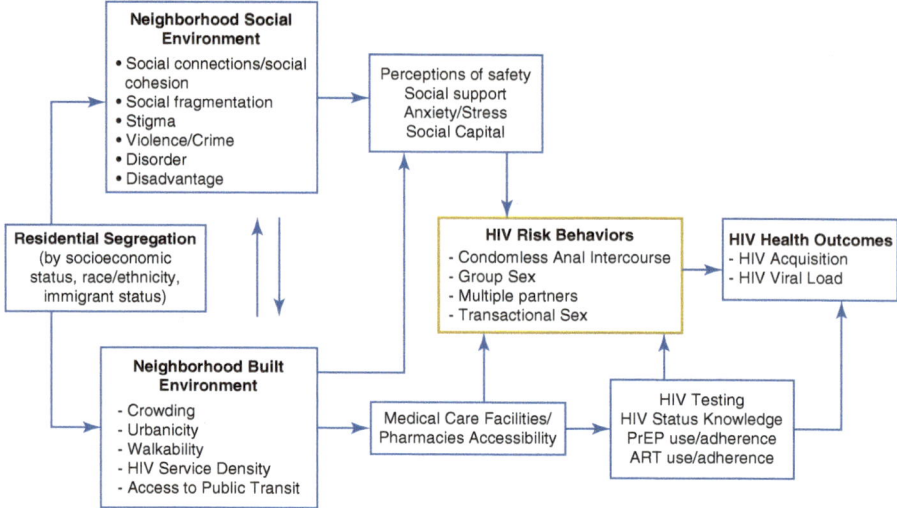

Fig. 9.1 Connecting social and built environmental characteristics of neighborhoods to HIV health outcomes

graffiti are associated with potential increased rate of HIV of neighborhoods [35]. Such neighborhood characteristics may be associated with HIV risk behaviors such as injecting drug use and sexual risk behavior, key risk factors for HIV acquisition.

In Fig. 9.1, we highlight how social and built environmental characteristics of neighborhoods may relate to HIV acquisition in communities of color in the United States. As an example, we highlight that racial residential segregation (discussed in detail below) often shapes the context of neighborhoods, including neighborhood-built environments such as access to public transit. Having easy access to buses and trains can influence one's HIV testing and knowledge of HIV status. For HIV-negative individuals, neighborhoods with increased access to public transit can also facilitate increased PrEP uptake and adherence. For HIV-positive individuals, neighborhoods with increased access to public transit can facilitate increased ART uptake and adherence.

While we have not conducted a systematic review of the literature on neighborhoods and HIV-related outcomes, we review seminal studies in this chapter. The vast majority of studies on neighborhoods and HIV focus on social environmental factors. As such, we start with residential segregation as a social environmental characteristic of neighborhoods.

Social Environment

Residential Segregation

Segregation, defined as separation of individuals into specific groups based on their membership in socially constructed categories such as race, ethnicity, gender, or religion, is a ubiquitous phenomenon in most of US cities. Residential segregation, one type of segregation that occurs where individuals live in residential space, may have short- and long-term influences on various health outcomes and behaviors, thus referred to as a fundamental determinant of health disparities [36]. Social/physical deprivation, limited access to health promoting resources, neighborhood stigma and related stress, and decreased social capital and social network are potential reasons for poor health outcomes and behaviors in segregated neighborhoods. Despite prevailing residential segregation in the United States, measures of segregation differ by methodologies, dimension, and geographic scale [37]. To illustrate, level of residential segregation would be differed by neighborhood definition and scale [38]. While there is wide range of measures of segregation, virtually all studies identified have been found to influences health outcomes and behaviors, especially among communities of color.

Among various health consequences of segregation, infectious diseases, of which HIV is one, can be susceptible to various social factors including residential segregation [39]. Studies have also investigated how HIV-related health outcomes and behavioral factors, such as HIV infection, HIV/AIDS prevalence, and sexual risk behaviors, may also be associated with residential segregation. In the following, we discuss specific studies on residential segregation and HIV-related health outcomes.

A longitudinal study of heterosexually-identified Black adults and adolescents in 95 large US metropolitan statistical areas (MSAs) in 2008–2015 found that racial residential segregation was associated with HIV infection [40]. In particular, a one standard deviation decrease in baseline isolation was associated with a 16.2% reduction in the rate of new HIV diagnoses, while one standard deviation reduction in isolation over time was associated with 4.6% decrease in the rate of new HIV diagnoses. Another cross-sectional study with national representative sample collected between 2006 and 2010 reported that core-based statistical area (CBSA) level racial residential segregation was associated with risky sexual behavior among non-Hispanic Blacks [41]. CBSAs with absolute centralization as well as relatively high concentration of non-Hispanic Black had approximately twofold risk of sexual risk behaviors (e.g., a greater number of sexual partners and condomless sex).

Also relevant to communities of color generally, studies of neighborhood sociodemographic and HIV have increasingly attended to racial composition. Even when accounting for differences in socioeconomic status, one study found that Black men living in areas highly concentrated with other Black people had higher rates of delayed HIV diagnoses than those in less concentrated areas [42] (CITE). This study also found that neighborhoods with highest (relative to lowest) Black racial concentration had higher relative risk of late HIV diagnosis among men (RR = 1.86; 95%CI = 1.15, 3.00) and women (RR = 5.37; 95%CI = 3.16, 10.43) independent of income inequality and socioeconomic deprivation [42]. In addition, in an analysis of four census tracts in Philadelphia, compared to the predominantly white high HIV prevalence tract, both the predominantly Black high and low HIV prevalence tracts had greater odds of HIV transmission via injection drug use and heterosexual contact than male-to-male sexual contact [43]. Among Blacks, there were greater than 15 new cases of HIV infection reported among the census tracts. Moreover, among a total of HIV positive participants ($n = 319$), $n = 27$ were Hispanic (not White) and n = 151 Black. In regard to HIV care, one study in Florida between 2000 and 2014 found that consistent trends of increased risks of nonretention in HIV care and viral load suppression among people who lived in neighborhood with high concentration of non-Hispanic Blacks [44].

Neighborhood HIV Prevalence

Once a neighborhood has a high prevalence of HIV, one could assume that living or socializing in such high HIV prevalence area increases the chances of an individual acquiring HIV. To illustrate, in a cohort study of 600 young MSM (15% Black, 38% Hispanic, 18% Mixed/Other and 29% White) in New York City who were aged 18–19 years at baseline, incidence of HIV infections (7.2%) was marginally higher among those residing in neighborhoods with higher rates of HIV prevalence [45]. In addition, among a racially and ethnically diverse sample of MSM in Chicago, one study found that Black young MSM had a significantly greater proportion of their sexual partners from high HIV prevalence neighborhoods than Latino, White, and Other young MSM [46]. In addition, a cross-sectional study in San Francisco reported that Black MSM had lower socioeconomic scores and are more likely to live in areas of higher HIV prevalence and lower income when compared to White MSM [47]. Further, it was found the Black MSM were more likely to report sero-discordant partnerships and higher numbers of potentially serodiscordant unprotected sex acts and increasing neighborhood HIV prevalence predicted an increase in the number of potentially serodiscordant unprotected sex acts among trans-females and Black MSM but only significantly so for transfemales. One longitudinal study of 396 African American adolescent females in high HIV prevalence neighborhood was less likely to have HIV test compared to them in low HIV prevalence area [48].

Gay Neighborhoods and Other Neighborhood Sociodemographics

Neighborhood socioeconomic (dis)advantage is only one, albeit a key, example of a neighborhood characteristic that has been examined relative to HIV. Overall, a number of other neighborhood sociodemographic factors (beyond segregation-related constructs discussed earlier) may relate to the prevention and management of HIV.

Relative to HIV, demographers and public health researchers have long-studied the unique settlement patterns of gay and bisexual men, focusing on neighborhoods with high population concentrations these populations often referred to as "gayborhoods" [49]. While conceptually it makes sense that gayborhoods may influence HIV prevention and management, such a relationship is anything but straightforward. Notably, studies have variously found living in a gayborhood to be associated with more condomless anal sex among MSM [50], less condomless sex [51], or have not found an association whatsoever [52]. These disparate findings suggest that any relationship between gayborhoods and HIV risk practices is either locally very specific (perhaps due to specific social norms) or of greater complexity than can be captured through a direct association. Interestingly, researchers have consistently linked the use of illicit drugs to living in neighborhoods with high concentrations of gay and bisexual men [50, 53–55].

It must be noted that gayborhood proximity is a rather crude associative marker of HIV risk. Someone who lives in a gayborhood is not necessarily part of those communities and, conversely, men who do not live in traditional gayborhoods may still spend much of their social lives immersed within them. This contention is supported by research that additionally assessed social networks, finding that while living in a gayborhood may not be directly linked to condomless sex among MSM, such a relationship is mediated by how socially connected men are to other gay men [55]. Nevertheless, attention to neighborhoods of gay and bisexual men remains important, including because HIV-related services are often situated within such neighborhoods [56] and gay men who live within them report greater exposure to media used to deliver HIV and safer sex messaging [52], which could at least partly explain why MSM living in gayborhoods report higher rates of HIV testing [52].

From an intersectional perspective, research also sought to understand how racial composition interacts with concentrations of gay and bisexual populations, noting that MSM of color are less likely to live in these areas than their White peers [52]. One study found that for MSM of color, living in a gayborhood was not associated with linkage to HIV care nor to viral suppression [57] while another observed that living in a gayborhood was associated with more consistent condom use among Black MSM after accounting for neighborhood concentrations of Black people [51].

In addition, higher neighborhood-level educational attainment was associated with less PrEP awareness among a sample of 618 young Black MSM in Chicago [58]. Increasingly, researchers have come to understand that the key to understanding how sociodemographic factors affect HIV outcomes is not so much *who* lives in a particular neighborhood but *how* they live there. As discussed, social networks are one mediating factor. Further, mixed-methods research has powerfully highlighted the significance of connection between neighborhood residents—defined often along lines of race and sexual orientation—can shape MSM of color's experiences of HIV risk and prevention [59].

By studying the examples presented here, it seems clear that the sociodemographics of one's neighborhood in concert with how individuals engage (or not) with that composition is far more useful for understanding HIV prevention and management than focusing on sociodemographics alone. Further, the unique intersectional positions produced by sexual orientation and race demand special attention to how different types of neighborhood characteristics interact relative to HIV outcomes and, importantly, how those interactions are mediated by configurations of social networks, social cohesion, and social capital (discussed below).

Neighborhood Disadvantage

Neighborhood disadvantage is one of the earliest and most studied neighborhood dimensions [1]. While many parameters are often used to define neighborhood disadvantage, the term neighborhood disadvantage typically refers to the socioeconomic disadvantage of a neighborhood (including disadvantage by education, income and occupation). Previous research found that under-resourced neighborhoods have greater exposure to crime, violence, disorder, and limited social cohesion predominantly because of poverty. Neighborhood disadvantage has been associated with HIV-related outcomes among different populations. Of relevance, living in a disadvantaged neighborhood also affects access and utilization of health services [60], further contributing to a higher HIV prevalence. Interestingly, neighborhood disadvantage is important to consider in population health research as it may influence health independently of individual's socioeconomic status [60]. Consequently, it is with utmost importance to conduct research investigating the complex relationships between neighborhood disadvantage and health outcomes, including HIV, among people of color.

Emerging research has been focusing on employing a lens on communities of colors when studying neighborhood disadvantage and HIV risk, including transactional sex. Transactional sex is directly linked to the informational economic sector, usually referred to as "the street economy". For instance, among a cross-sectional sample of young MSM living in Detroit ($n = 319$; aged 18–29 years; 50% Black, 25% white, 15% Latino, 9% other race/ethnicity; 9% HIV-positive), those who reported living in neighborhoods with greater socioeconomic disadvantage also reported more transactional sex [2]. These findings are consistent with a study focused exclusively on Black MSM [61]. A cross-sectional study in San Francisco ($n = 521$) reported that Black MSM have lower socioeconomic scores and were more likely to live in areas of lower income when compared to White MSM. In addition, it was found the Black MSM were more likely to report serodiscordant partnerships and higher numbers of potentially serodiscordant unprotected sex acts [47]. Furthermore, another study in focused on African American adults in Atlanta, GA, investigated the effect of changes in exposure to neighborhood characteristics, including neighborhood economic disadvantage, and several risk behaviors of HIV [62]. Data came from data a predominately substance-misusing cohort of African-American adults relocating from US public housing complexes and this study found that individuals who experienced improvements in economic conditions within their neighborhoods were likely to experience greater reduction in perceived partner risk (e.g., using an index to measure perceived partner risk, which measures the risk of a partner using dimensions like HIV/AIDS status, sexually transmitted infections (STIs) status, drug use, and number of partners for the other partner). Residing in neighborhood with high unemployment rate (a parameter for neighborhood disadvantage) was also associated with late HIV diagnosis for Latino males [63]. However, in another longitudinal study conducted among urban African American youth followed from adolescence into young adulthood ($n = 369$; 51% female) in multiple areas, contrary results regarding HIV testing were reported. It was found that individuals residing in neighborhoods of greater disadvantage were more likely to test for HIV. This could be attributable to public health campaigns designed for such communities [48]. In another study including a diverse sample of individuals from an HIV clinical cohort in the southern United States, residing in the most adverse neighborhood socioeconomic context was associated with lack of viral suppression [64]. Moreover, and in a non-US context, Massari et al. demonstrated that socioeconomic status, migration origin, and neighborhood disadvantage were barriers to HIV testing in the Paris (France) metropolitan area [65]. This reiterates the notion that people residing in disadvantaged neighborhoods and people of ethnic minorities (e.g., foreigners and people born to foreign parents in France) may have less access to health services and thus HIV-testing facilities.

Neighborhood Disorder and Neighborhood Violence

Neighborhood disorder is a neighborhood feature that includes multiple dimensions for its measurement, including both social and physical disorders. Examples of social disorder include verbal harassment on the street, open solicitation for prostitution, public intoxication, neighborhood violence and crime, and rowdy groups of young males in public, while physical disorder includes graffiti, abandoned cars, broken windows, and garbage in the streets [66]. Research has investigated the association between neighborhood disorder and sexual health outcomes, including HIV. Additionally, communities of color have been a special interest in this type of research as they are more likely to be residing in disordered neighborhoods.

Among social neighborhood disorders, neighborhood crime has been associated with increased HIV-related risk-taking behavior, including condomless sex, multiple concurrent relationships, and indirect concurrency [62, 67–69]. Additional studies demonstrated this relationship among adolescents, highlighting the impact of witnessing community violence on early sexual debut and sexual risk behaviors [70–74]. The findings on the association between neighborhood violence and/or crime with HIV risk behaviors are consistent with other research in the literature on communities of color, particularly African American populations. Among Black men living with HIV, neighborhood crime has been associated with having multiple HIV-negative or unknown-serostatus sexual partners [75]. This causes a concern in regard to HIV risk transmission behavior among sexually active Black individuals living with HIV. Furthermore, neighborhood threats and verbal harassment were also shown to be associated with various sexual risk behaviors among a sample of heterosexually-identified Black men (e.g., condom use, number of sexual partners) [76]. Among a sample of HIV-positive Black MSM in Chicago, community violence had significantly higher rates of condomless anal intercourse in the previous 6 months. Also, exposure to community violence was positively associated with psychological distress, hard drug use, and use of marijuana as a sex drug. Adherence to HIV antiretroviral medication was negatively associated with community violence [77].

Additionally, among a sample of African, Caribbean, and Black youth residents, it was found that those residing in more socially disordered neighborhoods endorsed stigmatizing beliefs more often with regard to HIV [78]. This may result in increased stigma towards individuals living with HIV in those neighborhoods. Related, in another study, African American MSM with HIV who resided in neighborhoods marked by disorder (e.g., vandalism, people selling drugs) were likely to experience more discrimination and hate crimes [79]. Experiencing interpersonal discrimination and stigma can possibly aggravate the effects of violence and harassment experiences within the neighborhood.

Although less prominently, research also investigated physical neighborhood disorders. A cross-sectional study among young Black MSM demonstrated that the presence of vacant building was associated with HIV infection among the neighborhood's residents [80]. Although the mechanism in which this association occurs remain unclear, several theories are suggested, including the link between vacant building and crime or low collective efficacy [81, 82]. Additionally, presence of vacant buildings can be associated with destabilization of community infrastructure [83] and an indicator of the lack of stability in housing and employment, which are also associated with HIV risk behaviors [84].

It is important to note that to date, the literature regarding neighborhood disorder and HIV risk has been inconsistent. For instance, some studies found social disorder to be associated with less anal intercourse and condomless anal intercourse [85]. Other studies found mixed association between indicators of neighborhood physical disorder and HIV risk behaviors among MSM of color and White MSM [86].

Neighborhood Social Capital and Income Inequality

Social capital theory is a theoretical perspective that emphasizes resources and norms of behaviors that are located external to individuals [87]. Within the neighborhood context and health, neighborhood social capital, such as shared values, neighborhood social network, and participation in local community organizations, influences individual's engagement in health behaviors. Social capital of neighborhoods could be translated into social norm, collective efficacy, or social cohesion; however, income inequality can erode social capital and weaken social ties in neighborhoods [88]. Social capital is defined in different ways in the fields of social science and public health, and measuring social capital has several modes. Robert Putnam examined participation in civic or social organization and trust among neighbors as indicators of social capital, which is frequently employed in surveys [89]. Collective efficacy or engagement which refers to social structure to achieve certain ends is another measure of social capital defined by James Coleman. Coleman's definition uses social participants and experience of collaboration with neighbors to sanction deviance and social norm as indicators of social capital [90].

A large body of literature has demonstrated the associations between neighborhood social capital and health behaviors and outcomes, including HIV risk. HIV risk behaviors, including sexual risk behaviors and drug use, were found to be correlated with neighborhood social capital. Neighborhoods with low social capital may have less access to relevant HIV knowledge and educational resources, thereby leading to high prevalence of HIV risk behaviors and HIV rate [91]. Epidemiologic studies have found empirical evidence of associations between social capital and STI including HIV [92]. Ransome and colleagues found a high prevalence of HIV and STI in neighborhoods with low social capital and income inequality in Philadelphia, using spatial statistics [93]. One cross-sectional multi-level analysis found that voting rate, one of proxies of social capital, was negatively associated with STI prevalence [94]. In one study of Latino MSM, researchers found that neighborhood-level social cohesion was associated with lower rates of condomless anal sex [95]. A study of MSM in Swaziland (Africa) demonstrated that high social capital predicted high HIV testing [96]. Another study in Chicago also revealed that collective efficacy, measured by self-reported neighborhood characteristics, was negatively associated with number of sexual partners among adolescents [97]. In addition, drawing on cross-sectional data collected in three Kansas City jails, one study described the social, neighborhood-based context of sexual health risk prior to incarceration for 290 women. Living in a neighborhood that was perceived to have low social capital was also associated with sexually transmitted infection history [98].

In an ecological study in New York City, low neighborhood social capital was associated with late HIV diagnosis [99]. To illustrate, low to high political participation and social cohesion corresponded with significant decreasing trend in late HIV diagnosis. One state-level ecological study examined inverse correlation between social capital and adolescents' sexual risk behaviors, such as more than five sexual partners and condomless sex [100]. In a multi-level study with 378 participants in New York City demonstrated that neighborhood income inequality is associated with more exchange sex, crack use, and membership in high HIV prevalence drug network [101]. Another study examined income inequality (using the GINI indices of inequality) at the community level and HIV prevalence in a sample of persons who inject drugs (PWID) in Thai Nguyen, Vietnam, and found a higher GINI coefficient at the community level was associated with higher odds of individual HIV infection in PWID (OR = 1.46 per 0.01, $p = 0.003$), while higher personal income was associated with reduced odds of infection (OR = 0.98 per \$10, $p = 0.022$) [102].

In addition to social norms in neighborhoods, HIV studies have examined social and sexual networks of neighborhoods. In one study, sexual network members residing in the same neighborhood as the participants and discussions around avoiding HIV acquisition with confidants were associated with greater PrEP awareness among a sample of Black MSM in Chicago [58].

Built Environment

In the next section of the chapter, we focus on the built environment, including availability of HIV testing locations.

Neighborhood Built Environment, Including Availability of HIV Testing Locations

Neighborhood access to HIV health services theoretically can influence HIV outcomes, as we briefly described earlier in the chapter. Conceptually, living in a neighborhood, or in close proximity, to HIV testing locations may facilitate one getting tested for HIV. These relationships may be more nuanced, however. HIV stigma, for example, can facilitate an individual not wanting to get tested for HIV in their "home" neighborhoods, including in communities of color, where HIV is still heavily stigmatized.

In a study of MSM in Chicago, higher Walk Score clusters [22] were less likely to contain HIV-positive individuals [80]. This is one of few studies that have examined associations between neighborhood walkability and HIV outcomes. Greater primary care density was associated with greater PrEP awareness among a sample of 618 young Black MSM in Chicago; however, greater neighborhood alcohol outlet density was associated with less PrEP awareness among the same sample of young Black MSM in Chicago [58]. In another study, participants living in areas with higher PrEP clinic density were significantly more willing to use PrEP (one standard deviation higher density of PrEP clinics per 10,000 population was associated with 16% higher willingness [adjusted prevalence ratio = 1.16, 95% CI: 1.03–1.31]) [103]. However, a study in Chicago found that areas where young Black MSM reside typically have low HIV service densities. HIV service density also corresponded poorly to some ZIP codes in which young Black MSM who report high rates of condomless sexual behavior reside [104]. This is in contrast to a recent geographic analysis of PrEP services in New York City, where we found no race-based neighborhood differences in where PrEP services were located; unsurprisingly, though, PrEP services were located in neighborhoods with high HIV prevalence rates [105]. In another counterintuitive study, greater access to public transit, shorter distance to medical care, and longer distance to pharmacies were associated with residence in a poor retention hotspots among a retrospective cohort in Philadelphia of 1404 persons newly diagnosed with HIV in 2008–2009 followed for 24 months after linkage to care [106]. Unexpectedly, shorter distance to pharmacies was associated with residence in poor viral suppression hotspots.

Limitations of Existing Research

The existing literature on neighborhoods and HIV and related outcomes is limited in a number of ways, including use of cross-sectional designs in most studies. Indeed, like the vast majority of neighborhoods and health research [1, 13], neighborhoods research focused on HIV is largely cross-sectional. Because most studies of neighborhoods and HIV outcomes have utilized cross-sectional designs, causal inference is limited. In addition, the vast majority of neighborhoods research on HIV-related outcomes focused on sexual health behaviors and HIV infection, while there is a broader range of HIV-related outcomes to be examined. A number of studies have used self-reported outcomes, including HIV infection. Consequently, social desirability bias is a concern with self-reported studies. In studies where the neighborhood characteristic is also self-report, same-source bias is a concern.

Future Research Directions on Neighborhoods and HIV

We recognize that certain neighborhood characteristics remain under-studied or not studied at all, including neighborhood-level incarceration. We are aware of only one study that found women who lived in urban neighborhoods, which had the highest density of our incarcerated participants, were three times as likely to report a history of trading sex for money, drugs, or life necessities compared to women who lived elsewhere in the city [98]. We are not aware of any research examining relationships between neighborhood stigma and HIV-related outcomes. Spatial stigma can include a negative image of the neighborhood in the media, negative perceptions of neighborhood's residents by others, and feelings of judgment by others because they live in a particular neighborhood [107]. Further, future studies need to incorporate both the built and social environment in the study design either as predictors of substantive interest, confounding covariates or effect modifiers. In addition to using objective measures of neighborhood characteristics (e.g., GIS measures), studies are needed to define more accurate neighborhood contexts, including GPS activity space neighborhoods. Our work and others show that GPS methods are feasible among Black populations in the United States [108, 109].

Additional studies are needed to focus on HIV prevention and HIV treatment behaviors and outcomes, including PrEP uptake. We have a study in the field (named The Neighborhoods and Networks [N2] Cohort Study) that, in part, is examining the impact of neighborhoods on PrEP uptake among Black MSM in Chicago, IL, Jackson, MS and New Orleans, LA. We also believe that studies need to examine other communities of color most impacted by HIV, including transgender women of color [110]. When we discuss race and ethnicity, we recognize that communities of color are *not* homogenous and, as discussed earlier in the chapter, attention to how intersectional positions of individuals, communities, and neighborhoods is essential. Some research has already started to do this among MSM of color in particular, but attention to factors beyond sexual orientation—including those relevant to heterosexual communities (e.g., nativity)—would be useful for future research, especially with the inclusion of moderating factors.

In terms of study designs, observational (cross-sectional and longitudinal) studies are fundamental to build the evidence base in a given area of research; however, stronger study studies design such as experiments and quasi-experimental studies permit causal inference by reducing threats to internal validity [111]. There are a handful of longitudinal studies connecting neighborhoods and HIV outcomes and ever increasing. As we discussed, while studies utilizing longitudinal designs are needed to facilitate causal inference, studies using experimental and quasi-experimental study designs are also needed. Finally, studies using agent-based models can facilitate causal inference and overcome the limitations of implementing a quasi-experiment for example. There is a clear paucity of evidence of neighborhood-level HIV-related interventions. However, the findings from observational studies suggest that neighborhood-level interventions can improve sexual health and related HIV outcomes, and therefore should be explored.

Conclusion

President Trump stated in February 2019 that he aims to end the US HIV epidemic in 10 years [112]. In order to meet this goal, studies (and the interventions that follow) must include factors beyond those of the individual. Because neighborhoods can impact HIV outcomes, including in communities of color, we need to focus research and intervention efforts on targeting restructuring neighborhoods and behavioral interventions need to account for the neighborhood context. However, additional research is indeed, including understanding the pathways connecting neighborhoods and HIV health outcomes in different communities of color.

Acknowledgments Dr. Dustin Duncan was supported in part by grants from the National Institute on Minority Health and Health Disparities (Grant Number R01MD013554), National Institute on Mental Health (Grant Number R01MH112406), National Institute on Drug Abuse (Grant Number R03DA039748), and the Centers for Disease Control and Prevention (Grant Number U01PS005122). We thank John Francois for contributing to the literature review for this chapter.

References

1. Duncan DT, Kawachi I. Neighborhoods and health. Oxford: Oxford University Press; 2018.
2. Bauermeister JA, Connochie D, Eaton L, Demers M, Stephenson R. Geospatial indicators of space and place: a review of multilevel studies of HIV prevention and care outcomes among young men who have sex with men in the United States. J Sex Res. 2017;54(4–5):446–64.
3. Singh S, Song R, Johnson AS, McCray E, Hall HI. HIV incidence, prevalence, and undiagnosed infections in US men who have sex with men. Ann Intern Med. 2018;168(10):685–94.

4. Howe CJ, Siegel H, Dulin-Keita A. Neighborhood environments and sexual risk behaviors for HIV infection among US women: a systematic review. AIDS Behav. 2017;21(12):3353–65.

5. Card KG, Lachowsky NJ, Althoff KN, Schafer K, Hogg RS, Montaner JS. A systematic review of the geospatial barriers to antiretroviral initiation, adherence and viral suppression among people living with HIV. Sex Health. 2018;16(1):1–17.

6. Bowleg L. The problem with the phrase women and minorities: intersectionality—an important theoretical framework for public health. Am J Public Health. 2012;102(7):1267–73.

7. Julia C, Valleron A-J. Louis-René Villermé (1782–1863), a pioneer in social epidemiology: re-analysis of his data on comparative mortality in Paris in the early 19th century. J Epidemiol Community Health. 2011;65(8):666–70.

8. Kim D. Blues from the neighborhood? Neighborhood characteristics and depression. Epidemiol Rev. 2008;30(1):101–17.

9. Ding D, Gebel K. Built environment, physical activity, and obesity: what have we learned from reviewing the literature? Health Place. 2012;18(1):100–5.

10. Grasser G, Van Dyck D, Titze S, Stronegger W. Objectively measured walkability and active transport and weight-related outcomes in adults: a systematic review. Int J Public Health. 2013;58(4):615–25.

11. Yen IH, Michael YL, Perdue L. Neighborhood environment in studies of health of older adults: a systematic review. Am J Prev Med. 2009;37(5):455–63.

12. Boardman JD, Finch BK, Ellison CG, Williams DR, Jackson JS. Neighborhood disadvantage, stress, and drug use among adults. J Health Soc Behav. 2001;42:151–65.

13. Arcaya MC, Tucker-Seeley RD, Kim R, Schnake-Mahl A, So M, Subramanian SV. Research on neighborhood effects on health in the United States: a systematic review of study characteristics. Soc Sci Med. 2016;168:16–29.

14. Roux AVD, Merkin SS, Arnett D, Chambless L, Massing M, Nieto FJ, et al. Neighborhood of residence and incidence of coronary heart disease. N Engl J Med. 2001;345(2):99–106.

15. Evans GW. The environment of childhood poverty. Am Psychol. 2004;59(2):77.

16. Feldman PJ, Steptoe A. How neighborhoods and physical functioning are related: the roles of neighborhood socioeconomic status, perceived neighborhood strain, and individual health risk factors. Ann Behav Med. 2004;27(2):91–9.

17. Pickett KE, Pearl M. Multilevel analyses of neighbourhood socioeconomic context and health outcomes: a critical review. J Epidemiol Community Health. 2001;55(2):111–22.

18. Leal C, Bean K, Thomas F, Chaix B. Multicollinearity in associations between multiple environmental features and body weight and abdominal fat: using matching techniques to assess whether the associations are separable. Am J Epidemiol. 2012;175(11):1152–62.

19. Cohen DA, Inagami S, Finch B. The built environment and collective efficacy. Health Place. 2008;14(2):198–208.

20. Dong H. Does walkability undermine neighbourhood safety? J Urban Des. 2017;22(1):59–75.

21. Duncan DT, Goedel WC, Chunara R. Quantitative methods for measuring neighborhood characteristics in neighborhood health research. In: Neighborhoods and health. Oxford: Oxford University Press; 2018. p. 57.

22. Duncan DT. What's your walk score(R)?: web-based neighborhood walkability assessment for health promotion and disease prevention. Am J Prev Med. 2013;45(2):244–5.

23. De Choudhury M, Sharma S, Kiciman E, editors. Characterizing dietary choices, nutrition, and language in food deserts via social media. Proceedings of the 19th ACM conference on computer-supported cooperative work & social computing. San Francisco, CA: ACM; 2016.

24. Cawkwell PB, Lee L, Weitzman M, Sherman SE. Tracking hookah bars in New York: utilizing yelp as a powerful public health tool. JMIR Public Health Surveill. 2015;1(2):e19.

25. Duncan DT, Regan SD, Chaix B. Operationalizing neighborhood definitions in health research: spatial misclassification and other issues. In: Neighborhoods and health. Oxford: Oxford University Press; 2018. p. 19–56.

26. Duncan DT, Kawachi I, Subramanian SV, Aldstadt J, Melly SJ, Williams DR. Examination of how neighborhood definition influences measurements of youths' access to tobacco retailers: a methodological note on spatial misclassification. Am J Epidemiol. 2014;179(3):373–81.

27. Duncan DT, Tamura K, Regan SD, Athens J, Elbel B, Meline J, et al. Quantifying spatial mis-classification in exposure to noise complaints among low-income housing residents across New York City neighborhoods: a Global Positioning System (GPS) study. Ann Epidemiol. 2017;27(1):67–75.
28. Harrison F, Burgoine T, Corder K, van Sluijs EM, Jones A. How well do modelled routes to school record the environments children are exposed to? A cross-sectional comparison of GIS-modelled and GPS-measured routes to school. Int J Health Geogr. 2014;13:5.
29. Boruff BJ, Nathan A, Nijënstein S. Using GPS technology to (re)-examine operational defini-tions of 'neighbourhood' in place-based health research. Int J Health Geogr. 2012;11(1):22.
30. Hirsch JA, Winters M, Clarke P, McKay H. Generating GPS activity spaces that shed light upon the mobility habits of older adults: a descriptive analysis. Int J Health Geogr. 2014;13:51.
31. Mooney SJ, Sheehan DM, Zulaika G, Rundle AG, McGill K, Behrooz MR, et al. Quantifying distance overestimation from global positioning system in urban spaces. Am J Public Health. 2016;106(4):651–3.
32. Chaix B, Meline J, Duncan S, Merrien C, Karusisi N, Perchoux C, et al. GPS tracking in neighborhood and health studies: a step forward for environmental exposure assessment, a step backward for causal inference? Health Place. 2013;21:46–51.
33. Tamura K, Elbel B, Athens JK, Rummo PE, Chaix B, Regan SD, et al. Assessments of resi-dential and global positioning system activity space for food environments, body mass index and blood pressure among low-income housing residents in New York City. Geospat Health. 2018;13(2). https://doi.org/10.4081/gh.2018.712. PMID: 30451471.
34. Zenk SN, Schulz AJ, Matthews SA, Odoms-Young A, Wilbur J, Wegrzyn L, et al. Activity space environment and dietary and physical activity behaviors: a pilot study. Health Place. 2011;17(5):1150–61.
35. Latkin CA, German D, Vlahov D, Galea S. Neighborhoods and HIV: a social ecological approach to prevention and care. Am Psychol. 2013;68(4):210.
36. Williams DR, Collins C. Racial residential segregation: a fundamental cause of racial dispari-ties in health. Public Health Rep. 2016;116:404.
37. Kramer MR. Residential segregation and health. In: Neighborhoods and health. Oxford: Oxford University Press; 2018. p. 321–56.
38. Kramer MR, Cooper HL, Drews-Botsch CD, Waller LA, Hogue CR. Do measures matter? Comparing surface-density-derived and census-tract-derived measures of racial residential segregation. Int J Health Geogr. 2010;9(1):29.
39. Acevedo-Garcia D. Residential segregation and the epidemiology of infectious diseases. Soc Sci Med. 2000;51(8):1143–61.
40. Ibragimov U, Beane S, Adimora A, Friedman S, Williams L, Tempalski B, et al. Relationship of racial residential segregation to newly diagnosed cases of HIV among black heterosexuals in US Metropolitan Areas, 2008-2015. J Urban Health. 2018;96:856.
41. Lutfi K, Trepka MJ, Fennie KP, Ibanez G, Gladwin H. Racial residential segregation and risky sexual behavior among non-Hispanic blacks, 2006–2010. Soc Sci Med. 2015;140:95–103.
42. Ransome Y, Kawachi I, Braunstein S, Nash D. Structural inequalities drive late HIV diagno-sis: the role of black racial concentration, income inequality, socioeconomic deprivation, and HIV testing. Health Place. 2016;42:148–58.
43. Brawner BM, Guthrie B, Stevens R, Taylor L, Eberhart M, Schensul JJ. Place still matters: racial/ethnic and geographic disparities in HIV transmission and disease burden. J Urban Health. 2017;94(5):716–29.
44. Sheehan DM, Fennie KP, Mauck DE, Maddox LM, Lieb S, Trepka MJ. Retention in HIV care and viral suppression: individual-and neighborhood-level predictors of racial/ethnic dif-ferences, Florida, 2015. AIDS Patient Care STDs. 2017;31(4):167–75.
45. Halkitis P, Kapadia F, Ompad D. Incidence of HIV infection in young gay, bisexual, and other YMSM: the P18 Cohort Study. J Acquir Immune Defic Syndr (1999). 2015;69(4):466.

46. Mustanski B, Birkett M, Kuhns LM, Latkin CA, Muth SQ. The role of geographic and network factors in racial disparities in HIV among young men who have sex with men: an egocentric network study. AIDS Behav. 2015;19(6):1037–47.
47. Raymond HF, Chen Y-H, Syme SL, Catalano R, Hutson M, McFarland W. The role of individual and neighborhood factors: HIV acquisition risk among high-risk populations in San Francisco. AIDS Behav. 2014;18(2):346–56.
48. Johns MM, Bauermeister JA, Zimmerman MA. Individual and neighborhood correlates of HIV testing among African American youth transitioning from adolescence into young adulthood. AIDS Educ Prev. 2010;22(6):509–22.
49. Brown M. Gender and sexuality II: there goes the gayborhood? Prog Hum Geogr. 2014;38(3):457–65.
50. Buttram ME, Kurtz SP. Risk and protective factors associated with gay neighborhood residence. Am J Mens Health. 2013;7(2):110–8.
51. Frye V, Koblin B, Chin J, Beard J, Blaney S, Halkitis P, et al. Neighborhood-level correlates of consistent condom use among men who have sex with men: a multi-level analysis. AIDS Behav. 2010;14(4):974–85.
52. Mills TC, Stall R, Pollack L, Paul JP, Binson D, Canchola J, et al. Health-related characteristics of men who have sex with men: a comparison of those living in "gay ghettos" with those living elsewhere. Am J Public Health. 2001;91(6):980.
53. Carpiano RM, Kelly BC, Easterbrook A, Parsons JT. Community and drug use among gay men: the role of neighborhoods and networks. J Health Soc Behav. 2011;52(1):74–90.
54. Egan JE. Gays in the neighborhood: how neighborhood and context impact HIV and substance use risks and resiliencies of gay, bisexual and other men who have sex with men in New York City. Ph.D. Dissertation, University of Pittsburgh. 2015.
55. Kelly BC, Carpiano RM, Easterbrook A, Parsons JT. Sex and the community: the implications of neighbourhoods and social networks for sexual risk behaviours among urban gay men. Sociol Health Illn. 2012;34(7):1085–102.
56. Fulcher C, Kaukinen C. Mapping and visualizing the location HIV service providers: an exploratory spatial analysis of Toronto neighborhoods. AIDS Care. 2005;17(3):386–96.
57. Mauck DE, Sheehan DM, Fennie KP, Maddox LM, Trepka MJ. Role of gay neighborhood status and other neighborhood factors in racial/ethnic disparities in retention in care and viral load suppression among men who have sex with men, Florida, 2015. AIDS Behav. 2018;22(9):2978–93.
58. Chen Y-T, Kolak M, Duncan DT, Schumm P, Michaels S, Fujimoto K, et al. Neighbourhoods, networks and pre-exposure prophylaxis awareness: a multilevel analysis of a sample of young black men who have sex with men. Sex Transm Infect. 2019;95(3):228–35.
59. Egan JE, Frye V, Kurtz SP, Latkin C, Chen M, Tobin K, et al. Migration, neighborhoods, and networks: approaches to understanding how urban environmental conditions affect syndemic adverse health outcomes among gay, bisexual and other men who have sex with men. AIDS Behav. 2011;15(Suppl 1):S35–50.
60. Hu J, Kind AJ, Nerenz D. Area deprivation index predicts readmission risk at an urban teaching hospital. Am J Med Qual. 2018;33(5):493–501.
61. Stevens R, Icard L, Jemmott JB, O'leary A, Rutledge S, Hsu J, et al. Risky trade: individual and neighborhood-level socio-demographics associated with transactional sex among urban African American MSM. J Urban Health. 2017;94(5):676–82.
62. Cooper HL, Linton S, Haley DF, Kelley ME, Dauria EF, Karnes CC, et al. Changes in exposure to neighborhood characteristics are associated with sexual network characteristics in a cohort of adults relocating from public housing. AIDS Behav. 2015;19(6):1016–30.
63. Sheehan DM, Trepka MJ, Fennie KP, Prado G, Madhivanan P, Dillon FR, et al. Individual and neighborhood determinants of late HIV diagnosis among Latinos, Florida, 2007–2011. J Immigr Minor Health. 2017;19(4):825–34.

64. Rebeiro PF, Howe CJ, Rogers WB, Bebawy SS, Turner M, Kheshti A, et al. The relationship between adverse neighborhood socioeconomic context and HIV continuum of care outcomes in a diverse HIV clinic cohort in theSouthern United States. AIDS Care. 2018;30(11):1426–34.

65. Massari V, Lapostolle A, Cadot E, Parizot I, Dray-Spira R, Chauvin P. Gender, socio-economic status, migration origin and neighbourhood of residence are barriers to HIV testing in the Paris metropolitan area. AIDS Care. 2011;23(12):1609–18.

66. Sampson RJ, Raudenbush SW. Systematic social observation of public spaces: a new look at disorder in urban neighborhoods. Am J Sociol. 1999;105(3):603–51.

67. Voisin DR. Victims of community violence and HIV sexual risk behaviors among African American adolescent males. J HIV/AIDS Prev Educ Adolesc Child. 2003;5(3–4):87–110.

68. Latkin CA, Curry AD, Hua W, Davey MA. Direct and indirect associations of neighborhood disorder with drug use and high-risk sexual partners. Am J Prev Med. 2007;32(6):S234–S41.

69. Wilson HW, Woods BA, Emerson E, Donenberg GR. Patterns of violence exposure and sexual risk in low-income, urban African American girls. Psychol Violence. 2012;2(2):194.

70. Albus KE, Weist MD, Perez-Smith AM. Associations between youth risk behavior and exposure to violence: implications for the provision of mental health services in urban schools. Behav Modif. 2004;28(4):548–64.

71. Voisin DR, Neilands TB. Community violence and health risk factors among adolescents on Chicago's southside: does gender matter? J Adolesc Health. 2010;46(6):600–2.

72. Voisin DR, Crosby R, Yarber WL, Salazar LF, DiClemente RJ, Staples-Horne M. Witnessing community violence and health-risk behaviors among detained adolescents. Am J Orthopsychiatry. 2007;77(4):506–13.

73. Brady SS. Lifetime community violence exposure and health risk behavior among young adults in college. J Adolesc Health. 2006;39(4):610–3.

74. Brady SS, Tschann JM, Pasch LA, Flores E, Ozer EJ. Violence involvement, substance use, and sexual activity among Mexican-American and European-American adolescents. J Adolesc Health. 2008;43(3):285–95.

75. Ojikutu BO, Bogart LM, Klein DJ, Galvan FH, Wagner GJ. Neighborhood crime and sexual transmission risk behavior among black men living with HIV. J Health Care Poor Underserved. 2018;29(1):383.

76. Bowleg L, Neilands TB, Tabb LP, Burkholder GJ, Malebranche DJ, Tschann JM. Neighborhood context and Black heterosexual men's sexual HIV risk behaviors. AIDS Behav. 2014;18(11):2207–18.

77. Quinn K, Voisin DR, Bouris A, Schneider J. Psychological distress, drug use, sexual risks and medication adherence among young HIV-positive Black men who have sex with men: exposure to community violence matters. AIDS Care. 2016;28(7):866–72.

78. Kerr J, Northington T, Sockdjou T, Maticka-Tyndale E. Perceived neighborhood quality and HIV-related stigma among African diasporic youth; results from the African, Caribbean, and Black Youth (ACBY) study. J Health Care Poor Underserved. 2018;29(2):651–63.

79. Dale SK, Bogart LM, Galvan FH, Wagner GJ, Pantalone DW, Klein DJ. Discrimination and hate crimes in the context of neighborhood poverty and stressors among HIV-positive African-American men who have sex with men. J Community Health. 2016;41(3):574–83.

80. Phillips G, Birkett M, Kuhns L, Hatchel T, Garofalo R, Mustanski B. Neighborhood-level associations with HIV infection among young men who have sex with men in Chicago. Arch Sex Behav. 2015;44(7):1773–86.

81. Garvin E, Branas C, Keddem S, Sellman J, Cannuscio C. More than just an eyesore: local insights and solutions on vacant land and urban health. J Urban Health. 2013;90(3):412–26.

82. Sampson RJ. Great American city: Chicago and the enduring neighborhood effect. Chicago: University of Chicago Press; 2012.

83. Buitrago K. Deciphering blight: vacant buildings data collection in the Chicago six county region. Chicago: Woodstock Institute; 2013.

84. German D, Latkin CA. Social stability and HIV risk behavior: evaluating the role of accumulated vulnerability. AIDS Behav. 2012;16(1):168–78.

85. Haley DF, Haardörfer R, Kramer MR, Adimora AA, Wingood GM, Goswami ND, et al. Associations between neighborhood characteristics and sexual risk behaviors among HIV-infected and HIV-uninfected women in the southern United States. Ann Epidemiol. 2017;27(4):252–9.e1.
86. Frye V, Nandi V, Egan JE, Cerda M, Rundle A, Quinn JW, et al. Associations among neighborhood characteristics and sexual risk behavior among black and white MSM living in a major urban area. AIDS Behav. 2017;21(3):870–90.
87. Kawachi I. Social capital and community effects on population and individual health. Ann N Y Acad Sci. 1999;896(1):120–30.
88. Kawachi I, Subramanian SV, Kim D. Social capital and health. New York: Springer; 2008. p. 1–26.
89. Putnam RD. Bowling alone: America's declining social capital. In: Crothers L, Lockhart C (eds). Culture and Politics. New York: Palgrave Macmillan; 2000. p. 223–34.
90. Coleman JS. Social capital in the creation of human capital. Am J Sociol. 1988;94:S95–S120.
91. Jesmin SS, Chaudhuri S. Why do some women know more? An exploration of the association of community socioeconomic characteristics, social capital, and HIV/AIDS knowledge. Women Health. 2013;53(7):669–92.
92. Holtgrave DR, Crosby RA. Social capital, poverty, and income inequality as predictors of gonorrhoea, syphilis, chlamydia and AIDS case rates in the United States. Sex Transm Infect. 2003;79(1):62–4.
93. Ransome Y, Dean LT, Crawford ND, Metzger DS, Blank MB, Nunn AS. How do social capital and HIV/AIDS outcomes geographically cluster and which sociocontextual mechanisms predict differences across clusters? J Acquir Immune Defic Syndr (1999). 2017;76(1):13–22.
94. Haley DF, Edmonds A, Schoenbach VJ, Ramirez C, Hickson DA, Wingood GM, et al. Associations between county-level voter turnout, county-level felony voter disenfranchisement, and sexually transmitted infections among women in the Southern United States. Ann Epidemiol. 2019;29:67–73.e1.
95. O'Donnell L, Agronick G, San Doval A, Duran R, Myint UA, Stueve A. Ethnic and gay community attachments and sexual risk behaviors among urban Latino young men who have sex with men. AIDS Educ Prev. 2002;14(6):457–71.
96. Grover E, Grosso A, Ketende S, Kennedy C, Fonner V, Adams D, et al. Social cohesion, social participation and HIV testing among men who have sex with men in Swaziland. AIDS Care. 2016;28(6):795–804.
97. Browning CR, Burrington LA, Leventhal T, Brooks-Gunn J. Neighborhood structural inequality, collective efficacy, and sexual risk behavior among urban youth. J Health Soc Behav. 2008;49(3):269–85.
98. Ramaswamy M, Kelly PJ. Sexual health risk and the movement of women between disadvantaged communities and local jails. Behav Med. 2015;41(3):115–22.
99. Ransome Y, Galea S, Pabayo R, Kawachi I, Braunstein S, Nash D. Social capital is associated with late HIV diagnosis: an ecological analysis. J Acquir Immune Defic Syndr (1999). 2016;73(2):213.
100. Crosby RA, Holtgrave DR, DiClemente RJ, Wingood GM, Gayle JA. Social capital as a predictor of adolescents' sexual risk behavior: a state-level exploratory study. AIDS Behav. 2003;7(3):245–52.
101. Rudolph AE, Crawford ND, Latkin C, Fowler JH, Fuller CM. Individual and neighborhood correlates of membership in drug using networks with a higher prevalence of HIV in New York City (2006–2009). Ann Epidemiol. 2013;23(5):267–74.
102. Lim TW, Frangakis C, Latkin C, Ha TV, Le Minh N, Zelaya C, et al. Community-level income inequality and HIV prevalence among persons who inject drugs in Thai Nguyen, Vietnam. PloS One. 2014;9(3):e90723.
103. Ojikutu BO, Bogart LM, Mayer KH, Stopka TJ, Sullivan PS, Ransome Y. Spatial access and willingness to use pre-exposure prophylaxis among Black/African American individuals in the United States: cross-sectional survey. JMIR Public Health Surveill. 2019;5(1):e12405.

104. Pierce SJ, Miller RL, Morales MM, Forney J. Identifying HIV prevention service needs of African American men who have sex with men: an application of spatial analysis techniques to service planning. J Public Health Manag Pract. 2007;13:S72–S9.
105. Kim B, Callander D, DiClemente R, Trinth-Chevrin C, Thorpe L, Duncan DT. Location of pre-exposure prophylaxiz (PrEP) services across New York City neighborhoods: do neighborhood socio-demographic characteristics and HIV prevalence matter? AIDS Behav. 2019;23(10):2795–802.
106. Eberhart MG, Yehia BR, Hillier A, Voytek CD, Fiore DJ, Blank M, et al. Individual and community factors associated with geographic clusters of poor HIV care retention and poor viral suppression. J Acquir Immune Defic Syndr (1999). 2015;69(01):S37.
107. Duncan DT, Ruff RR, Chaix B, Regan SD, Williams JH, Ravenell J, et al. Perceived spatial stigma, body mass index and blood pressure: a global positioning system study among low-income housing residents in New York City. Geospat Health. 2015;11(2):164–73.
108. Duncan DT, Chaix B, Regan SD, Park SH, Draper C, Goedel WC, et al. Collecting mobility data with GPS methods to understand the HIV environmental riskscape among young black men who have sex with men: a multi-city feasibility study in the deep south. AIDS Behav. 2018;22(9):3057–70.
109. Zenk SN, Schulz AJ, Odoms-Young AM, Wilbur J, Matthews S, Gamboa C, et al. Feasibility of using global positioning systems (GPS) with diverse urban adults: before and after data on perceived acceptability, barriers, and ease of use. J Phys Act Health. 2012;9(7):924–34.
110. Herbst JH, Jacobs ED, Finlayson TJ, McKleroy VS, Neumann MS, Crepaz N, et al. Estimating HIV prevalence and risk behaviors of transgender persons in the United States: a systematic review. AIDS Behav. 2008;12(1):1–17.
111. Schmidt NM, Nguyen QC, Osypuk TL. Experimental and quasi-experimental designs in neighborhood health effects research: neighborhoods and health. Oxford: Oxford University Press; 2018.
112. Fauci AS, Redfield RR, Sigounas G, Weahkee MD, Giroir BP. Ending the HIV epidemic: a plan for the United States. JAMA. 2019;321(9):844–5.

Chapter 10
Substance Use Disorder and HIV

Deepika Slawek and Chinazo Cunningham

Introduction

From the beginning of the HIV epidemic, the link between HIV and substance use has been well established. Substance use is directly and indirectly related to HIV transmission [1]. It is also associated with poor HIV outcomes among people living with HIV (PLWH) including poor engagement in care, suboptimal antiretroviral (ARV) adherence, and subsequent treatment failure [2, 3]. Communities of color are disproportionately affected by both substance use [4] and HIV [5] due to poor access to care, stigma, and social, environmental, and economic risk factors [6].

This chapter discusses the prevalence of drug use among PLWH, link between HIV and substance use, substance use treatment as HIV prevention and treatment, and integration of HIV and substance use treatment. These concepts are all discussed with particular attention to race and ethnicity.

Defining Terms and Principles

For all addictive substances, there is a continuum of use that ranges from no use (abstinence) to a substance use disorder (SUD) with very high-risk behaviors. Between these two extremes, other points exist on the continuum of substance use. These points include: use of a substance without problems, hazardous or problematic use of a substance without a SUD, and a SUD. In addition, within this continuum includes relatively low-risk behaviors (e.g., ingesting a legal substance) to very high-risk behaviors (e.g., injecting an illicit substance with shared injection equipment). While this chapter focuses primarily on SUDs, it is important to recognize

D. Slawek (✉) · C. Cunningham
Department of Medicine, Albert Einstein College of Medicine, Bronx, NY, USA
e-mail: dslawek@montefiore.org; ccunning@montefiore.org

© Springer Nature Switzerland AG 2021
B. O. Ojikutu, V. E. Stone (eds.), *HIV in US Communities of Color*,
https://doi.org/10.1007/978-3-030-48744-7_10

that most substance use does not result in a SUD. Like other medical illnesses, it is critical to diagnose the appropriate condition, as doing so has important implications in terms of treatment and prognosis.

SUD is defined as continued substance use despite significant substance-related negative consequences [7]. SUD is diagnosed via the American Psychiatric Association's *Diagnostic and Statistical Manual of Mental Disorders, Fifth edition* (DSM-5) criteria for SUD. These 11 criteria describe problematic use of an intoxicating substance within a 12-month period. They focus on continuous and compulsive substance use leading to negative social, occupational, psychological, and physical consequences, including comorbid conditions. It is important to note that physical dependence to a substance is included in these criteria, but physical dependence alone does not meet the criteria for SUD. Previous iterations of the DSM separated "substance abuse" and "substance dependence" as two different diagnoses. Dependence could be interpreted either as uncontrolled drug-seeking behavior, as the DSM intended, or as a physiologic phenomenon. Due to the confusion created by this terminology, these terms are no longer used and instead substance use disorder severity is delineated [8]. Severity is defined by the number of criteria endorsed—two to three criteria met is "mild substance use disorder," four to five criteria met is "moderate substance use disorder," and six or more criteria met is "severe substance use disorder" [7].

SUDs are chronic medical conditions that have no cure. SUDs often include periods of remission and relapse. In general, treatment or management of SUDs are long term, and treatment often improves medical and social outcomes, including improving survival. For most SUDs, pharmacologic treatment is superior to behavioral treatment alone. However, for some people with SUDs, the combination of pharmacologic and behavioral treatment can lead to optimal outcomes. In this chapter, we separately discuss common substance use disorders (opioids, alcohol, stimulants, tobacco, cannabis) and their treatment, emphasizing evidence-based treatment. Subsequently, we discuss behavioral treatments in general for substance use disorders.

Language used to describe people who use drugs has a history of being incredibly stigmatizing. Stigma exacerbates barriers to care by creating social isolation and deters individuals from seeking out care. This results in further disenfranchisement of people with substance use disorder. It is important to be mindful about use of language and refrain from using terms such as "junkie" or "addict." Throughout this chapter, person-first language is used to focus on maintaining respect and dignity of individuals [9].

Prevalence of Substance Use Disorder Among People with or at Risk of HIV in Communities of Color

In 2016, approximately 20 million people aged 12 or older (8%) had a SUD in the past year. These include 15 million who had an alcohol use disorder and 7.4 million who had an illicit drug use disorder. In addition, 63 million people (24%) used tobacco products, and 137 million (51%) used alcohol in the past 30 days [4].

Substance use among PLWH is common. In 2015, national surveillance data among adult PLWH estimated that 29% used non-injection drugs and 3% injected drugs. Sixty-two percent reported alcohol use, and 57% reported tobacco use [10]. Other estimates of drug and alcohol use have been far higher than these, ranging from 50% to 80% [11–13]. These estimates used different survey methods, and some reported past 30-day, past 3-month, past year, and lifetime substance use. Despite differing estimates, it is evident that substance use is prevalent in PLWH. Evidence-based tools are available for the screening of substance use and substance use disorders in PLWH [14]. Several population-level studies have established that in people living without HIV and in PLWH, substance use and SUDs are proportionally higher in communities of color than in white populations [4, 15].

Link Between Substance Use and HIV

Opioids

Prevalence

Opioids are a group of substances that are chemically of a similar structure and include prescription pain relievers (e.g., hydrocodone, oxycodone, morphine, and fentanyl) and heroin. Opioids can be illicit (e.g., heroin) or prescribed for the treatment of pain, anesthesia, or the management of opioid use disorder. Illicit opioids can be snorted, smoked, ingested, or injected; the latter route of administration tends to lead to the most serious complications. The opioid crisis in the United States has escalated in three interrelated waves since 1999. The first was attributed to increased prescribing of opioids in the 1990s leading to opioid overdose deaths; the second wave began in 2010 due to heroin; and the third began in 2013 with increases in overdose deaths involving synthetic opioids such as fentanyl [16]. The number of opioid overdose deaths in 2017 was six times higher than in 1999 [16].

Opioid prescribing almost doubled between 1999 and 2010 [17] which was accompanied by a growing number of individuals misusing prescription and illicit opioids [4]. The majority of opioid use in 2017 was misuse of prescription opioids, and the remainder used both prescription opioids and heroin or heroin alone [4]. PLWH have experienced similar trends, with the majority misusing prescription opioids, and a smaller proportion using heroin [18].

From 2008 to 2014, HIV diagnoses in people who inject drugs have declined by 48%, which is attributed to aggressive prevention programs. One in 10 HIV diagnoses are among people who inject drugs. The epidemiology of the opioid epidemic has shifted in recent years with a growing number of people who inject drugs in non-urban settings. From 2005 to 2015, the proportion of black people who inject drugs has declined by half, and a larger proportion are now white. Increases in prescription opioid misuse have subsequently led to more injection drug use. The shift in the geography and epidemiology of the opioid epidemic has presented new prevention challenges [19].

Injection drug use and HIV transmission are examples of racial and ethnic disparities in the United States. This has been illustrated in the HIV epidemic among people who inject drugs in New York City. After HIV was introduced to the injection drug-using community, large disparities emerged—HIV was twice as prevalent in black and Latinx people who inject drugs as it was in white people who inject drugs [20]. Though prevalence of HIV has dropped among people who inject drugs in New York City through implementation of harm reduction programs, racial and ethnic disparities remain. Compared to white people, black and Latinx people who inject drugs have higher odds of HIV infection [21].

Risk Behaviors

PLWH who use opioids are at increased risk for multiple medical complications, including overdose, transmission of HIV, and other blood-borne infections such as viral hepatitis, sexually transmitted infections (STIs), and bacterial infections involving the skin, blood, and heart.

Over 70,000 drug overdose deaths occurred in the United States in 2017, driven by opioid overdose, specifically the synthetic opioid, fentanyl. Increases in overdose deaths have been across multiple demographic groups, with increases in fatal opioid overdoses among white, black, and Latinx people. The largest opioid overdose death rate is among men aged 25–44 years [22]. In 2017, the largest increase in opioid overdose rates were among black people. In addition, Native Americans have experienced larger increases in overdose deaths than the general population [23].

Risk of acquiring HIV is increased by high-risk practices such as sharing needles, syringes, and other injection equipment. The average risk of acquiring HIV among people who inject drugs and share needles is 1 in 160 [24]. In addition to increased risk of HIV, these risk behaviors increase the likelihood of transmission of viral hepatitis, such as hepatitis B and hepatitis C viruses. Likelihood of HIV transmission is higher among young people who inject drugs than those who are older because they are more likely to share needles and engage in high-risk sexual behaviors.

Injecting opioids can reduce inhibitions, leading to increased high-risk sexual behaviors. Condom-less sex with an HIV-discordant partner is common among people who inject drugs, with as much as a quarter reporting doing so. This is more common among people living without than in PLWH who inject drugs. Additionally, one-third of people who inject drugs report having sex in exchange for money or drugs. These high-risk sexual behaviors place individuals at increased risk of acquiring other STIs in addition to HIV and viral hepatitis. STIs can also increase the likelihood of acquiring and transmitting HIV. Bacterial STIs including *Neisseria gonorrhea*, *Chlamydia trachomatis*, and syphilis are more common in PLWH who inject drugs than in living without HIV who inject drugs. High-risk sexual behaviors are particularly common among black and Latinx men who have sex with men who use opioids [19].

Community-based outreach with peer educators reduces risky behaviors by reaching people who use drugs in non-clinical settings to offer education on risk reduction, referring individuals to substance use treatment, and other prevention services. Use of community-based outreach can be a strategy to build trust between people who use drugs and healthcare providers [25].

HIV Outcomes

Once in a lifetime HIV testing is recommended for the general population and annual testing is recommended for high-risk populations, including people who inject drugs and their partners, and those with high-risk sexual behaviors [26]. Stigma, discrimination, and distrust of the healthcare system among people who use opioids limit disclosure of their drug use to healthcare providers and subsequently reduce testing for HIV or hepatitis C virus. Lack of disclosure about drug use often slows diagnosis and impedes engagement in care, and can additionally increase the risk of transmission of HIV or hepatitis C virus. Increased HIV testing in emergency departments, drug treatment programs, jails, and prisons are strategies to increase diagnosis of HIV and facilitate linkage to care [27].

People who use drugs, particularly people who inject drugs, link to and stay engaged in HIV care at far lower rates than non-users. After linkage to care, initiation of ARV therapy in a timely manner is essential. There is also lower uptake of ARV treatment, adherence to treatment, and poorer overall clinical outcomes in PLWH who use drugs than those who do not use drugs [28, 29]. This could be for several reasons, including structural barriers such as low health literacy, socioeconomic status, lack of health insurance, unstable housing, and intermittent incarceration. Those who are engaged in substance use treatment are more likely to link to and engage in HIV care, and adhere to HIV treatment [30, 31]. Integration of HIV treatment and substance use treatment offers a means to improve both HIV and substance use outcomes [32].

Opioid Use Disorder Treatment

Treatment of opioid use disorder leads to many positive outcomes, including improved survival, quality of life, neonatal outcomes in infants born to women who use opioids, social outcomes such as criminal activity, and high-risk behaviors that could put individuals at risk for HIV transmission [33, 34]. National practice guidelines for the treatment of opioid use disorder focus on the use of three pharmacologic treatments: methadone, buprenorphine, and naltrexone. The most effective treatment for opioid use disorder is pharmacologic treatment [35].

Methadone treatment is delivered in opioid treatment programs, which are highly monitored and regulated by federal and state laws. Methadone is a full opioid agonist that is dosed daily, and behavioral treatment is recommended in conjunction with methadone. Individuals receiving methadone treatment typically must visit methadone programs nearly daily for observed administration of medication [35]. Because clinically significant drug-drug interactions between methadone and a number of ARVs exist, potential interactions should be checked before initiating or changing treatment.

Buprenorphine treatment can be provided in various settings outside of opioid treatment programs (e.g., it can be provided in primary care settings, emergency departments, community-based settings, and jails). Buprenorphine is a partial opioid agonist and often co-formulated with naloxone to reduce the likelihood of diversion. Buprenorphine is often dosed daily or twice daily, and medication can be obtained from community-based pharmacies [35]. Few drug-drug interactions between buprenorphine and ARVs exist, and most are not clinically significant.

Naltrexone is an opioid antagonist used to prevent relapse of opioid use disorder in patients who have completed detoxification from opioids. It can be administered as a daily oral formulation or as an extended release injection every 4 weeks. It has only been found to be effective in conjunction with behavioral treatment, whereas buprenorphine and methadone are both effective with or without behavioral treatment. When selecting treatment for OUD, many factors should be considered, including patient's preferences, location and intensity of treatment setting, availability of medication, comorbidities, prior experience with treatment modalities, and drug-drug interactions [35]. Of the three medications to treat OUD, methadone is well known to have many drug-drug interactions with ARVs [36].

Behavioral treatment for the management of opioid use disorder is effective when used in addition to medication-assisted treatment; however, when behavioral treatment is used alone, it is much less effective than pharmacologic treatment. Several different behavioral treatments have been studied in conjunction with pharmacologic treatment, including behavioral drug and HIV risk reduction counseling, contingency management, general supportive counseling, cognitive behavioral therapy, and motivational interviewing, among others. These approaches are effective in improving treatment outcomes, but no single behavioral treatment strategy is superior to another [37].

All patients with opioid use disorder should be given naloxone and trained in its use for opioid overdose reversal. Patient's family members and significant others should also be given naloxone [35].

Alcohol

Prevalence

Alcohol use is common and among the substances most frequently used among PLWH. In one large survey, over one-third of PLWH reported alcohol use [38]. Nationally, more than 14% of PLWH report binge drinking in the past 30 days, and 6% report daily alcohol use [10]. Alcohol use disorder is prevalent in 12–14% of PLWH [39].

Populations who are risk for both HIV and heavy alcohol use or alcohol use disorder include men who have sex with men, racial and ethnic minorities [40], people who inject drugs, people who have sex in exchange for money or drugs, and individuals of low socioeconomic status [41, 42].

Risk Behaviors

There is a strong association between alcohol use and HIV incidence [42]. Alcohol consumption is associated with high-risk sexual behaviors, including increased sexual activity, increased number of sex partners, unprotected sex, and engagement in sex in exchange for money or drugs [38, 41, 43, 44]. These same high-risk behaviors increase the risk of STIs, such as *Neisseria gonorrhea*, *Chlamydia trachomatis*, and syphilis.

Behavioral interventions aimed to reduce alcohol use to subsequently reduce high-risk sexual behaviors have been successful in reducing alcohol use and in increasing condom use [45].

HIV Outcomes

Compared to those who do not use alcohol, those with alcohol use have a lower likelihood of being tested for HIV and therefore delays of entry into care. Independent from a delay in diagnosis, alcohol use is also associated with delayed engagement in care, poor retention in HIV care, and poor ARV adherence. Missed doses of ARVs could be due to complex dosing regimens, intoxication, or concerns about potential interactions between ARVs and alcohol. Alcohol use is associated with reduced viral load suppression and progression of HIV disease.

Alcohol Use Disorder Treatment

All patients engaged in care should be screened for alcohol use using an evidence-based practice of screening, brief intervention, and referral to treatment (SBIRT). This model is used to identify, reduce, and prevent problematic alcohol use. Several evidence-based screening tools exist to determine the risk of alcohol use [46]. In patients with problematic alcohol use, hazardous use, or binge use, but who do not meet criteria for alcohol use disorder, healthcare providers should conduct a brief intervention which provides personalized feedback about the risks and consequences of excessive drinking [47]. Brief interventions improve many outcomes, including reducing unhealthy alcohol use, and reducing emergency room visits and days hospitalized [48].

Patients who have alcohol use disorder should receive pharmacologic treatment. Treatment for alcohol use disorder can lead to many positive outcomes, including improved viral load suppression, improved survival, improved mental health, and

slowed progression of chronic diseases. National guidelines recommend pharmacologic treatment of moderate to severe alcohol use disorder in combination with
motivational interviewing or cognitive behavioral therapy [49, 50].

In patients with moderate to severe alcohol use disorder, acomprosate or naltrexone
are recommended as first-line treatment. Acamprosate is an oral medication administered three times per day and initiated after abstaining from alcohol use for several days.
Because of frequent dosing, acamprosate may pose adherence challenges. Naltrexone
can be used for the treatment of both alcohol use disorder and opioid use disorder. It is
administered either orally daily, or intramuscularly every 4 weeks. It reduces the likelihood that an individual will use alcohol after a period of abstinence [49].

In patients with moderate to severe alcohol use disorder who do not tolerate
acamprosate or naltrexone, disulfiram is a treatment option. When consistently
taken, disulfiram causes an unpleasant physiological reaction if alcohol is con-
sumed. This reaction includes tachycardia, flushing, headache, nausea, and vomit-
ing. The anticipation of these symptoms is a deterrent to alcohol use. Disulfiram
may interact with ARVs; thus, medication interactions should be checked prior to
initiating treatment. Other medications that are not approved by the Food and Drug
Administration but improve abstinence are topiramate and gabapentin [49].

Stimulants

Prevalence

Stimulants, including cocaine, crack, amphetamine, and methamphetamines are
used often by PLWH, and play a role in the HIV epidemic. Stimulants can be
injected, smoked, or snorted. In a 2015 national survey, when asked about non-
injection drug use, 5% of PLWH reported using cocaine, 5% methamphetamine,
and 1% amphetamine. When asked about injection drug use, 2% reported injecting
methamphetamine [10]. In another study targeting individuals at risk for HIV, stimulant use was much more common, with 40% reporting cocaine use and 14% reporting methamphetamine or amphetamine use [51]. Among people at risk for HIV,
stimulant use is disproportionately prevalent among men who have sex with men
[52, 53]. In estimates of stimulant use among black and Latinx men who have sex
with men, 15–50% reported cocaine or methamphetamine use [54–56].

Risk Behaviors

Use of stimulants is associated with increased HIV risk, especially high-risk sexual
behaviors. Stimulant use has been associated with unprotected anal and vaginal sex, a
large number of sex partners [57], sero-discordant sex, exchange or money or drugs for
sex, use of other drugs and alcohol, and drug use before or during sex [58]. These high-
risk sexual behaviors increase the risk of HIV and STI acquisition and transmission.

HIV Outcomes

Stimulant use is associated with poor HIV outcomes. Compared to those who do not use stimulants, PLWH who use stimulants are less likely to have access to healthcare [59], less likely to engage with primary care providers [59], and more likely to have worse healthcare utilization. PLWH who use cocaine are less likely to initiate and continue ARVs than those who use other drugs [60–62]. They are more likely to have poor ARV adherence and unsuppressed VL, than those who do not use stimulants [57, 63, 64]. Many of these effects are reversible with treatment of the stimulant use disorder [65, 66].

Stimulant Use Disorder Treatment

No pharmacologic therapies are available for the management of stimulant use disorder. Behavioral therapies are associated with reduction in stimulant use and high-risk sexual behavior. Contingency management and cognitive-behavioral therapy are two behavioral interventions that are efficacious in treatment of cocaine use disorder. These therapies are not well studied for the treatment of other stimulant use disorders [67].

Tobacco

Prevalence

Tobacco use among PLWH remains highly prevalent despite a significant reduction in tobacco use in the general population. Tobacco use prevalence in PLWH is estimated to be over 40%, which is approximately twice the prevalence of smoking in the United States. Tobacco use is more common among PLWH over the age of 40 years than in those under 29 years of age, and is more common among white and black PLWH than in Latinx PLWH. Among PLWH, homelessness, incarceration, low education level, non-injection substance use, and binge alcohol use are associated with tobacco use [68].

HIV and Other Health Outcomes

While PLWH with unsuppressed viral loads are more likely to use tobacco [68], there is no evidence that tobacco use leads to HIV disease progression [69]. PLWH who use tobacco have a higher risk of all-cause mortality than those who do not use tobacco, and almost double the risk of all-cause mortality compared with people who use tobacco who do not have HIV. Tobacco-related mortality in PLWH is primarily due to cardiovascular disease, respiratory conditions, and malignancies [70].

Among people who use tobacco, cardiovascular disease is more common in PLWH than people without HIV. Chronic-obstructive pulmonary disease is also more common among PLWH compared to people living without HIV. This is likely due to the high prevalence of tobacco use in PLWH. Tobacco use is also associated with bacterial pneumonia in PLWH. The risk of malignancy in PLWH is twice that of people living without HIV, and includes AIDS-related cancers (e.g., Kaposi sarcoma and cervical cancer), and non-AIDS related cancers (e.g., lung cancer). In PLWH who use tobacco, lung cancer risk is significantly increased compared to those who do not use tobacco. This relationship remains, even when taking into account immunodeficiency [70], with abstinence from tobacco use, the risk of cardiovascular events, chronic obstructive pulmonary disease, and lung cancer all diminish over time [70, 71].

Tobacco Use Disorder Treatment

All patients engaged in care should be screened for tobacco use. National guidelines recommend that all clinicians ask about tobacco use, advise cessation, assess readiness to quit, assist people who use tobacco in quitting, and arrange follow-up visits [72]. Treatment of tobacco use disorder involves both non-pharmacologic and pharmacologic interventions. Non-pharmacologic therapy focuses on counseling to encourage cessation and can occur in-person or by innovative methods using technology [70]. Motivational interviewing, in which clinicians help individuals explore barriers to cessation, has been found to be more effective than brief counseling interventions [73].

Pharmacologic treatment options for tobacco use disorder include varenicline, bupropion, and nicotine replacement therapy. Each treatment option is more effective in combination with counseling than without counseling [74]. Nicotine replacement therapy works by alleviating cravings and nicotine withdrawal symptoms. Bupropion works by impacting the nicotine reward pathway by way of inhibiting dopamine. Varenicline acts as a partial agonist at the nicotinic receptor to reduce cravings and diminish the rewarding symptoms of tobacco use. National guidelines recommend two regimens for the treatment of tobacco use disorder: nicotine therapy with behavioral therapy, or varenicline with behavioral therapy. If one of these fails, then the other should be tried prior to using a different pharmacologic therapy. Providers and patients should be aware that relapse is common, but should not be a deterrent from continued quit attempts and use of pharmacotherapy [75].

Cannabis

Prevalence

Cannabis use is common among PLWH. In national surveys, 10% of individuals aged 12 years or older report cannabis use [4]. By contrast, national estimates of cannabis use among PLWH range from 25% to 38%. In PLWH, young age and male sex are associated with increased likelihood of using cannabis. In some national surveys, Latinx and black PLWH are less likely to use cannabis compared to white PLWH [57]. In the general population, cannabis use is most common among blacks, followed by whites, and Latinx [76].

In longitudinal analyses of cannabis use of PLWH, the prevalence of current cannabis use has decreased over time; however, those with current cannabis use are using cannabis more frequency. More PLWH who use cannabis are using cannabis daily [77].

Risk Behaviors

Cannabis use is associated with high-risk sexual behavior in people with and at-risk for HIV. Compared to people who have never used cannabis, people who currently or formerly use cannabis are more likely to have high numbers of recent sexual partners and low frequency of condom use [57, 78]. Among black men who have sex with men, cannabis use in the context of sexual encounters is associated with high-risk sexual behaviors such as unprotected sex [79].

HIV Outcomes

Studies evaluating the impact of cannabis use on HIV outcomes have had mixed findings. Compared to PLWH who do not use cannabis, those who use cannabis have similar engagement in HIV care and initiation of ARVs [80]. In regard to viral load suppression, studies have reported inconsistent findings, including cannabis use being associated with improved, worsened, and no change in viral load suppression [80–83]. Similar patterns are reported with ARV adherence, with some studies showing worse ARV adherence and others showing no change in ARV adherence [81, 83–91].

Cannabis Use Disorder Treatment

There are no FDA-approved pharmacologic therapies for the treatment of cannabis use disorder, and clinicians should refer patients for behavioral therapies. Cognitive-behavioral therapy, motivational enhancement therapy, and contingency management are all efficacious in reducing frequency and severity of cannabis use [92].

Behavioral Treatments of Substance Use Disorders

Behavioral treatment can be used for treatment of substance use disorder. It is used in conjunction with evidence-based pharmacotherapy for opioid use disorder, alcohol use disorder, and tobacco use disorder, or alone if effective pharmacotherapy is not available.

Brief Interventions have been established for use in problematic alcohol use and tobacco use disorder, but have been adapted to use substance use disorders. Brief interventions tend to be 5–15-minute interventions designed to help express the risk of substance use and to encourage patients to reduce their use or achieve abstinence. Brief Interventions are cost-effective and reduce alcohol use by 20–30%. In patients with alcohol use disorder, brief interventions are inadequate; patients with alcohol use disorder should receive more intensive treatment in addition to pharmacotherapy [93].

Motivational interviewing uses empathetic and reflective listening to support self-efficacy and optimism in making positive changes. It is studied most extensively in problematic alcohol use and alcohol use disorder, and is effective in reducing alcohol use in problematic alcohol use. Motivational interviewing can reduce use in other substance use disorders, and should be combined with available pharmacotherapies [93].

Contingency management utilizes an incentive-based system for abstinence from substance use. Typically, financial incentives are provided for specific behaviors such as urine drug screens without evidence of drug use. Contingency management is effective in many different populations, and has been shown to improve other co-occurring psychiatric symptoms, such as depression and emotional distress. Contingency management can be particularly useful for initial abstinence from substance use [94].

Cognitive-behavioral therapy teaches individuals strategies to prevent recurrent substance use after a period of abstinence. Individuals are taught how to identify triggers and strategies to avoid them, as well as strategies to cope with sequelae of substance use [95]. Cognitive behavioral therapy has demonstrated positive effects in alcohol, cannabis, stimulants, opioids, and other injection drug use [93].

Treatment Considerations for HIV at Risk Who Have SUD

Harm Reduction

Harm reduction is an approach that focuses on to reducing negative consequences or harms of substance use. Harm reduction approaches include providing accessible, convenient, low-threshold, non-judgmental services in which the person who uses drugs is central in deciding goals of treatment. In the United States, while traditional teaching and historical approaches have been focused solely on abstinence, for many individuals and situations, abstinence-only approaches may be ineffective. Because achieving abstinence can be challenging for many people with substance use disorders, focusing on abstinence as the only worthy goal can set people up for failure and ignore other important outcomes. Treatment that focuses on reducing substance use, rather than abstinence only, can be effective in reducing negative consequences of substance use. Nicotine replacement therapy for tobacco use disorder, opioid agonist treatment for opioid use disorder, naloxone for prevention of opioid overdose death, and messaging around responsible alcohol use (drink responsibly, don't drink and drive) are some examples in which harm reduction principles are demonstrated [96]. Across the world, harm reduction approaches have been broadly applied to many aspects of substance use disorders, and have been effective in several contexts [96].

One of the best-known harm reduction strategies is syringe exchange programs. In these programs, injection equipment is collected in exchange for sterile injection equipment. These programs are often accompanied by peer referrals, HIV prevention education and risk reduction, and referrals to medical, mental health, and drug treatment. Syringe exchange programs are effective in reducing HIV risk behavior and transmission of HIV and hepatitis C virus, without increasing frequency of injection [97–100]. Resources to find local syringe exchange programs can be found at www.nasen.org.

Supervised injection facilities (also referred to as safe consumption sites or overdose prevention sites) is another harm reduction approach that has gained attention in the United States because of the opioid epidemic. These sites provide a safe space where people can bring drugs to use safely. Hundreds of these sites exist in many countries around the world. In these facilities, well-lit stalls, sterile injection equipment, and medical supervision offer interventions to limit HIV and hepatitis C virus transmission, bacterial infections, and overdose [101].

Pre-exposure Prophylaxis

HIV prevention is possible using pre-exposure prophylaxis (PrEP) with a combination tenofovir disoproxil fumarate/emtricitabine pill taken once daily. PrEP is recommended to reduce the likelihood of HIV transmission in people living without HIV and at high-risk for acquiring HIV. This includes individuals at high risk for HIV transmission secondary to high-risk sexual behaviors and injection drug use behaviors [102].

Role of Race in the Approach to Treatment of SUD

Systemic differences in the approach to substance use have led to disparities in the treatment of substance use disorder among people of color. Despite a similar prevalence of drug use in white people and people of color, drug offense sentencing enacted in the 1980s led to large increases in incarceration of black people for drug-related crimes. Prison sentences were longer and more punitive for possession of drugs that were used with more frequency in communities of color (e.g., crack cocaine) than in white communities (e.g., powder cocaine). This differential treatment in the legal system was further exacerbated by differences in pharmaceutical marketing of prescribed medications and treatments for substance use disorder [103].

The treatment of opioid use disorder provides a clear example of how race and treatment of substance use disorders are intertwined. In general, prior to the opioid epidemic, opioid use disorder was viewed as a criminal justice problem, and for decades, people of color were incarcerated for their opioid use disorder. As the opioid epidemic grew and white people experienced unprecedented increases in opioid use disorder and opioid overdoses, the approach to opioid use disorder began to shift. Opioid use disorder started to be viewed as a medical condition that required medical treatment, rather than a criminal justice issue that required incarceration.

Until 2002, methadone was the only FDA-approved medication for the treatment of opioid use disorder. Methadone treatment is restricted to opioid treatment programs that are highly regulated. Examples of regulated elements of methadone treatment include the number of patients receiving treatment, directly observed dosing, methadone dose, frequency of nearly daily visits, and frequency of counseling and urine drug tests. In addition, opioid treatment programs are heavily concentrated in black and Latinx communities.

In contrast to methadone, buprenorphine, which was FDA-approved in 2002, can be offered in any treatment setting. Thus, buprenorphine treatment can occur in less stigmatizing, more accessible, and more private clinical settings. In addition, although buprenorphine is regulated, it is much less regulated than methadone. For example, the frequency of visits, urine drug tests, and counseling are not regulated. In addition, buprenorphine is dispensed in community pharmacies and can be refilled. Given the substantial difference in how buprenorphine and methadone treatment are delivered, it is not surprising that substantial disparities exist in who receives each type of treatment. It is well documented that people of color are more likely to receive methadone treatment, while white people are more likely to receive buprenorphine treatment [104].

Though this example is specific to the treatment of opioid use disorder, similar structural and societal barriers exist in the management of all substance use disorders, resulting in disparities in care.

Stigma

HIV-related stigma is associated with many negative consequences, including being labeled and stereotyped, social isolation, loss of social status, and experiencing discrimination and prejudice. Health-related consequences of stigma include depression, anxiety, suicidal ideations, and poor ARV adherence. Stigma directed toward PLWH can come from family and friends, workplace interactions, healthcare providers, and government policies [105].

PLWH who use drugs experience additional stigma related to their substance use as well. Stigma toward substance use disorder is more severe than stigma toward other mental illnesses. Individuals with substance use are often judged to be more violent and dangerous, they are more likely to be judged in social relationships, and they are likely to be discriminated against in employment, housing, and governmental policy [106].

Stigma associated with both HIV and substance use can be compounded and lead to deleterious mental health outcomes, such as depression [107]. The effects of stigma are exacerbated further by social identity, such as race and social class. Structural interventions are needed to reduce stigma for PLWH who use drugs. One such proposed intervention has been the use of substance use treatment in less stigmatizing settings, such as primary care. Despite this, drug treatment options that are less stigmatizing are not readily available to PLWH of color [108].

Integration of HIV and SUD Treatment

The integration of treatment for HIV and opioid use disorder with buprenorphine has been well studied. Integrating HIV and buprenorphine treatment is feasible and associated with improved outcomes, including engagement in HIV treatment, improved CD4 counts, initiation of ARVs, suppressed viral loads, decreased opioid use, and improved quality of life [31, 109]. HIV care integrated into methadone clinics also leads to high retention in care and improved HIV outcomes [110, 111].

Integrating HIV and substance use treatment increases substance use and HIV detection, provides support and interventions for treatment adherence, enhances continuity of care, and reduces likelihood of drug-drug interactions. Though positive outcomes have been found from integration of HIV and substance use treatment, barriers to integrating treatment remain. Implementing buprenorphine treatment in HIV care settings requires training providers and meets challenges in combining differing clinical practices and navigating appropriate financing [32].

Conclusion

HIV and substance use are intricately intertwined. Patients with substance use disorders are at increased risk for acquiring HIV and having poor HIV outcomes. SUDs are chronic illnesses that require long-term treatment. Among PLWH with substance use disorders, the provision of evidence-based treatment improves both SUD and HIV outcomes. Integrating SUD and HIV treatment is a particularly promising strategy to improve health outcomes. Harm reduction approaches, including measuring success beyond abstinence, is one important strategy to improve outcomes. Stigma and disparities in care for HIV and substance use disorders continue to be challenges, particularly for people of color. Despite this, existing treatment and treatment approaches have the potential to improve the lives of people of color living with HIV and substance use disorders.

References

1. Strathdee SA, Stockman JK. Epidemiology of HIV among injecting and non-injecting drug users: current trends and implications for interventions. Curr HIV/AIDS Rep. 2010;7(2):99–106.
2. Westergaard RP, Hess T, Astemborski J, Mehta SH, Kirk GD. Longitudinal changes in engagement in care and viral suppression for HIV-infected injection drug users. AIDS. 2013;27(16):2559–66.
3. Celentano DD, Galai N, Sethi AK, Shah NG, Strathdee SA, Vlahov D, et al. Time to initiating highly active antiretroviral therapy among HIV-infected injection drug users. AIDS. 2001;15(13):1707–15.
4. SAMHSA. Key substance use and mental health indicators in the United States: results from the 2016 National Survey on Drug Use and Health. In: HHS, editor. Rockland: Center for Behavioral Health Statistics and Quality; 2017.
5. Center for Disease Control and Prevention. HIV surveillance report, 2016; vol. 28. http://www.cdc.gov/hiv/library/reports/hiv-surveillance.html. Published November 2017. Accessed 25 Jan 2019.
6. Vilsaint CL, NeMoyer A, Fillbrunn M, Sadikova E, Kessler RC, Sampson NA, et al. Racial/ethnic differences in 12-month prevalence and persistence of mood, anxiety, and substance use disorders: variation by nativity and socioeconomic status. Compr Psychiatry. 2018;89:52–60.
7. American Psychiatric Association. Substance-related and addictive disorders. In: Diagnostic and statistical manual of mental disorders. 5th ed. Washington, D.C.: American Psychiatric Association; 2013.
8. O'Brien C. Addiction and dependence in DSM-V. Addiction. 2011;106(5):866–7.
9. Broyles LM, Binswanger IA, Jenkins JA, Finnell DS, Faseru B, Cavaiola A, et al. Confronting inadvertent stigma and pejorative language in addiction scholarship: a recognition and response. Subst Abus. 2014;35(3):217–21.
10. Center for Disease Control and Prevention. Behavioral and clinical characteristics of persons with diagnosed HIV infection—medical monitoring project, United State, 2015 cycle (June 2015-May 2016). HIV Surveillance Report 20. 2018.
11. Bing EG, Burnam MA, Longshore D, Fleishman JA, Sherbourne CD, London AS, et al. Psychiatric disorders and drug use among human immunodeficiency virus-infected adults in the United States. Arch Gen Psychiatry. 2001;58(8):721–8.
12. Durvasula R. HIV/AIDS in older women: unique challenges, unmet needs. Behav Med. 2014;40(3):85–98.
13. Dawson-Rose C, Draughon JE, Zepf R, Cuca YP, Huang E, Freeborn K, et al. Prevalence of substance use in an HIV primary care safety net clinic: a call for screening. J Assoc Nurses AIDS Care. 2017;28(2):238–49.
14. National Institute on Drug Abuse. Drug screening and assessment resources. Chart of evidence-based screening & assessment tools for adults and adolescents. June 2018. Available from: https://www.drugabuse.gov/nidamed-medical-health-professionals/tool-resources-your-practice/additional-screening-resources.
15. Grigoryan A, Hall HI, Durant T, Wei X. Late HIV diagnosis and determinants of progression to AIDS or death after HIV diagnosis among injection drug users, 33 US States, 1996-2004. PLoS One. 2009;4(2):e4445.
16. Center for Disease Control and Prevention. Annual surveillance report of drug-related risks and outcomes—United States, 2017. Surveillance Special Report 1. Center for Disease Control and Prevention, U.S. Department of Health and Human Services. Published August 31, 2017. Accessed from: https://www.cdc.gov/drugoverdose/pdf/pubs/2017-cdc-drug-surveillance-report.pdf.
17. Becker WC, Gordon K, Edelman EJ, Kerns RD, Crystal S, Dziura JD, et al. Trends in any and high-dose opioid analgesic receipt among aging patients with and without HIV. AIDS Behav. 2016;20(3):679–86.

18. Lemons A, DeGroote N, Perez A, Craw J, Nyaku M, Broz D, et al. Opioid misuse among HIV-positive adults in medical care: results from the Medical Monitoring Project, 2009-2014. J Acquir Immune Defic Syndr. 2019;80(2):127–34.
19. Center for Disease Control and Prevention. HIV infection, risk, prevention, and testing behaviors among persons who inject drugs—National HIV Behavioral Surveillance: Injection Drug Use, 20 U.S.Cities, 2015. HIV Surveillance Special Report 18. 2015.
20. Friedman SR, Chapman TF, Perlis TE, Rockwell R, Paone D, Sotheran JL, et al. Similarities and differences by race/ethnicity in changes of HIV seroprevalence and related behaviors among drug injectors in New York City, 1991-1996. J Acquir Immune Defic Syndr. 1999;22(1):83–91.
21. Des Jarlais DC, Arasteh K, McKnight C, Feelemyer J, Tross S, Perlman D, et al. Racial/ethnic disparities at the end of an HIV epidemic: persons who inject drugs in New York City, 2011-2015. Am J Public Health. 2017;107(7):1157–63.
22. Scholl L, Seth P, Kariisa M, Wilson N, Baldwin G. Drug and opioid-involved overdose deaths - United States, 2013-2017. MMWR Morb Mortal Wkly Rep. 2018;67(5152):1419–27.
23. Joshi S, Weiser T, Warren-Mears V. Drug, opioid-involved, and heroin-involved overdose deaths among American Indians and Alaska natives - Washington, 1999-2015. MMWR Morb Mortal Wkly Rep. 2018;67(50):1384–7.
24. Patel P, Borkowf CB, Brooks JT, Lasry A, Lansky A, Mermin J. Estimating per-act HIV transmission risk: a systematic review. AIDS. 2014;28(10):1509–19.
25. Center for Disease Control and Prevention. Integrated prevention services for HIV infection, viral hepatitis, sexually transmitted diseases, and tuberculosis for persons who use drugs illicitly: summary guidance from CDC and The U.S. Department of Health and Human Services. Morb Mortal Wkly Rep Recomm Rep. 2012;61:1–43.
26. Branson BM, Handsfield HH, Lampe MA, Janssen RS, Taylor AW, Lyss SB, et al. Revised recommendations for HIV testing of adults, adolescents, and pregnant women in health-care settings. Morb Mortal Wkly Rep Recomm Rep. 2006;55(RR-14):1–17; quiz CE1-4.
27. Meyer JP, Althoff AL, Altice FL. Optimizing care for HIV-infected people who use drugs: evidence-based approaches to overcoming healthcare disparities. Clin Infect Dis. 2013;57(9):1309–17.
28. Altice FL, Kamarulzaman A, Soriano VV, Schechter M, Friedland GH. Treatment of medical, psychiatric, and substance-use comorbidities in people infected with HIV who use drugs. Lancet. 2010;376(9738):367–87.
29. Joseph B, Kerr T, Puskas CM, Montaner J, Wood E, Milloy MJ. Factors linked to transitions in adherence to antiretroviral therapy among HIV-infected illicit drug users in a Canadian setting. AIDS Care. 2015;27(9):1128–36.
30. Gardner LI, Marks G, Strathdee SA, Loughlin AM, Del Rio C, Kerndt P, et al. Faster entry into HIV care among HIV-infected drug users who had been in drug-use treatment programs. Drug Alcohol Depend. 2016;165:15–21.
31. Altice FL, Bruce RD, Lucas GM, Lum PJ, Korthuis PT, Flanigan TP, et al. HIV treatment outcomes among HIV-infected, opioid-dependent patients receiving buprenorphine/naloxone treatment within HIV clinical care settings: results from a multisite study. J Acquir Immune Defic Syndr. 2011;56(Suppl 1):S22–32.
32. Haldane V, Cervero-Liceras F, Chuah FL, Ong SE, Murphy G, Sigfrid L, et al. Integrating HIV and substance use services: a systematic review. J Int AIDS Soc. 2017;20(1):21585.
33. Gowing L, Farrell MF, Bornemann R, Sullivan LE, Ali R. Oral substitution treatment of injecting opioid users for prevention of HIV infection. Cochrane Database Syst Rev. 2011;(8):CD004145.
34. Larochelle MR, Bernson D, Land T, Stopka TJ, Wang N, Xuan Z, et al. Medication for opioid use disorder after nonfatal opioid overdose and association with mortality: a Cohort Study. Ann Intern Med. 2018;169(3):137–45.
35. Kampman K, Jarvis M. American Society of Addiction Medicine (ASAM) National Practice Guideline for the use of medications in the treatment of addiction involving opioid use. J Addict Med. 2015;9(5):358–67.

36. Fanucchi L, Springer SA, Korthuis PT. Medications for treatment of opioid use disorder among persons living with HIV. Curr HIV/AIDS Rep. 2019;16:1–6.
37. Dugosh K, Abraham A, Seymour B, McLoyd K, Chalk M, Festinger D. A systematic review on the use of psychosocial interventions in conjunction with medications for the treatment of opioid addiction. J Addict Med. 2016;10(2):93–103.
38. Scott-Sheldon LA, Walstrom P, Carey KB, Johnson BT, Carey MP, Team MR. Alcohol use and sexual risk behaviors among individuals infected with HIV: a systematic review and meta-analysis 2012 to early 2013. Curr HIV/AIDS Rep. 2013;10(4):314–23.
39. Bensley KM, McGinnis KA, Fortney J, KCG C, Dombrowski JC, Ornelas I, et al. Patterns of alcohol use among patients living with HIV in urban, large rural, and small rural areas. J Rural Health. 2018;35:330.
40. Delker E, Brown Q, Hasin DS. Alcohol consumption in demographic subpopulations: An epidemiologic overview. Alcohol Res. 2016;38(1):7–15.
41. Hall HI, Geduld J, Boulos D, Rhodes P, An Q, Mastro TD, et al. Epidemiology of HIV in the United States and Canada: current status and ongoing challenges. J Acquir Immune Defic Syndr. 2009;51(Suppl 1):S13–20.
42. Williams EC, Hahn JA, Saitz R, Bryant K, Lira MC, Samet JH. Alcohol use and human immunodeficiency virus (HIV) infection: current knowledge, implications, and future directions. Alcohol Clin Exp Res. 2016;40(10):2056–72.
43. Scott-Sheldon LA, Carey KB, Cunningham K, Johnson BT, Carey MP, Team MR. Alcohol use predicts sexual decision-making: a systematic review and meta-analysis of the experimental literature. AIDS Behav. 2016;20(Suppl 1):S19–39.
44. Vagenas P, Ludford KT, Gonzales P, Peinado J, Cabezas C, Gonzales F, et al. Being unaware of being HIV-infected is associated with alcohol use disorders and high-risk sexual behaviors among men who have sex with men in Peru. AIDS Behav. 2014;18(1):120–7.
45. Scott-Sheldon LAJ, Carey KB, Johnson BT, Carey MP, Team MR. Behavioral interventions targeting alcohol use among people living with HIV/AIDS: a systematic review and meta-analysis. AIDS Behav. 2017;21(Suppl 2):126–43.
46. Substance Abuse and Mental Health Services Administration. SAMHSA-HRSA Center for integrated health solutions 2019. Available from: https://www.integration.samhsa.gov/clinical-practice/screening-tools.
47. Moyer VA, Preventive Services Task Force. Screening and behavioral counseling interventions in primary care to reduce alcohol misuse: U.S. preventive services task force recommendation statement. Ann Intern Med. 2013;159(3):210–8.
48. O'Connor EA, Perdue LA, Senger CA, Rushkin M, Patnode CD, Bean SI, et al. Screening and Behavioral Counseling interventions to reduce unhealthy alcohol use in adolescents and adults: updated evidence report and systematic review for the US Preventive Services Task Force. JAMA. 2018;320(18):1910–28.
49. Reus VI, Fochtmann LJ, Bukstein O, Eyler AE, et al. The American Psychiatric ASsociation practice guidelines for the pharmacologic treatment of patients with alcohol use disorder. Am J Psychiatry. 2018;175(1):86–90.
50. SAMHSA-NIAAA. In: SAMHSA, editor. Medication for the treatment of alcohol use disorder: a brief guide. Rockville: HHS Publication; 2015.
51. Sohler NL, Wong MD, Cunningham WE, Cabral H, Drainoni ML, Cunningham CO. Type and pattern of illicit drug use and access to health care services for HIV-infected people. AIDS Patient Care STDs. 2007;21(Suppl 1):S68–76.
52. Vu NT, Holt M, Phan HT, Le HT, La LT, Tran GM, et al. Amphetamine-type stimulant use among men who have sex with men (MSM) in Vietnam: results from a socio-ecological, community-based study. Drug Alcohol Depend. 2016;158:110–7.
53. Colfax G, Santos GM, Chu P, Vittinghoff E, Pluddemann A, Kumar S, et al. Amphetamine-group substances and HIV. Lancet. 2010;376(9739):458–74.
54. Young SD, Shoptaw S. Stimulant use among African American and Latino MSM social networking users. J Addict Dis. 2013;32(1):39–45.

55. Wohl AR, Frye DM, Johnson DF. Demographic characteristics and sexual behaviors associated with methamphetamine use among MSM and non-MSM diagnosed with AIDS in Los Angeles County. AIDS Behav. 2008;12(5):705–12.
56. Halkitis PN, Jerome RC. A comparative analysis of methamphetamine use: black gay and bisexual men in relation to men of other races. Addict Behav. 2008;33(1):83–93.
57. Mimiaga MJ, Reisner SL, Grasso C, Crane HM, Safren SA, Kitahata MM, et al. Substance use among HIV-infected patients engaged in primary care in the United States: findings from the Centers for AIDS research network of integrated clinical systems cohort. Am J Public Health. 2013;103(8):1457–67.
58. Mimiaga MJ, Reisner SL, Fontaine YM, Bland SE, Driscoll MA, Isenberg D, et al. Walking the line: stimulant use during sex and HIV risk behavior among Black urban MSM. Drug Alcohol Depend. 2010;110(1–2):30–7.
59. Cunningham CO, Sohler NL, Berg KM, Shapiro S, Heller D. Type of substance use and access to HIV-related health care. AIDS Patient Care STDs. 2006;20(6):399–407.
60. Kalichman SC, Graham J, Luke W, Austin J. Perceptions of health care among persons living with HIV/AIDS who are not receiving antiretroviral medications. AIDS Patient Care STDs. 2002;16(5):233–40.
61. Metsch LR, McCoy HV, McCoy CB, Miles CC, Edlin BR, Pereyra M. Use of health care services by women who use crack cocaine. Women Health. 1999;30(1):35–51.
62. Metsch LR, Pereyra M, Brewer TH. Use of HIV health care in HIV-seropositive crack cocaine smokers and other active drug users. J Subst Abus. 2001;13(1–2):155–67.
63. Baum MK, Rafie C, Lai S, Sales S, Page B, Campa A. Crack-cocaine use accelerates HIV disease progression in a cohort of HIV-positive drug users. J Acquir Immune Defic Syndr. 2009;50(1):93–9.
64. Arnsten JH, Demas PA, Grant RW, Gourevitch MN, Farzadegan H, Howard AA, et al. Impact of active drug use on antiretroviral therapy adherence and viral suppression in HIV-infected drug users. J Gen Intern Med. 2002;17(5):377–81.
65. Palepu A, Tyndall MW, Joy R, Kerr T, Wood E, Press N, et al. Antiretroviral adherence and HIV treatment outcomes among HIV/HCV co-infected injection drug users: the role of methadone maintenance therapy. Drug Alcohol Depend. 2006;84(2):188–94.
66. Kapadia F, Vlahov D, Wu Y, Cohen MH, Greenblatt RM, Howard AA, et al. Impact of drug abuse treatment modalities on adherence to ART/HAART among a cohort of HIV seropositive women. Am J Drug Alcohol Abuse. 2008;34(2):161–70.
67. Harada T, Tsutomi H, Mori R, Wilson DB. Cognitive-behavioural treatment for amphetamine-type stimulants (ATS)-use disorders. Cochrane Database Syst Rev. 2018;12:CD011315.
68. Mdodo R, Frazier EL, Dube SR, Mattson CL, Sutton MY, Brooks JT, et al. Cigarette smoking prevalence among adults with HIV compared with the general adult population in the United States: cross-sectional surveys. Ann Intern Med. 2015;162(5):335–44.
69. Marshall MM, McCormack MC, Kirk GD. Effect of cigarette smoking on HIV acquisition, progression, and mortality. AIDS Educ Prev. 2009;21(3 Suppl):28–39.
70. Pacek LR, Cioe PA. Tobacco use, use disorders, and smoking cessation interventions in persons living with HIV. Curr HIV/AIDS Rep. 2015;12(4):413–20.
71. Shepherd L, Ryom L, Law M, Petoumenos K, Hatleberg CI, d'Arminio Monforte A, et al. Cessation of cigarette smoking and the impact on cancer incidence in HIV-positive persons: the data collection on adverse events of anti-HIV drugs study. Clin Infect Dis. 2018;68:650.
72. Public Health Service Guideline Update Panel L, Staff. Treating tobacco use and dependence: 2008 update U.S. Public Health Service Clinical Practice Guideline executive summary. Respir Care. 2008;53(9):1217–22.
73. Lindson-Hawley N, Thompson TP, Begh R. Motivational interviewing for smoking cessation. Cochrane Database Syst Rev. 2015;3:CD006936.
74. Rigotti NA. Clinical practice. Treatment of tobacco use and dependence. N Engl J Med. 2002;346(7):506–12.

75. Shields PG, Herbst RS, Arenberg D, Benowitz NL, Bierut L, Luckart JB, et al. Smoking cessation, version 1.2016, NCCN clinical practice guidelines in oncology. J Natl Compr Cancer Netw. 2016;14(11):1430–68.
76. The health effects of cannabis and cannabinoids: the current state of evidence and recommendations for research. The National Academies Collection: Reports funded by National Institutes of Health. Washington, D.C.; 2017.
77. Okafor CN, Cook RL, Chen X, Surkan PJ, Becker JT, Shoptaw S, et al. Prevalence and correlates of marijuana use among HIV-seropositive and seronegative men in the Multicenter AIDS Cohort Study (MACS), 1984-2013. Am J Drug Alcohol Abuse. 2017;43(5):556–66.
78. Andrade LF, Carroll KM, Petry NM. Marijuana use is associated with risky sexual behaviors in treatment-seeking polysubstance abusers. Am J Drug Alcohol Abuse. 2013;39(4):266–71.
79. Morgan E, Skaathun B, Michaels S, Young L, Khanna A, Friedman SR, et al. Marijuana use as a sex-drug is associated with HIV risk among black MSM and their network. AIDS Behav. 2016;20(3):600–7.
80. Lake S, Kerr T, Capler R, Shoveller J, Montaner J, Milloy MJ. High-intensity cannabis use and HIV clinical outcomes among HIV-positive people who use illicit drugs in Vancouver, Canada. Int J Drug Policy. 2017;42:63–70.
81. Furler MD, Einarson TR, Millson M, Walmsley S, Bendayan R. Medicinal and recreational marijuana use by patients infected with HIV. AIDS Patient Care STDs. 2004;18(4):215–28.
82. Milloy MJ, Marshall B, Kerr T, Richardson L, Hogg R, Guillemi S, et al. High-intensity cannabis use associated with lower plasma human immunodeficiency virus-1 RNA viral load among recently infected people who use injection drugs. Drug Alcohol Rev. 2015;34(2):135–40.
83. Abrams DI, Hilton JF, Leiser RJ, Shade SB, Elbeik TA, Aweeka FT, et al. Short-term effects of cannabinoids in patients with HIV-1 infection: a randomized, placebo-controlled clinical trial. Ann Intern Med. 2003;139(4):258–66.
84. D'Souza G, Matson PA, Grady CD, Nahvi S, Merenstein D, Weber KM, et al. Medicinal and recreational marijuana use among HIV-infected women in the Women's Interagency HIV Study (WIHS) cohort, 1994-2010. J Acquir Immune Defic Syndr. 2012;61(5):618–26.
85. Bredt BM, Higuera-Alhino D, Shade SB, Hebert SJ, McCune JM, Abrams DI. Short-term effects of cannabinoids on immune phenotype and function in HIV-1-infected patients. J Clin Pharmacol. 2002;42(S1):82S–9S.
86. Harris GE, Dupuis L, Mugford GJ, Johnston L, Haase D, Page G, et al. Patterns and correlates of cannabis use among individuals with HIV/AIDS in Maritime Canada. Can J Infect Dis Med Microbiol. 2014;25(1):e1–7.
87. Slawson G, Milloy MJ, Balneaves L, Simo A, Guillemi S, Hogg R, et al. High-intensity cannabis use and adherence to antiretroviral therapy among people who use illicit drugs in a Canadian setting. AIDS Behav. 2015;19(1):120–7.
88. de Jong BC, Prentiss D, McFarland W, Machekano R, Israelski DM. Marijuana use and its association with adherence to antiretroviral therapy among HIV-infected persons with moderate to severe nausea. J Acquir Immune Defic Syndr. 2005;38(1):43–6.
89. Bonn-Miller MO, Oser ML, Bucossi MM, Trafton JA. Cannabis use and HIV antiretroviral therapy adherence and HIV-related symptoms. J Behav Med. 2014;37(1):1–10.
90. Tucker JS, Burnam MA, Sherbourne CD, Kung FY, Gifford AL. Substance use and mental health correlates of nonadherence to antiretroviral medications in a sample of patients with human immunodeficiency virus infection. Am J Med. 2003;114(7):573–80.
91. Wilson KJ, Doxanakis A, Fairley CK. Predictors for non-adherence to antiretroviral therapy. Sex Health. 2004;1(4):251–7.
92. Gates PJ, Sabioni P, Copeland J, Le Foll B, Gowing L. Psychosocial interventions for cannabis use disorder. Cochrane Database Syst Rev. 2016;5:CD005336.
93. Jhanjee S. Evidence based psychosocial interventions in substance use. Indian J Psychol Med. 2014;36(2):112–8.

94. Schierenberg A, van Amsterdam J, van den Brink W, Goudriaan AE. Efficacy of contingency management for cocaine dependence treatment: a review of the evidence. Curr Drug Abuse Rev. 2012;5(4):320–31.
95. Penberthy JK, Ait-Daoud N, Vaughan M, Fanning T. Review of treatment for cocaine dependence. Curr Drug Abuse Rev. 2010;3(1):49–62.
96. Logan DE, Marlatt GA. Harm reduction therapy: a practice-friendly review of research. J Clin Psychol. 2010;66(2):201–14.
97. Wodak A, Cooney A. Do needle syringe programs reduce HIV infection among injecting drug users: a comprehensive review of the international evidence. Subst Use Misuse. 2006;41(6–7):777–813.
98. Turner KM, Hutchinson S, Vickerman P, Hope V, Craine N, Palmateer N, et al. The impact of needle and syringe provision and opiate substitution therapy on the incidence of hepatitis C virus in injecting drug users: pooling of UK evidence. Addiction. 2011;106(11):1978–88.
99. Fernandes RM, Cary M, Duarte G, Jesus G, Alarcao J, Torre C, et al. Effectiveness of needle and syringe Programmes in people who inject drugs - An overview of systematic reviews. BMC Public Health. 2017;17(1):309.
100. Fisher DG, Fenaughty AM, Cagle HH, Wells RS. Needle exchange and injection drug use frequency: a randomized clinical trial. J Acquir Immune Defic Syndr. 2003;33(2):199–205.
101. Potier C, Laprevote V, Dubois-Arber F, Cottencin O, Rolland B. Supervised injection services: what has been demonstrated? A systematic literature review. Drug Alcohol Depend. 2014;145:48–68.
102. Choopanya K, Martin M, Suntharasamai P, Sangkum U, Mock PA, Leethochawalit M, et al. Antiretroviral prophylaxis for HIV infection in injecting drug users in Bangkok, Thailand (the Bangkok Tenofovir Study): a randomised, double-blind, placebo-controlled phase 3 trial. Lancet. 2013;381(9883):2083–90.
103. Netherland J, Hansen H. White opioids: pharmaceutical race and the war on drugs that wasn't. BioSocieties. 2017;12(2):217–38.
104. EuroQol G. EuroQol--a new facility for the measurement of health-related quality of life. Health Policy. 1990;16(3):199–208.
105. Galvan FH, Davis EM, Banks D, Bing EG. HIV stigma and social support among African Americans. AIDS Patient Care STDs. 2008;22(5):423–36.
106. Birtel MD, Wood L, Kempa NJ. Stigma and social support in substance abuse: implications for mental health and well-being. Psychiatry Res. 2017;252:1–8.
107. Earnshaw VA, Smith LR, Cunningham CO, Copenhaver MM. Intersectionality of internalized HIV stigma and internalized substance use stigma: implications for depressive symptoms. J Health Psychol. 2015;20(8):1083–9.
108. Hansen HB, Siegel CE, Case BG, Bertollo DN, DiRocco D, Galanter M. Variation in use of buprenorphine and methadone treatment by racial, ethnic, and income characteristics of residential social areas in New York City. J Behav Health Serv Res. 2013;40(3):367–77.
109. Korthuis PT, Tozzi MJ, Nandi V, Fiellin DA, Weiss L, Egan JE, et al. Improved quality of life for opioid-dependent patients receiving buprenorphine treatment in HIV clinics. J Acquir Immune Defic Syndr. 2011;56(Suppl 1):S39–45.
110. Simeone C, Shapiro B, Lum PJ. Integrated HIV care is associated with improved engagement in treatment in an urban methadone clinic. Addict Sci Clin Pract. 2017;12(1):19.
111. Selwyn PA, Feingold AR, Iezza A, Satyadeo M, Colley J, Torres R, et al. Primary care for patients with human immunodeficiency virus (HIV) infection in a methadone maintenance treatment program. Ann Intern Med. 1989;111(9):761–3.

Chapter 11
HIV Prevention, Care, and Treatment for Transgender Communities of Color

Tonia Poteat and Asa E. Radix

Introduction

This chapter focuses on unique considerations in HIV prevention, care, and treatment for transgender people of color. Given the disproportionate burden of HIV among Black and Latinx transgender people, it is important for providers engaged in HIV prevention and care to be knowledgeable about the specific needs of trans communities of color. Transgender people can be broadly defined as those whose gender identity differs from their assigned sex at birth [1, 2]. In this chapter, we use the term "transgender" (trans) to describe individuals whose gender identity and/or presentation differs from the sex they were assigned on their original birth certificate, inclusive of people who do not identify with a binary sex of male or female. Trans people vary in whether they modify their bodies to affirm their gender. Some people make no anatomical changes while others undergo hormone therapy, surgical interventions, and/or other body modifications.

In addition to this physical diversity, the terms trans people use to describe themselves vary over time and place. This diversity in terminology poses a challenge to the systematic collection of data about trans populations [3, 4]. No sampling frame exists for all trans people, making probability sampling difficult; therefore, most studies use convenience samples. Inclusion and exclusion criteria for trans study participants vary widely between studies, and it is often unclear how study participants were recruited or identified [5]. Clinical studies are often limited by small sample sizes as well as lack of clarity about the hormonal and surgical histories that

T. Poteat (✉)
Department of Social Medicine, University of North Carolina Chapel Hill,
Chapel Hill, NC, USA
e-mail: Tonia_Poteat@med.unc.edu

A. E. Radix
Callen-Lorde Community Health Center, New York, NY, USA
e-mail: ARadix@callen-lorde.org

© Springer Nature Switzerland AG 2021
B. O. Ojikutu, V. E. Stone (eds.), *HIV in US Communities of Color*,
https://doi.org/10.1007/978-3-030-48744-7_11

may impact HIV risk and outcomes. Despite these limitations, the preponderance of data indicate that trans people of color, particularly Black and Latinx trans women, experience a disproportionate burden of HIV when compared with cisgender people or White trans people.

Terminology

The terminology used to describe trans people continues to evolve over time and across geographical and cultural contexts [6]. Terms used to describe women who were assigned male at birth include transgender women, trans women, trans feminine individuals, and women of trans experience. Terms for men assigned female at birth include transgender men, trans men, trans masculine individuals, and men of trans experience. Some individuals do not identify as male or female, using words such as gender non-binary and gender non-conforming to describe themselves. Other individuals may not have a fixed sense of their gender and may move back and forth among different gender identities, and are described as gender fluid. Agender persons do not identify with having any gender, and may use other terms such as null-gender or neutrois.

Gender affirmation describes processes whereby a person receives social recognition, value, and support for their gender identity and expression [7]. Gender affirmation occurs across multiple dimensions, including social (e.g., use of pronouns, names, or clothing that align with gender identity), medical (e.g., use of hormones and/or surgery), legal (e.g., legal change of name and/or gender markers on identity documents), and psychological (e.g., the degree of self-acceptance) [8]. Gender affirmation has been shown to improve mental health and well-being among trans individuals [9, 10].

Epidemiology

Accurate data are necessary to advance understanding of the diverse health needs of trans people and to respond to that diversity in clinical care [11]. Trans communities are leading movements to replace pathologization of gender with an understanding of gender diversity as a normal variation of human existence [12]. This is reflected in current trends to count trans people in population data sets based on self-identity rather than using psychological diagnostic criteria or counting only trans people who seek gender-affirming medical interventions [13–16].

The UCSF Center of Excellence for Transgender Health currently recommends using a two-step method to identify trans people. One step queries sex assigned at birth (male or female), while the other step asks for current gender identity – including male/man, female/woman, transgender man, transgender woman, and gender non-binary among others [17, 18]. While this is considered a best practice in quantitative data collection, it has limited ability to capture the growing number and complexities of emerging gender identities, particularly among youth [19]. Widespread stigma has been well-documented and may prevent trans people from sharing their gender identities or gender histories with others, even on anonymous surveys and in confidential medical records [20, 21]. However, routine collection of gender identity data is important for planning clinical services and may signal to trans patients and clients that they are welcome [22].

Prevalence of Trans Identities

The US Behavioral Risk Factor Surveillance Study (BRFSS) collects data via interviews with more than 400,000 adults each year in all 50 states as well as the District of Columbia, Puerto Rico, Palau, Guam, American Samoa, and the US Virgin Islands, making it the largest continuously conducted health survey system in the world [23]. In 2014, 19 states began to include the question, "Do you consider yourself to be transgender?" The Williams Institute, a sexual orientation and gender identity law and public policy think tank, has analyzed BRFSS data and estimates that 1.4 million adults (0.6% of the US population) identify as transgender [24] as well as 150,000 US youth (0.7% of the population aged 13–17 years) [25]. The population of trans adults is more racially and ethnically diverse than the US general population: 55% identify as White, 16% identify as African-American or Black, 21% identify as Latinx or Hispanic, and 8% identify as another race or ethnicity. Adults who are African-American or Black (0.8%), Latinx or Hispanic (0.8%), and of another race or ethnicity (0.6%) are more likely than White adults (0.5%) to identify as transgender [26].

National, population-based estimates of the numbers of gender non-binary people (who may or may not consider themselves to be transgender) are not available. However, 31% of the 27,715 people who completed the 2015 US Transgender Survey (USTS) identified as gender non-binary [27]. A recent meta-analysis identified 5 population-based national surveys with 20 waves of data collection that reported on trans identities between 2006 and 2016 [28]. A meta-regression of these data suggests that the number and proportion of people who identify as trans has been rising and will continue to rise over time.

HIV Prevalence

HIV prevalence among trans people in the United States is estimated to be 13.7%: 18.8% among trans women and 2% among trans men [29] with the highest burden among Black (44.2%) and Latinx (25.8%) trans women [29]. Data on HIV prevalence among non-binary individuals is limited. Of the non-binary individuals who completed the 2015 USTS, 0.4% self-reported living with HIV, including 1% of participants assigned male at birth and 0.2% assigned female at birth [27].

In the first national-level analysis of trans people with diagnosed HIV infection, the National HIV Surveillance system identified 2351 trans people with newly diagnosed HIV infection during 2009–2014: 84.0% were trans women, 15.4% were trans men, and 0.7% were additional gender identity [30]. The majority of trans women (50.8%) and trans men (58.4%) with newly diagnosed HIV were Black/African-American. Almost half of newly diagnosed trans people resided in the South (44.4%) and 18.2% had AIDS at the time of diagnosis based on the Centers for Disease Control and Prevention (CDC) case definition [30, 31].

In 2017, the Ryan White HIV/AIDS Program provided services for 8811 trans people living with HIV, representing 1.8% of Ryan White clients living with HIV. Of these trans clients, 7837 (89%) were trans women, 853 (10%) were trans men, and 121 (1%) were trans with current gender unknown. The majority were Black [5081 (57.6%)] or Latinx [2619 (29.7%)] [32].

HIV Vulnerability

The elevated burden of HIV among Black and Latinx trans people is driven by multiple, intersecting factors. Black and Latinx trans people in the United States live within the context of structural, social, and interpersonal racism, ethnocentrism, cissexism, transphobia, and widespread HIV stigma. As a result, they face disproportionate rates of poverty, unemployment, housing instability, and incarceration as well as associated survival sex work, substance use, and psychological distress [27, 29]. Independently and synergistically, these factors increase vulnerability to HIV and present barriers to condom use, PrEP uptake and persistence, and engagement in HIV care and treatment.

Engagement in Biomedical HIV Prevention

Data on PrEP acceptability and willingness among trans people have been limited to trans women, are typically derived from studies designed for cisgender men who have sex with men, include relatively small numbers of trans women [33–35], and often fail to disaggregate findings by gender identity [36–39]. Research in Latin America and Asia suggest high acceptability, willingness, and uptake of PrEP among trans women [40–43]; however, data from the United States are less promising, demonstrating low PrEP acceptability and uptake [44–46]. Trans-specific barriers to PrEP identified in qualitative studies with trans women include stigma, exclusion of trans women in advertising, concerns about drug interactions with feminizing hormones, and lack of research on trans women and PrEP [44, 45, 47]. Even among Black and Latinx trans women willing to take PrEP, uptake has been low [48]. In order to effectively engage trans women who may be interested in PrEP, community-led strategies are essential [49, 50].

HIV Care Continuum

There are minimal data on the HIV care continuum among trans men and non-binary individuals, and existing data among trans women are mixed [51, 52]. Where disparities have been identified, trans women living with HIV, most of whom are Black or Latinx, are less likely to receive treatment, be adherent to treatment, and achieve viral suppression [53–56]. Trans people may experience numerous barriers to successful engagement along the HIV care continuum [27, 57]. For example, compared with Ryan White clients overall, trans clients were significantly less likely to have stable housing (76.8% vs. 87.1%), live above the federal poverty level (23.8% vs. 37.2%), and be virally suppressed (80.9% vs. 85.9%) [32]. Experiences of violence, discrimination, and other trauma are common among trans people and have been associated with treatment failure [27, 58].

Challenges to Engagement in HIV Care and Treatment

Trans people may avoid the healthcare system due to stigma and past negative experiences, such as being called the wrong name or pronoun, verbally harassed, asked invasive questions about being transgender, and having to teach their providers about trans people [27, 59–61]. For many trans people, gender-affirmation therapy is a greater priority than HIV treatment and care [62, 63]. Concerns about adverse interactions between antiretroviral drugs and hormone therapy are common [62]. One study found that 40% of trans women with HIV did not take their antiretroviral therapy (ART) as directed due to concerns about drug-drug interactions, yet less than half had discussed this concern with their providers [64]. A recent study found that Black and Latinx trans women living with HIV had a high prevalence of ART interruptions (57.3%) [65]. Unmet surgical needs and lack of current hormone use were significantly associated with ART interruptions, suggesting that unmet need for gender affirmation may inhibit successful, consistent engagement with HIV treatment and highlighting opportunities to mitigate care interruptions in alignment with community needs and goals.

Interventiovns to Facilitate HIV Care Engagement

Individuals are more likely to engage in HIV care when gender affirmation needs are met [7, 60]. Data from a national study of trans people with HIV found that participants with HIV care providers who affirm their gender were more likely to be virally suppressed [63]. Adherence to hormone therapy has been found to correlate with adherence to ART [66, 67]. However, making access to hormone therapy contingent upon ART adherence is associated with lower likelihood of viral suppression [63]. According to research with trans youth [60] and adults [62], integration of HIV care with gender care facilitates treatment. In addition to minimizing the number of provider visits and potentially stressful clinical interactions, care integration facilitates the ability to discuss any concerns about drug-drug interactions between HIV treatment and gender-affirming medications. Where integrated care is not feasible, referral and collaboration between the ART prescriber and the hormone therapy prescriber facilitates quality care. Peer navigation has been found to improve durable viral suppression among key populations, including trans women [68]. Research with youth and adults suggest that having visible trans staff in the clinical environment also facilitates engagement in care [60].

Provider-Patient Interaction and Affirming Language (Best Practices)

Positive provider interactions are essential to engaging trans people in healthcare. Trans individuals frequently cite negative experiences in healthcare and poor interactions with medical providers, in particular, as reasons for delaying both preventive and emergency healthcare services [27, 60, 69–71]. Some of these experiences include being refused care, needing to teach their providers about trans medicine, being treated disrespectfully (use of incorrect name or pronoun) as well as being asked unnecessary and intrusive questions about their bodies [27, 72, 73]. Anticipated stigma also keeps trans people out of care even when not witnessed firsthand. In fact knowing someone else who has had a bad experience is a strong predictor of not engaging in necessary services [71].

Gender-Affirming Medical Settings

Using affirming language is the first step to creating a trans-inclusive and welcoming environment. All patients should be asked for their pronouns before using terms such as "sir" or "ma'am". This starts even before the person enters the clinic or other health setting, e.g., when a patient speaks on the telephone, assumptions should never be made about gender based on their voice. At registration it is important to have forms that allow patients to use their name and gender even if there have not been legal name changes, or changes to insurance and identity documents. Transgender-inclusive forms have been found to be an important factor to improve the healthcare environment for trans people [74]. These forms should include options for gender identity as well as sex assigned at birth. This "two-step" question has been found to improve identification of trans people and is also essential for provision of preventive care that relies on knowledge of birth sex [75]. Other items include having healthcare workers who are also transgender, gender neutral restrooms, health promotion materials that include images of trans people and medical gender affirmation, including provision of hormones [6, 60, 76]. Reviews of best practices for providing trans-inclusive medical settings often prioritize medical knowledge and trainings [77]. However, improving medical provider interactions and cultural competence through trainings is not straightforward. Although trainings have been developed that result in improved knowledge of trans health topics or comfort treating trans patients [78–80], few have included validated measures to determine whether these result in improved patient care outcomes [81–84]. Since provider attitudes, especially transphobia, have been shown to be directly correlated with provider knowledge, a focus on explicit and implicit bias is an essential component for trainings in trans health [83]. Regardless, it is important for medical providers to be familiar with trans terminology, the essentials of hormone therapy, including monitoring of adverse effects, and how to manage hormones in patients with concurrent medical issues.

Provider Interactions

In addition to using the correct name and pronoun for patients, there are also other issues that providers should be aware of when interacting with trans patients. Medical history taking needs to include documentation of a patient's steps to gender affirmation – including legal, medical, and social. Understanding the ways that patients have affirmed their gender, including whether they have had a legal name change and/or updated identity documents, can help to identify the need for additional resources. Their history of hormone use should be documented, including whether hormones have been prescribed or obtained outside of medical settings. Many trans women have used silicone and other soft tissue fillers to enhance their appearance. Silicone use may lead to long-term health issues, such as silicone migration, granulomas, skin and soft tissue infections, pneumonitis, and rarely hypercalcemia and embolic phenomena [85–88]. Medical providers should note where in the body and how much silicone was injected.

The medical history should include any gender-affirming procedures undertaken (Table 11.1) and plans for future hormones or surgeries. Adverse effects or complications from gender-affirming surgeries or hormones should be noted. Medical

Table 11.1 Gender-affirming surgeries

Trans feminine	Trans masculine
Breast augmentation	Bilateral mastectomy
Vaginoplasty	Phalloplasty
Orchiectomy	Metoidioplasty
Chondrolaryngoplasty	Hysterectomy
Facial surgery	Oophorectomy
Feminization laryngoplasty	Facial surgery
	Masculinization laryngoplasty

providers should ask about sex work as many trans women have been or are sex workers, which has associated risk with HIV and STI risk, as well as risk for violence and incarceration [89, 90].

Sexual health interviewing is often challenging for trans patients. The CDC has recommended questions for sexual health history taking that includes asking about sexual partners, practices, protection from STDs, past history of STDs, and prevention of pregnancy (the 5 Ps). Trans patients often have diverse sexual partners [27], including cisgender men, cisgender women, trans men, trans women, and nonbinary or agender individuals. Medical providers should ask about the gender of sexual partners without making assumptions that their gender and anatomy will align. Appropriate lines of questioning might include "tell me about the gender(s) of your sexual partners" or "you told me that you have a boyfriend, was he assigned male or female at birth?"

Trans patients have often experienced high rates of intimate partner violence as well as sexual trauma, including child sex abuse and sexual assault [91–93]. Medical providers are often unfamiliar or uncomfortable asking questions about sexual trauma and frequently neglect to include this when obtaining a medical history [94]. Even when asked directly (e.g."when you were a child, did you ever have a sexual experience with an adult?"), disclosure may be hampered by feelings of shame or mistrust.

Physical Exam

Since many trans patients have had a history of avoiding medical settings and preventive care, medical providers should plan to spend additional time establishing rapport and explaining the reason for any examinations or procedures. Patients may also be more comfortable with a chaperone or friend during an exam.

Language Use

Medical providers should ask patients about language use, as some may prefer nonmedical terms to be used, or terms that better align with their gender identity. For example, "front hole" may be preferred to vagina and trans men will almost always prefer "chest" to "breasts", whether or not they have undergone "top surgery" or mastectomy. Nongendered terms, such as genitals and internal or external parts, will cover most organs examined during the sexual health exam.

Genital Examinations

Trans men who have been on testosterone may experience vaginal dryness or pain [1]. Conducting a pelvic exam may require a smaller speculum and lubrication. Some providers will offer patients vaginal estrogen 2 weeks prior to the exam to reduce discomfort [1]. For trans women who have a neovagina, a pediatric specu-lum or anoscope may be used for the exam. Trans women who have not had any genital surgeries may practice genital tucking – pulling the penis and scrotum back between the buttocks and pushing the testes into the inguinal canals. This is usually held in place with tape or cloth. The area should be carefully examined for skin irritation, fungal infections, and balanitis.

HIV Pre-exposure Prophylaxis: Screening and Prevention Recommendations

The CDC has recommended pre-exposure prophylaxis (PrEP) with a fixed dose combination of tenofovir disoproxil fumarate and emtricitabine (TDF/FTC) for pre-vention of HIV since 2011 [95]. The initial guidelines specifically addressed men who have sex with men, later expanded to heterosexuals at risk and did not address use in trans people. However, the most recent 2017 update and the 2019 USPSTF recommendation advocate the use of PrEP in all persons at risk of acquiring HIV sexually [96, 97]. The only clinical trial of PrEP to include trans people in signifi-cant numbers failed to show efficacy of TDF/FTC, thought to be due to very low adherence; however, no seroconversions occurred in those taking at least 4 pills per week, and the trans women who seroconverted had no evidence of the study drug in their blood [98]. In addition, a recent analysis revealed that differences in the base-line characteristics between the trans women and cisgender men in the study explained the observed effect difference [99]. A concern about a possible drug-drug interaction between estrogens and TDF has resulted in some small studies, which suggest that feminizing hormone therapy may result in lower plasma tenofovir lev-els (that are still within the therapeutic range) [100] as well as less favorable ratios of tenofovir metabolites and deoxynucleotides in rectal tissue, that may indicate lower potency [101]. These findings do not change the recommendation that trans women at risk should be offered PrEP. The greatest threat to PrEP efficacy in trans individuals is that many individuals are still not aware of PrEP, are not offered it by their providers, are worried about stigma, may have financial barriers to accessing it, and have concerns that TDF-FTC will interfere with hormones or cause side effects. Providers should be diligent about assessing all patients for PrEP, discussing risks and benefits, normalizing use, and for trans individuals, discussing the evi-dence that refutes any adverse impact of PrEP on hormones [45, 102].

Unique Treatment Considerations

All people living with HIV, regardless of gender identity, should receive antiretrovi-ral treatment (ART) to improve health outcomes and reduce the risk of HIV trans-mission [103]. There are additional considerations, however, for trans people related to hormone use and the impact of these on metabolic factors. The hormone regimens used by trans women include different formulations of estrogens and androgen blockers (usually spironolactone) and result in breast growth and softening of the skin and slowing of androgenetic hair loss [104]. Trans men may use testosterone, commonly either injectable or transdermal, that results in facial hair, deepening of the voice, and usually cessation of menses [104].

Hormones and ART

Most of the studies that have investigated interactions between hormone therapy and ART have focused on the effects of oral contraceptives, since ethinyl estradiol is metabolized through the cytochrome P450 system, also used by the protease inhibitors (PIs), non-nucleoside reverse trans criptase inhibitors (NNRTIs), and the boosters cobicistat and ritonavir [105]. The efficacy of ART is not expected to be influenced by hormone therapy. However, it is possible that some ART may increase or decrease hormone levels. In general, boosted PIs are thought to reduce estradiol levels. The NNRTIs efavirenz, etravirine, and nevirapine are thought to reduce both testosterone and estradiol levels. Medical providers who are prescribing hormone therapy should consider monitoring hormone levels before and after instituting ART to ensure that hormone levels remain in the recommended ranges of serum estradiol of 100–200 pg/mL for those receiving estrogens and 400–700 ng/dL for trans men on testosterone [104].

Estrogen therapy has an effect on lipids, causing high triglycerides [104]. Estrogens have been shown to increase the risk of venous thromboembolism and ischemic stroke. Trans women who are taking estrogens should be encouraged to reduce cardiovascular risk factors, including healthy eating and exercise and given assistance with smoking cessation. Trans women may have higher rates of osteopenia, even if they have never taken hormones [106], and all trans people are at risk for bone loss if they have removed their gonads, especially if hormones are stopped [107]. Adequate exercise, diet, smoking cessation, and vitamin D replacement are all recommended interventions. The choice of ART should take into account effects on lipids and bone health and whether enhanced screening needs to be undertaken.

Dolutegravir and Pregnancy

Currently dolutegravir (DTG), an integrase strand transfer inhibitor, is not recommended in early pregnancy and for those who might get pregnant, due to an elevated risk of neural tube defects (NTD). Trans and gender nonbinary people who are sexually active and can get pregnant should be counseled about the risk of NTD and offered effective contraception if they wish to use DTG. Trans masculine people on testosterone can still get pregnant. They should be advised that testosterone is not an effective method of contraception and provided with effective contraceptive options [108]. The current DHHS Perinatal Guidelines state that DTG should not be prescribed for individuals who are pregnant and within 12 weeks post-conception [109].

Conclusion

In summary, transgender communities of color face significant vulnerabilities to HIV and barriers to HIV prevention and care rooted in systemic, intersecting oppression (racism, cissexism, transphobia, HIV stigma). HIV prevention and care providers can facilitate the health of transgender communities by addressing structural barriers and engaging with community-led strategies for gender-affirming services.

References

1. Center of Excellence For Transgender Health DOFACM, University Of California San Francisco. Guidelines for the primary and gender-affirming care of transgender and gender nonbinary people. San Francisco: University of California San Francisco; 2016. Available from: www.Transhealth.Ucsf.Edu/.
2. Winter S, Diamond M, Green J, Karasic D, Reed T, Whittle S, et al. Transgender people: health at the margins of society. Lancet (London, England). 2016;388(10042):390–400.
3. Labuski C, Keo-Meier C. The (Mis)Measure of Trans. TSQ. 2015;2(1):13–33.
4. Glick JL, Theall K, Andrinopoulos K, Kendall C. For data's sake: dilemmas in the measurement of gender minorities. Cult Health Sex. 2018;20:1362.
5. Reisner SL, Poteat T, Keatley J, Cabral M, Mothopeng T, Dunham E, et al. Global health burden and needs of transgender populations: a review. Lancet (London, England). 2016;388(10042):412–36.
6. Reisner SL, Radix A, Deutsch MB. Integrated and gender-affirming transgender clinical care and research. J Acquir Immune Defic Syndr (1999). 2016;72(Suppl 3):S235–42.
7. Sevelius JM. Gender affirmation: a framework for conceptualizing risk behavior among transgender women of color. Sex Roles. 2013;68(11–12):675–89.
8. Glynn TR, Gamarel KE, Kahler CW, Iwamoto M, Operario D, Nemoto T. The role of gender affirmation in psychological well-being among transgender women. Psychol Sex Orientat Gend Divers. 2016;3(3):336–44.
9. Bauer GR, Scheim AI, Pyne J, Travers R, Hammond R. Intervenable factors associated with suicide risk in transgender persons: a respondent driven sampling study in Ontario, Canada. BMC Public Health. 2015;15:525.
10. Mahfouda S, Moore JK, Siafarikas A, Hewitt T, Ganti U, Lin A, et al. Gender-affirming hormones and surgery in transgender children and adolescents. Lancet Diabetes Endocrinol. 2018;7:484.
11. Singer TB. The profusion of things: the "transgender matrix" and demographic imaginaries in US Public Health. TSQ. 2015;2(1):58–76.
12. Meier SC, Labuski CM. The demographics of the transgender population. In: Baumle A, editor. The international handbook on the demography of sexuality. New York: Springer Press; 2013. p. 289–327.
13. Wiepjes CM, Nota NM, De Blok CJM, Klaver M, De Vries ALC, Wensing-Kruger SA, et al. The Amsterdam Cohort of Gender Dysphoria Study (1972-2015): trends in prevalence, treatment, and regrets. J Sex Med. 2018;15:582.
14. Mcfarland W, Wilson E, Fisher RH. How many transgender men are there in San Francisco? J Urban Health. 2017;95:129.
15. Johnston LG, Prybylski D, Raymond H, Mirzazadeh A, Manopaiboon C, Mcfarland W. Incorporating the service multiplier method in respondent-driven sampling surveys to estimate the size of hidden and hard-to-reach populations: case studies from around the world. Sex Transm Dis. 2013;40(4):129.

16. Yi SK, Steyvers M, Lee MD, Dry MJ. The wisdom of the crowd in combinatorial problems. Cogn Sci. 2012;36(3):452–70.
17. Tate CC, Ledbetter JN, Youssef CP. A two-question method for assessing gender categories in the social and medical sciences. J Sex Res. 2013;50(8):767–76.
18. Deutsch MB. Guidelines for the primary and gender-affirming care of transgender and gender nonbinary people. 2nd ed. San Francisco: University of California, San Francisco, Department of Family and Community Medicine Center of Excellence for Transgender Health; 2016. p. 199.
19. The Geniuss Group. In: Herman J, editor. Best practices for asking questions to identify transgender and other gender minority respondents on population-based surveys. Los Angeles: The Williams Institute; 2014.
20. Hughto JMW, Reisner SL, Pachankis JE. Transgender stigma and health: a critical review of stigma determinants, mechanisms, and interventions. Soc Sci Med. 2015;147:222–31.
21. Thompson HM. Patient perspectives on gender identity data collection in electronic health records: an analysis of disclosure, privacy, and access to care. Transgend Health. 2016;1(1):205–15.
22. Ingraham N, Pratt V, Gorton N. Counting trans∗ patients: a Community Health Center case study. TSQ. 2015;2(1):136–47.
23. Arnold EA, Sterrett-Hong E, Jonas A, Pollack LM. Social networks and social support among ball-attending African American men who have sex with men and transgender women are associated with HIV-related outcomes. Glob Public Health. 2018;13(2):144–58.
24. Flores AR, Herman JL, Gates GJ, Brown TNT. How many adults identify as transgender in the United States? Los Angeles: The Williams Institute; 2016. [Cited 2017 June 30]. Available From: Http://Williamsinstitute.Law.Ucla.Edu/Wp-Content/Uploads/How-Many-Adults-Identify-As-Transgender-In-The-United-States.Pdf.
25. Herman JL, Flores AR, Brown TN, Wilson BD, Conron KJ. Age of individuals who identify as transgender in the United States. Los Angeles: The Williams Institute; 2017.
26. Flores AR, Brown TN, Herman J. Race and ethnicity of adults who identify as transgender in the United States. Los Angeles: Williams Institute, UCLA School of Law; 2016.
27. James SE, Herman JL, Rankin S, Keisling M, Mottet L, Anafi M. The report of the 2015 U.S. transgender survey. Washington, D.C.: National Center For Transgender Equality; 2016.
28. Meerwijk EL, Sevelius JM. Transgender population size in the United States: a meta-regression of population-based probability samples. Am J Public Health. 2017;107(2):E1–8.
29. Becasen JS, Denard CL, Mullins MM, Higa DH, Sipe TA. Estimating the Prevalence of HIV and Sexual Behaviors Among the US Transgender Population: A Systematic Review and Meta-Analysis, 2006-2017. Am J Public Health. 2019;109(1):e1-e8. https://doi.org/10.2105/AJPH.2018.304727.
30. Clark H, Babu AS, Wiewel EW, Opoku J, Crepaz N. Diagnosed HIV infection in transgender adults and adolescents: results from the National HIV Surveillance System, 2009-2014. AIDS Behav. 2016;21:2774.
31. Selik RM, Mokotoff ED, Branson B, Owen SM, Whitmore S, Hall HI, et al. Revised surveillance case definition for HIV infection—United States, 2014. MMWR Recomm Rep. 2014;63(3):1–10.
32. Health Resources and Services Administration. Ryan White HIV/AIDS program annual client-level data report 2017. Published 2018 [Updated December 2018; Cited 15 December 2018]. Available from: Http://Hab.Hrsa.Gov/Data/Data-Reports.
33. Nunn AS, Brinkley-Rubinstein L, Oldenburg CE, Mayer KH, Mimiaga M, Patel R, et al. Defining the HIV pre-exposure prophylaxis care continuum. AIDS (London, England). 2017;31(5):731–4.
34. Calabrese SK. Interpreting gaps along the preexposure prophylaxis cascade and addressing vulnerabilities to stigma. Am J Public Health. 2018;108(10):1284–6.
35. Golub SA, Gamarel KE, Rendina HJ, Surace A, Lelutiu-Weinberger CL. From efficacy to effectiveness: facilitators and barriers to prep acceptability and motivations for adherence among MSM and transgender women in New York City. AIDS Patient Care STDs. 2013;27(4):248–54.

36. Grant RM, Anderson PL, Mcmahan V, Liu A, Amico KR, Mehrotra M, et al. Uptake of pre-exposure prophylaxis, sexual practices, and HIV incidence in men and transgender women who have sex with men: a cohort study. Lancet Infect Dis. 2014;14(9):820–9.
37. Poteat T, German D, Flynn C. The conflation of gender and sex: gaps and opportunities in HIV data among transgender women and MSM. Glob Public Health. 2016;11(7–8):835–48.
38. Eaton LA, Kalichman SC, Price D, Finneran S, Allen A, Maksut J. Stigma and conspiracy beliefs related to pre-exposure prophylaxis (Prep) and interest in using Prep among black and white men and transgender women who have sex with men. AIDS Behav. 2017;21(5):1236–46.
39. Garnett M, Hirsch-Moverman Y, Franks J, Hayes-Larson E, El-Sadr WM, Mannheimer S. Limited awareness of pre-exposure prophylaxis among black men who have sex with men and transgender women in New York City. AIDS Care. 2018;30(1):9–17.
40. Jalil EM, Grinsztejn B, Velasque L, Ramos Makkeda A, Luz PM, Moreira RI, et al. Awareness, willingness, and prep eligibility among transgender women in Rio De Janeiro, Brazil. J Acquir Immune Defic Syndr (1999). 2018;79(4):445–52.
41. Oldenburg CE, Le B, Toan T, Thien DD, Huyen HT, Friedman MR, et al. HIV pre-exposure prophylaxis indication and readiness among HIV-uninfected transgender women in Ho Chi Minh City, Vietnam. AIDS Behav. 2016;20(Suppl 3):365–70.
42. Wang Z, Lau JTF, Yang X, Cai Y, Gross DL, Ma T, et al. Acceptability of daily use of free oral pre-exposure prophylaxis (prep) among transgender women sex workers in Shenyang, China. AIDS Behav. 2017;21(12):3287–98.
43. Zalazar V, Aristegui I, Kerr T, Marshall BDL, Romero M, Sued O, et al. High willingness to use HIV pre-exposure prophylaxis among transgender women in Argentina. Transgend Health. 2016;1(1):266–73.
44. Restar AJ, Kuhns L, Reisner SL, Ogunbajo A, Garofalo R, Mimiaga MJ. Acceptability of anti-retroviral pre-exposure prophylaxis from a cohort of sexually experienced young transgender women in two U.S. cities. AIDS Behav. 2018;22:3649.
45. Rael C, Martinez M, Giguere R, Bockting W, Maccrate C, Mellman W, et al. Barriers and facilitators to oral Prep use among transgender women in New York City. AIDS Behav. 2018;22(11):3627–36.
46. Kuhns LM, Reisner SL, Mimiaga MJ, Gayles T, Shelendich M, Garofalo R. Correlates of Prep indication in a multi-site cohort of young HIV-uninfected transgender women. AIDS Behav. 2016;20(7):1470–7.
47. Sevelius JM, Keatley J, Calma N, Arnold E. 'I am not a man': trans-specific barriers and facilitators to Prep acceptability among transgender women. Glob Public Health. 2016;11(7–8):1060–75.
48. Poteat T, Wirtz A, Malik M, Cooney E, Cannon C, Hardy WD, et al. A gap between willingness and uptake: findings from mixed methods research on HIV prevention among Black and Latina transgender women. J Acquir Immune Defic Syndr (1999). 2019;82(2):131–40.
49. Brooks RA, Cabral A, Nieto O, Fehrenbacher A, Landrian A. Experiences of pre-exposure prophylaxis stigma, social support, and information dissemination among Black and Latina transgender women who are using pre-exposure prophylaxis. Transgend Health. 2019;4(1):188–96.
50. Poteat T, Wirtz AL, Reisner S. Strategies for engaging transgender populations in HIV prevention and care. Curr Opin HIV AIDS. 2019;14(5):393–400.
51. Beckwith CG, Kuo I, Fredericksen RJ, Brinkley-Rubinstein L, Cunningham WE, Springer SA, et al. Risk behaviors and HIV care continuum outcomes among criminal justice-involved HIV-infected transgender women and cisgender men: data from the seek, test, treat, and retain harmonization initiative. Plos One. 2018;13(5):E0197730.
52. Poteat T, Hanna DB, Rebeiro PF, Klein M, Silverberg MJ, Eron JJ, et al. Characterizing the human immunodeficiency virus care continuum among transgender women and cisgender women and men in clinical care: a retrospective time-series analysis. Clin Infect Dis. 2019;70(6):1131–8.
53. Kalichman SC, Hernandez D, Finneran S, Price D, Driver R. Transgender women and HIV-related health disparities: falling off the HIV treatment cascade. Sex Health. 2017;14(5):469–76.

54. Mizuno Y, Frazier E, Huang P, Skarbinski J. Characteristics of transgender women living with HIV receiving medical care in the United States. LGBT Health. 2015;2:228.
55. Santos GM, Wilson EC, Rapues J, Macias O, Packer T, Raymond HF. HIV treatment cascade among transgender women in a San Francisco respondent driven sampling study. Sex Transm Infect. 2014;90(5):430–3.
56. Baguso GN, Gay CL, Lee KA. Medication adherence among transgender women living with HIV. AIDS Care. 2016;28(8):976–81.
57. Mizuno Y, Beer L, Huang P, Frazier EL. Factors associated with antiretroviral therapy adherence among transgender women receiving HIV medical care in the United States. LGBT Health. 2017;4:181.
58. Machtinger EL, Haberer JE, Wilson TC, Weiss DS. Recent trauma is associated with antiretroviral failure and HIV transmission risk behavior among HIV-positive women and female-identified transgenders. AIDS Behav. 2012;16(8):2160–70.
59. Poteat T, German D, Kerrigan D. Managing uncertainty: a grounded theory of stigma in transgender health care encounters. Soc Sci Med (1982). 2013;84:22–9.
60. Dowshen N, Lee S, Franklin J, Castillo M, Barg F. Access to medical and mental health services across the HIV care continuum among young transgender women: a qualitative study. Transgend Health. 2017;2(1):81–90.
61. Sevelius JM, Carrico A, Johnson MO. Antiretroviral therapy adherence among transgender women living with HIV. J Assoc Nurses AIDS Care. 2010;21(3):256–64.
62. Sevelius JM, Patouhas E, Keatley JG, Johnson MO. Barriers and facilitators to engagement and retention in care among transgender women living with human immunodeficiency virus. Ann Behav Med. 2014;47(1):5–16.
63. Chung C, Kalra A, Mcbride B, Roebuck C, Sprague L. Some kind of strength: findings on health care and economic wellbeing from a national needs assessment of transgender and gender non-conforming people living with HIV. Oakland: Transgender Law Center; 2016.
64. Braun HM, Candelario J, Hanlon CL, Segura ER, Clark JL, Currier JS, et al. Transgender women living with HIV frequently take antiretroviral therapy and/or feminizing hormone therapy differently than prescribed due to drug-drug interaction concerns. LGBT Health. 2017;4(5):371–5.
65. Rosen JG, Malik M, Cooney EE, Wirtz AL, Yamanis T, Lujan M, et al. Antiretroviral treatment interruptions among Black and Latina transgender women living with HIV: characterizing co-occurring, multilevel factors using the gender affirmation framework. AIDS Behav. 2019;23:2588.
66. Crosby RA, Salazar LF, Hill BJ. Correlates of not using antiretroviral therapy among transwomen living with HIV: the unique role of personal competence. Transgend Health. 2018;3(1):141–6.
67. Sevelius JM, Saberi P, Johnson MO. Correlates of antiretroviral adherence and viral load among transgender women living with HIV. AIDS Care. 2014;26(8):976–82.
68. Cunningham WE, Weiss RE, Nakazono T, Malek MA, Shoptaw SJ, Ettner SL, et al. Effectiveness of a peer navigation intervention to sustain viral suppression among HIV-positive men and transgender women released from jail: the link La randomized clinical trial. JAMA Intern Med. 2018;178(4):542–53.
69. Sevelius JM, Fau PE, Keatley JG, Johnson MO. Barriers and facilitators to engagement and retention in care among transgender women living with human immunodeficiency virus. Ann Behav Med. 2014;47(1):5–16. (1532-4796 (Electronic)).
70. Jaffee KD, Shires DA, Stroumsa D. Discrimination and delayed health care among transgender women and men: implications for improving medical education and health care delivery. Med Care. 2016;54:1010.
71. Shipherd JC, Green KE, Abramovitz S. Transgender clients: identifying and minimizing barriers to mental health treatment. J Gay Lesbian Mental Health. 2010;14(2):94–108.
72. Shires DA, Jaffee K. Factors associated with health care discrimination experiences among a national sample of female-to-male transgender individuals. Health Soc Work. 2015;40(2):134–41.

73. Sperber J, Landers S, Lawrence S. Access to health care for transgendered persons: results of a needs assessment in Boston. Int J Transgend. 2005;8(2–3):75–91.
74. Dowshen N, Matone M, Luan X, Lee S, Belzer M, Fernandez MI, et al. Behavioral and health outcomes for HIV+ young transgender women (YTW) linked to and engaged in medical care. LGBT Health. 2016;3(2):162–7.
75. Cahill S, Singal R, Grasso C, King D, Mayer K, Baker K, et al. Do ask, do tell: high levels of acceptability by patients of routine collection of sexual orientation and gender identity data in four diverse American Community Health Centers. PLoS One. 2014;9(9):E107104.
76. Radix AE, Lelutiu-Weinberger C, Gamarel KE. Satisfaction and healthcare utilization of transgender and gender non-conforming individuals in Nyc: a community-based participatory study. LGBT Health. 2014;1(4):302–8.
77. Safer JD, Tangpricha V. Care of the transgender patient. Ann Intern Med. 2019;171(1):Itc1–Itc16.
78. Eriksson SE, Safer JD. Evidence-based curricular content improves student knowledge and changes attitudes towards transgender medicine. Endocr Pract. 2016;22(7):837–41.
79. Safer JD, Pearce EN. A simple curriculum content change increased medical student comfort with transgender medicine. Endocr Pract. 2013;19(4):633–7.
80. Vance SR Jr, Deutsch MB, Rosenthal SM, Buckelew SM. Enhancing pediatric trainees' and students' knowledge in providing care to transgender youth. J Adolesc Health. 2017;60(4):425–30.
81. Radix A, Maingi S. LGBT cultural competence and interventions to help oncology nurses and other health care providers. Semin Oncol Nurs. 2018;34(1):80–9.
82. Lelutiu-Weinberger C, Pollard-Thomas P, Pagano W, Levitt N, Lopez EI, Golub SA, et al. Implementation and evaluation of a pilot training to improve transgender competency among medical staff in an urban clinic. Transgend Health. 2016;1(1):45–53.
83. Stroumsa D, Shires DA, Richardson CR, Jaffee KD, Woodford MR. Transphobia rather than education predicts provider knowledge of transgender health care. Med Educ. 2019;53(4):398–407.
84. Braun HM, Garcia-Grossman IR, Quinones-Rivera A, Deutsch MB. Outcome and impact evaluation of a transgender health course for health profession students. LGBT Health. 2017;4(1):55–61.
85. Lungu E, Thibault-Lemyre A, Dominguez JM, Trudel D, Bureau NJ. A case of recurrent leg necrotic ulcers secondary to silicone migration in a transgender patient: radiographic, ultrasound and MRI findings. BJR Case Rep. 2016;2(1):20150309.
86. Leonardi NR, Compoginis JM, Luce EA. Illicit cosmetic silicone injection: a recent reiteration of history. Ann Plast Surg. 2016;77(4):485–90.
87. Agrawal N, Altiner S, Mezitis NH, Helbig S. Silicone-induced granuloma after injection for cosmetic purposes: a rare entity of calcitriol-mediated Hypercalcemia. Case Rep Med. 2013;2013:807292.
88. Soeroso NN, Rhinsilva E, Soeroso L. Acute pneumonitis following breast silicone liquid injection. Respirol Case Rep. 2018;6(6):E00335.
89. Poteat T, Wirtz AL, Radix A, Borquez A, Silva-Santisteban A, Deutsch MB, et al. HIV risk and preventive interventions in transgender women sex workers. Lancet (London, England). 2015;385(9964):274–86.
90. Nuttbrock LA, Hwahng SJ. Ethnicity, sex work, and incident HIV/STI among transgender women in New York City: a three year prospective study. AIDS Behav. 2017;21(12):3328–35.
91. Newcomb ME, Hill R, Buehler K, Ryan DT, Whitton SW, Mustanski B. High burden of mental health problems, substance use, violence, and related psychosocial factors in transgender, non-binary, and gender diverse youth and young adults. Arch Sex Behav. 2019;49:645.
92. Murchison GR, Agenor M, Reisner SL, Watson RJ. School restroom and locker room restrictions and sexual assault risk among transgender youth. Pediatrics. 2019;143(6):e20182902.
93. Griner SB, Vamos CA, Thompson EL, Logan R, Vázquez-Otero C, Daley EM. The Intersection of Gender Identity and Violence: Victimization Experienced by Transgender College Students [published online ahead of print, 2017 Aug 1]. J Interpers Violence. 2017;886260517723743. doi:10.1177/0886260517723743

94. Birkhoff EM, Krouwel EM, Nicolai MP, De Boer BJ, Beck JJ, Putter H, et al. Dealing with patients facing a history of sexual abuse: a cross-sectional survey among Dutch general practitioners. Eur J Gen Pract. 2016;22(2):126–33.

95. Centers for Disease Control and Prevention (CDC). Interim guidance: preexposure prophylaxis for the prevention of HIV infection in men who have sex with men. MMWR Morb Mortal Wkly Rep. 2011;60(3):65–8.

96. US Preventive Services Task Force. Preexposure prophylaxis for the prevention of HIV infection: US Preventive Services Task Force recommendation statement. JAMA. 2019;321(22):2203–13.

97. Centers for Disease Control and Prevention. US Public Health Service: Preexposure prophylaxis for the prevention of HIV infection in the United States—2017 Update: A clinical practice guideline. 2018. Available at https://www.cdc.gov/hiv/pdf/risk/prep/cdc-hiv-prep-guidelines-2017.pdf. Accessed June 3, 2020.

98. Deutsch MB, Glidden DV, Sevelius J, Keatley J, Mcmahan V, Guanira J, et al. HIV pre-exposure prophylaxis in transgender women: a subgroup analysis of the iprex trial. Lancet HIV. 2015;2(12):e512–9.

99. Mehrotra ML, Westreich D, Mcmahan VM, Glymour MM, Geng E, Grant RM, et al. Baseline characteristics explain differences in effectiveness of randomization to daily oral TDF/FTC prep between transgender women and cisgender men who have sex with men in the iprex trial. J Acquir Immune Defic Syndr (1999). 2019;81(3):E94.

100. Hiransuthikul A, Janamnuaysook R, Himmad K, Kerr SJ, Thammajaruk N, Pankam T, et al. Drug-drug interactions between feminizing hormone therapy and pre-exposure prophylaxis among transgender women: the ifact study. J Int AIDS Soc. 2019;22(7):E25338.

101. Cottrell ML, HMA P, Schauer AP, Sykes C, Maffuid K, Poliseno A, et al. Decreased tenofovir diphosphate concentrations in a transgender female cohort: implications for HIV pre-exposure prophylaxis (prep). Clin Infect Dis. 2019;69:2201.

102. Wood SM, Lee S, Barg FK, Castillo M, Dowshen N. Young transgender women's attitudes toward HIV pre-exposure prophylaxis. J Adolesc Health. 2017;60(5):549–55.

103. Panel on Antiretroviral Guidelines for Adults and Adolescents. Guidelines for the Use of Antiretroviral Agents in Adults and Adolescents with HIV. Department of Health and Human Services. Available at http://www.aidsinfo.nih.gov/ContentFiles/AdultandAdolescentGL.pdf. Accessed June 3, 2020.

104. Hembree WC, Cohen-Kettenis PT, Gooren L, Hannema SE, Meyer WJ, Murad MH, et al. Endocrine treatment of gender-dysphoric/gender-incongruent persons: an Endocrine Society∗ Clinical practice guideline. J Clin Endocrinol Metabol. 2017;102(11):3869–903.

105. Radix A, Sevelius J, Deutsch MB. Transgender women, hormonal therapy and HIV treatment: a comprehensive review of the literature and recommendations for best practices. J Int AIDS Soc. 2016;19(3 Suppl 2):20810.

106. Van Caenegem E, Taes Y, Wierckx K, Vandewalle S, Toye K, Kaufman JM, et al. Low bone mass is prevalent in male-to-female transsexual persons before the start of cross-sex hormonal therapy and gonadectomy. Bone. 2013;54(1):92–7.

107. Radix A, Deutsch MB. Bone health and osteoporosis. In: Deutsch MB, editor. Guidelines for the primary and gender-affirming care of transgender and gender nonbinary people. 2nd ed. San Francisco: Center of Excellence for Transgender Health, Department of Family and Community Medicine, University of California San Francisco; 2016.

108. Light A, Wang LF, Zeymo A, Gomez-Lobo V. Family planning and contraception use in transgender men. Contraception. 2018;98(4):266–9.

109. Department Of Health And Human Services. Recommendations for the use of antiretroviral drugs in pregnant women with HIV infection and interventions to reduce perinatal HIV transmission in the United States 2018. Available from: Https://Aidsinfo.Nih.Gov/Guidelines/Html/3/Perinatal-Guidelines/0.

Chapter 12
Medical Mistrust, Discrimination, and the Domestic HIV Epidemic

Laura M. Bogart, Sae Takada, and William E. Cunningham

Introduction

Medical mistrust is distrust of the healthcare system, providers, and treatments, and is regarded as a key contributor to racial/ethnic health and healthcare disparities in the United States, including for HIV [1]. Medical mistrust is conceptualized as the absence of trust that healthcare providers and organizations genuinely care for patients' interests, are honest, practice confidentiality, and have the competence to produce the best achievable results [2–5]. Medical mistrust has multiple dimensions, including general mistrust of healthcare providers and systems (e.g., that hospitals have experimented on patients without their knowledge, that providers have ulterior motives), trust in providers' competence or values, and race-related mistrust (e.g., that racial discrimination is common in healthcare) [6]. Medical mistrust specific to HIV has been termed "HIV conspiracy beliefs," defined as medical mistrust about the origin, prevention, and treatment of HIV [7, 8]. In the United States, medical mistrust is thought to arise from experiences of historical and contemporary, ongoing discrimination within healthcare [9, 10] and is more prevalent among people of color than among White Americans. In representative samples of areas of the United States as well as patients in specific healthcare settings (e.g., set of clinics), Black Americans have been found to be less trusting of healthcare providers compared to Whites [11–17].

William E. Cunningham deceased at the time of publication.

L. M. Bogart (✉)
RAND Corporation, Santa Monica, CA, USA
e-mail: lbogart@rand.org

S. Takada · W. E. Cunningham
Division of General Internal Medicine, Department of Medicine, University of California Los Angeles (UCLA), Los Angeles, CA, USA
e-mail: STakada@mednet.ucla.edu

© Springer Nature Switzerland AG 2021   207
B. O. Ojikutu, V. E. Stone (eds.), *HIV in US Communities of Color*,
https://doi.org/10.1007/978-3-030-48744-7_12

In the US general population, medical mistrust has been associated with health services underutilization [6, 18], including not adhering to medical advice or filling prescriptions [19], delaying age-appropriate cancer screening and other preventive services [16, 20–22], and low engagement in primary care [11, 15, 16, 21, 23], especially among Black and Latinx Americans [11, 15, 16, 20, 23–25]. Mistrust can be a barrier to participating in biomedical research among Black Americans [26–28], leading to their underrepresentation in efforts to develop new treatments and therapies. The present chapter focuses on the origins and implications of medical mistrust, both general mistrust and HIV conspiracy beliefs, for HIV prevention, care, and treatment outcomes in communities of color.

Medical Mistrust and HIV

General Medical Mistrust A handful of studies have considered medical mistrust and HIV-related behaviors and outcomes, and more research has examined HIV treatment–related behaviors than HIV prevention behaviors in relation to mistrust. Medical mistrust has been associated with decreased uptake of pre-exposure prophylaxis (PrEP), which can potentially eliminate new HIV infections among communities with high HIV incidence [29]. A qualitative study found that sexual minority men who were sex workers showed high medical mistrust (evidenced in terms of, for example, perceptions that doctors are motivated by money and are unreceptive to patients' self-diagnoses or expertise), as well as nondisclosure of sex with men or with transactional (sex work) partners to medical providers – both of which could potentially impede access to PrEP [30]. In addition, a study of women receiving care in Planned Parenthood found that Black women had higher levels of medical mistrust compared to White women, which was in turn associated with lower comfort in discussing PrEP with a provider [31].

Regarding HIV treatment–related behaviors and mistrust, lower levels of antiretroviral therapy (ART) adherence were associated with distrust in one's provider in a nationally representative sample of people in care for HIV, and general levels of medical mistrust among HIV-positive Black men [32, 33]. For example, in a longitudinal convenience sample of Black men with HIV, Dale and colleagues found that 92% agreed with at least one general medical mistrust item and 80% agreed with at least one racism-related medical mistrust item on a validated scale [6], and general medical mistrust, but not racism-related mistrust, predicted lower ART adherence over time [32]. Encounters with healthcare during incarceration can lead to mistrust and compromised access to care. A qualitative study among incarcerated people of color with HIV showed that negative healthcare experiences during incarceration (e.g., unsupportive providers who did not provide sufficient information about HIV and treatment) fostered mistrust of providers and suspicion toward ART, and affected engagement in care after release [34]. Furthermore, results of a national sample of adults with HIV in the United States showed that discriminatory healthcare experiences were associated with greater healthcare provider mistrust, which in turn were associated with weaker beliefs about the benefits of ART and, consequently, lower adherence [33]. Similarly, research indicates that beliefs about the necessity, efficacy, and adverse effects of ART (e.g., "My health, at present, depends on my medicine" or "Having to take my medications worries me") partially account for (i.e., mediate, or explain) the relationship between medical mistrust and ART nonadherence [35–37]. Thus, general medical mistrust may affect how patients think about medications specifically, which in turn may impact motivation (or lack of motivation) to take them, leading to nonadherence and consequent adverse health outcomes. Consistent with this line of thinking, medical mistrust was associated with detectable HIV viral load in a convenience sample of HIV-positive Black sexual minority men [38].

HIV-Specific Medical Mistrust (HIV Conspiracy Beliefs) The majority of studies on medical mistrust and HIV have focused on HIV conspiracy beliefs [7, 8]. A conspiracy belief is defined here as an effort to explain the causes of an event, practice, or circumstances by reference to the actions of powerful people who attempt to conceal their role [39, 40]. Note that this definition takes an objective perspective, such that a conspiracy belief is not necessarily false, harmful, unjustified, or irrational.

HIV conspiracy beliefs have received the most research attention among Black Americans, given the history of structural and interpersonal discrimination, including racial segregation, and mistreatment in housing and healthcare, and restricted economic opportunities [41]. HIV conspiracy beliefs involve genocidal beliefs and treatment-related beliefs [7, 8, 42] and include both benign-neglect theories (e.g., that actors are not intentionally harming communities but, rather, are indifferent or careless) and malicious-intent theories (that malevolent actors aim to harm communities); benign-neglect theories tend to be more highly endorsed [43]. Genocidal HIV conspiracy beliefs (which tend to be malicious-intent theories) commonly attribute HIV disparities to government actors (e.g., the CIA) who are intentionally withholding a cure and/or created HIV in a government laboratory as a form of genocide against people of color. Treatment-related HIV conspiracy beliefs (which can be either malicious-intent or benign-neglect theories) are focused on medications related to HIV, such as that the medications are poison or ineffective, or can cause AIDS, or that people who take ART are serving as laboratory animals in experiments for the government.

HIV conspiracy beliefs are highest among Black Americans compared to Latinx and White Americans, and Latinx people show higher conspiracy beliefs than do Whites [31, 44–49]. High levels of conspiracy beliefs have persisted over time in nationally representative samples of Black Americans. For example, the 2016 National Survey on HIV in the Black Community, a nationally representative email survey of Black individuals aged 18–50 in the United States, found that 31% (of 868 participants) agreed strongly or agreed that "HIV is a man-made virus," 40% that "there is a cure for HIV but the government is withholding it from the poor," and 33% that "the medicine that doctors prescribe to treat HIV is poison" [50]. Although some research indicates differences by socio-demographic characteristics in endorsement of conspiracy beliefs (e.g., that Black Americans of lower socio-economic status are more likely to endorse conspiracy beliefs), these differences are typically small or non-significant [43, 51, 52], suggesting that conspiracy beliefs are not isolated to sub-groups of Black Americans.

Much research in this area has recruited convenience samples of people living with and at-risk for HIV; this research shows similarly high levels of conspiracy beliefs as representative samples, especially among racial/ethnic minority individuals [8, 48, 53–57]. In a study of 214 HIV-positive Black men (most of whom were sexual minority men), 75% agreed with at least one conspiracy belief; the most frequently endorsed belief (among 52%) was "HIV is a manmade virus" [54]. Qualitative research with samples of primarily Black individuals has similarly found belief in conspiracies among many or most participants [41, 58, 59]. Furthermore, conspiracy beliefs extend to PrEP: a convenience sample of 285 HIV-negative Black and White sexual and gender minorities indicated that 42% agreed with conspiracy beliefs about PrEP (e.g., that drug companies are lying or taking advantage of people regarding PrEP), with greater endorsement among Black than White participants [44].

Endorsement of conspiracy beliefs has been associated with HIV prevention behaviors and ART adherence [7, 8, 30, 31, 38, 42, 44, 45, 50, 54, 59–62]. In terms of prevention behaviors, belief in HIV conspiracies has been associated with condomless sex among Black men in general [42], Black men with HIV [54], and racial/ethnic minority sexual minority men (including Asian American, Black, Native American, and Latinx men) [45]. Belief in HIV conspiracies has also been associated with lower likelihood of PrEP awareness among Black and Latinx sexual minority men [48] and lower intention to adopt PrEP among Black sexual minority men [56] quantitatively.

In contrast, research conducted in the United States has generally found a positive association between HIV conspiracy beliefs and HIV testing: belief in HIV conspiracies has been associated with higher odds of HIV testing among socially vulnerable, racially/ethnically diverse men and women in Los Angeles [60], among Black individuals in low-income, high drug use neighborhoods [55], and in the 2016 National Survey on HIV in the Black community [50]. The 2016 National Survey on HIV in the Black community additionally found that greater HIV risk partially explained (i.e., mediated) the association between HIV conspiracy beliefs and HIV testing. Although people who endorse conspiracies may mistrust the government regarding the origin of HIV, they may also believe that HIV is a serious disease, based on the observed effects of HIV in their communities, as well as community-based messaging around HIV, and thus may believe that people who are at risk should be tested. Alternately, people who believe that the government intentionally created HIV as a harmful agent as a form of genocide may also be impelled to protect themselves from HIV, starting with HIV testing. Nevertheless, research has also found that organizational suspicion (e.g., distrust of HIV-related medical services) predicted lower likelihood of having been tested for HIV among racial/

ethnic minority men but not among White sexual minority men [45] – suggesting that different forms of mistrust may have different effects on HIV testing. More research is needed to fully understand the association between medical mistrust and HIV testing.

Several studies indicate significant associations between medical mistrust and HIV conspiracy beliefs with lower ART adherence among Black Americans. A systematic review showed that belief in conspiracies about HIV and its treatment was correlated with nonadherence among Black individuals [63]. For example, in a longitudinal study of HIV-positive Black men, belief in treatment-related HIV conspiracy theories was associated with nonadherence to ART [8], but belief in genocidal conspiracies were not. Research also has indicated that treatment-related HIV conspiracy beliefs are associated with detectable viral load among HIV-positive Black sexual minority men [38]. Qualitative interviews with US Black veterans similarly suggest that suspicions about ART (e.g., that they speed progression to AIDS and death) may lead to low adherence [59].

A handful of studies have indicated non-significant associations between HIV conspiracy beliefs or mistrust and HIV care behaviors. A study of a diverse racial/ ethnic sample of Black, Asian, Latinx, White, and multiracial/ethnic patients at public health centers did not find significant associations between conspiracy beliefs and access to care, retention in care, or adherence to ART [64], and a small study of young Black, Latinx, and Asian HIV-positive sexual minority men found that conspiracy beliefs were not significantly associated with diagnosis, linkage to, or engagement in care [53]. These results are consistent with qualitative research indicating that HIV-positive Black and Latinx people who were not engaged in care felt that their belief in HIV conspiracies was not a barrier to seeking care, because they prioritized managing their HIV and overall health, regardless of the origins of HIV and whether a cure was being withheld [65]. A limitation of these studies is that they combined responses of Black participants with those of other racial/ethnic groups. Given the history of unethical treatment and discrimination within healthcare, and research indicating that Black individuals show higher levels of mistrust than do individuals of other racial/ethnic groups, it is likely that effects of medical mistrust (including HIV conspiracy beliefs) are stronger among Black Americans. Thus, combining responses among races/ethnicities could lead to weaker or non-significant effects of mistrust.

In sum, research indicates high levels of medical mistrust in general and HIV conspiracy beliefs specifically among people of color, as well as robust associations between mistrust and health outcomes and behaviors related to HIV prevention, testing, and ART nonadherence. Nevertheless, most of this research is among Black individuals, and Latinx and other minority racial/ethnic subgroups have been understudied [25]. Furthermore, data are needed on associations of mistrust with other important HIV-related outcomes across the HIV prevention and care continuum (e.g., PrEP use and adherence over time), as well as outcomes related to sexually transmitted infections and HIV comorbidities (e.g., cardiovascular disease).

Psychological Perspectives on the Origins of Mistrust

Given the profound impact of medical mistrust on the health of people at risk for and living with HIV, understanding the individual, interpersonal, and structural origins of medical mistrust is critical for developing ways to address medical mistrust and subsequent health outcomes. Much of the psychological research on the origins of mistrust views trust as a reflection of individuals' psychological disposition [66–68]. Consistent with this perspective, research on conspiracy beliefs indicates that some people have a personality type or tendency toward conspiratorial thinking [69, 70], such that those who believe in one conspiracy theory are more likely to believe in other conspiracy theories, regardless of content [71]. Research in this vein indicates that higher levels of conspiracy beliefs are associated with mistrust (of other people and authority) [69, 71, 72], as well as other traits such as low self-esteem [72], paranoia, delusion, and belief in the paranormal [69, 73, 74], biased, illogical, disordered cognitions or irrationality [69, 71], and narcissism [75]. However, suggesting ways to "persuade," "silence," and "cure" people who promote conspiracy beliefs [39] (as is stated in some of the psychological literature) delegitimizes individuals' perspectives rather than helps to understand how these beliefs may be rooted in historical and contemporary experiences of discrimination and injustice.

The psychological literature also suggests that the individual tendency to mistrust is a product of early life experiences with peers, parents, and teachers [76, 77], as well as experiences with discrimination across the lifespan [67, 77]. The sociological literature describes how the interplay between the physical and social environments create beliefs and behaviors that drive racial disparities [78]. Individuals who live in disadvantaged neighborhoods may be less trusting because high levels of disorder in their neighborhoods engender a sense of powerlessness that leads to social alienation and suspicion of others [79]. Children may be socialized by family members to be prepared to experience racial bias [80], which may help children to understand discrimination and may engender mistrust as a coping mechanism [81]. These factors may explain why many Black Americans and some other populations of color show higher levels of medical mistrust. In this chapter, we take the perspective that multiple levels of influence work in tandem to produce and maintain mistrust in communities.

Why Is Mistrust Associated with HIV Outcomes? A Multilevel Perspective

To understand the phenomenon of mistrust specifically among Black Americans and the effects of mistrust on HIV disparities, one must take into account context and use a multilevel social determinants approach in which individuals are embedded within social networks in communities and in the larger society, which creates, sustains, and reinforces mistrust [82]. According to our proposed model (Fig. 12.1),

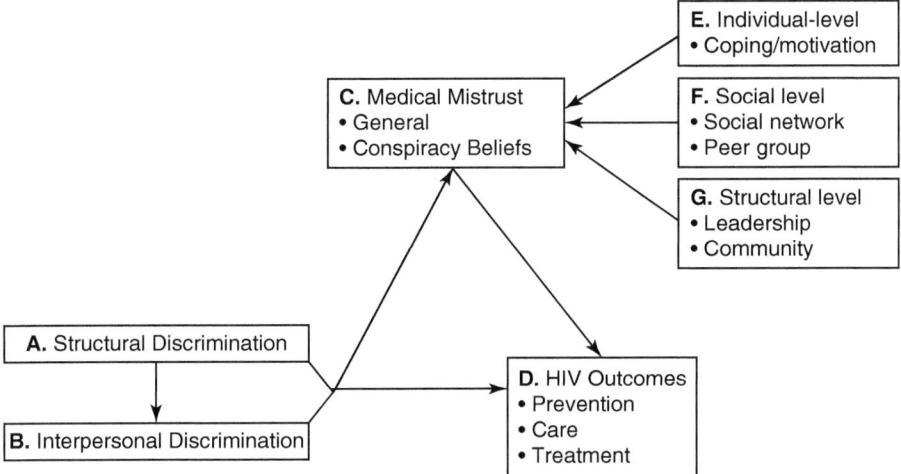

Fig. 12.1 Conceptual model of discrimination, medical mistrust, and HIV outcomes

current, ongoing structural discrimination (both at the societal level and within healthcare) has led to the development, spread, and maintenance of medical mistrust and HIV conspiracy beliefs within communities and social networks, and has additionally amplified the association between mistrust and health behaviors. Because inequities and mistreatment have continued, mistrust continues to be sustained in communities disproportionately affected by HIV [10].

Discrimination leads to mistrust (Boxes A, B, and C) The model begins with discrimination as the origin of mistrust: Structural discrimination (Box A) manifests historically and currently as policies and practices in society in general and in institutions (such as healthcare systems), and leads to interpersonal discrimination (Box B) by individuals (including healthcare providers) whose stereotypes and prejudicial beliefs may be directly influenced by societal/cultural beliefs and social network norms. General medical mistrust as well as HIV conspiracy beliefs (Box C) in turn stem from these experiences of discrimination at the structural and interpersonal levels, which in turn can affect HIV prevention, care, and treatment outcomes (Box D).

In support of the structural discrimination pathway, mistrust among Black Americans is thought to stem from knowledge of current and historical injustices in health care and US society in general, such as (but not limited to) unethical medical experimentation (e.g., the Tuskegee syphilis study) [83–89]. Empirically, knowledge of historical racial mistreatment and racism in the United States has been associated with greater belief in the plausibility of anti-Black conspiracies [90]. Notably, this association was shown among Black Americans in an observational study (who had greater historical knowledge about racial mistreatment and awareness of past racism such as the Tuskegee syphilis study, and therefore greater belief in conspiracy), as well as experimentally among White Americans (who were randomized to read information about historical racism such as Tuskegee syphilis study vs. about non-racial conspiracies such as the Iran–Contra affair) [90]. Furthermore, a mixed geographic and survey data analysis demonstrated that older Black men who lived closer to Macon County, Alabama (which contains Tuskegee), showed increased medical mistrust, substantially reduced inpatient and outpatient healthcare utilization, and increased mortality from before 1972 to after 1972 (when the Tuskegee syphilis study was publicly disclosed), controlling for changes in public health expenditures and hospital service availability during the two timeframes; the effect declined with greater distance from Macon County [86]. In addition, possibly because of their greater awareness of Black culture and the history of oppression, in another study, Black individuals who had a stronger sense of racial identity (i.e., racial centrality) reported higher discrimination in healthcare and medical mistrust compared to Black individuals who have a weaker sense of racial identity, and perceived discrimination mediated the association between racial identity and mistrust [91].

In support of the interpersonal discrimination pathway, research has found a direct association between discrimination (both anticipated and experienced) and medical mistrust [21, 33, 92–95]. Galvan and colleagues found that HIV-positive Latinx sexual minority men who experienced discrimination due to being HIV-positive or discrimination due to being Latinx were less likely to adhere to ART, and both of these associations were explained by general medical mistrust [94]. Another study of HIV-negative Black sexual minority men indicated that general medical mistrust mediated the association between healthcare-related perceived discrimination around sexual orientation and race (e.g., "I have been mistreated by healthcare providers because of my sexual orientation [race]") and longer time since last physical exam [96].

Mistrust is spread and sustained in individuals and communities via individual-, interpersonal-, and structural-level mechanisms (Boxes E, F, and G) When individuals and communities are faced with the external threat of discrimination, individual-, interpersonal-, and structural-level processes provide mechanisms by which mistrust arises and is maintained. At the *individual-level*, mistrust (including conspiracy beliefs) can serve as a functional coping mechanism that helps individuals to maintain a sense of meaning, control, and empowerment when in a state of threat or uncertainty [97, 98], allowing for the ability to respond better to unexpected situations [99]. This may be especially relevant for Black individuals, whose mistrust may serve as a protective and adaptive survival mechanism, or resilience resource, in the face of oppression [100]. Specifically, conspiracy beliefs have been conceptualized as coping strategies that fulfill epistemic, existential, and social psychological motivations [40, 98, 101]. *Epistemic motivation* is the desire for understanding when faced with uncertainty, such as when there is no clear, official explanation for complex events. *Existential motivation* is the desire for control and security when feeling threatened or powerless, such as when feeling alienated from official structures and the political system due to expectations of future mistreatment stemming from experiences with or awareness about current and historical mistreatment [72]. *Social motivation* is the desire to maintain a positive view of self or one's ingroup, including making external attributions to discrimination, to explain why one's group is low-status or underprivileged. Consistent with this motivational approach, correlational and experimental research indicates that conspiracy beliefs are associated with feelings of powerlessness and alienation [71, 72], need for cognitive closure (a drive toward order and structure and away from ambiguity and uncertainty, to restore and maintain perceived control) [102], and perceived lack of control [52, 70, 97, 98, 103]. Thus, conspiracy beliefs can help Black individuals to understand poverty, crime, health disparities, and other issues disproportionately affecting Black communities, as well as provide a sense of control, safety, empowerment, and racial pride against the threat of HIV, by attributing HIV to the external force of structural discrimination, including benign neglect and malicious intent by public officials (i.e., "system blame" of an unjust social system) [102, 104]; such attributions can in turn provide resilience and coping resources against discrimination.

At the *interpersonal level*, *social networks* are thought to be key factors in the origin and spread of conspiracies [39, 57, 105]. In the case of HIV, especially in communities with heightened medical mistrust, people may seek advice about HIV from social network members, who understand the context of discrimination and have reason to be suspicious of healthcare, and therefore are believed to be more credible sources than healthcare providers. Reliance on social network members may be especially relevant for Black communities, in which support from kin and trusted others is a key coping mechanism in the face of oppression [100]. For example, in a study examining HIV conspiracy beliefs within the social networks of Black individuals with HIV, Bogart and colleagues found that expression of conspiracy beliefs by similar others in the network (in terms of age, gender, HIV status, sexual orientation, and race/ethnicity) was associated with ART nonadherence [57]. Thus, mistrust may be especially influential when expressed by similar social network members. Moreover, conspiracy beliefs are more difficult to change in communities and social networks in which those who hold alternate viewpoints are unwilling to share their beliefs publicly due to fear of censure [106]. When alternate viewpoints are not discussed, individuals may believe that more people endorse conspiracies than actually do (a false consensus), which in turn can encourage more people to believe in conspiracies as an accepted perceived norm [39]. Thus, in Black communities, due to residential racial segregation as well as avoidance of external communities and other places where discrimination is anticipated [107], conspiracy beliefs may be more likely to be spread and be maintained. Addressing conspiracy beliefs by providing accurate information (e.g., about the biological origin of HIV or the effectiveness of ART) may not be effective, because such information comes from biomedical researchers and the public health system, which are the same entities believed to be conspiring against Black communities.

Mistrust and conspiracy beliefs also may be created and maintained through *societal structures*. Formal leaders, including elected officials and religious leaders, and informal popular opinion leaders such as artists may inject mistrust-related beliefs into communities through the media, popular culture (e.g., music), and the Internet, as well as in person through lectures and speeches (e.g., church sermons) [40, 108]. A particularly striking (non-US) example is the advancement of HIV conspiracy beliefs by the South African government, especially President Mbeki (e.g., that HIV does not cause AIDS and that the treatment is ineffective or harmful), and the government's subsequent failure to provide adequate treatment, which is estimated to have led to 330,000 deaths and 35,000 babies being born with HIV from 2000–2005 [109]. In the United States, research in Louisiana found that Black leaders (i.e., locally elected officials) were as likely to endorse HIV conspiracy beliefs as church congregants – and thus may serve as reinforcers of such beliefs in communities [43, 52]. In terms of the popular culture, well-known musicians have popularized HIV conspiracy theories in their lyrics, while others have used music as a medium to promote HIV knowledge and prevention [110]. Under our model (Fig. 12.1), we propose that formal and informal community leaders can infuse conspiracy beliefs and other forms of mistrust into communities; moreover, such beliefs may be maintained if community members have awareness of and direct experience with structural-level discrimination, and individual-level coping mechanisms support the motivation for such beliefs. Conversely, formal and informal leaders can also work to promote and infuse HIV prevention messages into popular culture in order to counteract inaccurate beliefs about HIV.

In sum, mistrust may be spread and maintained at the individual, interpersonal, and structural levels. These mechanisms are critical to understand as they suggest potential strategies to address mistrust.

Potential Intervention Approaches to Address Medical Mistrust

Our model of the mistrust process in Fig. 12.1 shows a number of possible intervention points to address mistrust at the individual, social, and structural levels. Importantly, any intervention to address medical mistrust would need to acknowledge first the historical and current context of discrimination in the United States as the root cause of such beliefs. Individual-level interventions can empower individuals to leverage their innate resilience resources to improve health in the face of real and persistent discrimination, and provide an outlet for individuals to discuss concerns and process experiences with discrimination. Individual-level interventions need to be conducted in a sensitive way that does not explicitly or implicitly blame the target of discrimination. Simultaneously, structural-level interventions are needed as a long-term strategy to enact societal change. The need for both individual- and structural-level interventions can be conceptualized with an analogy to a "burning building". If a building is on fire, it is necessary both to rescue the people inside (an individual-level intervention) and to extinguish the fire (a structural-level intervention); it is not sufficient only to rescue the people or only to extinguish the fire. Individual-level interventions are as necessary as structural-level interventions to address discrimination and mistrust at a societal level.

Overall, few interventions have been developed to improve trust in healthcare systems and providers, or reduce conspiracy beliefs, and much of those that exist have not been fully tested in randomized controlled trials and/or have shown small or non-significant effects. Below we review interventions that have been developed that have potential to be refined and tested in fully powered randomized controlled trials.

Individual-Level Interventions Individual-level interventions can provide a mechanism for individuals to process, discuss, and become aware of the harmful effects of discrimination and mistrust on their mental and physical health. We identified three interventions that address mistrust among people with HIV. These interventions are currently being tested or have yet to be tested for effects on mistrust; although results on mistrust are not yet available as of the writing of this chapter, we describe them as examples of how mistrust can be addressed using social or clinical psychological strategies for behavior change. Of note, none of the interventions aim to reduce levels of medical mistrust. The interventions implicitly or explicitly acknowledge mistrust as a survival mechanism and rational response to structural and interpersonal discrimination, and thus instructing participants to have less mistrust would be invalidating. Rather, these individual-level interventions attempt to disassociate mistrust and health outcomes by raising awareness about the effects of mistrust on health, and replacing inaccurate cognitions about care and treatment with accurate ones.

Rise is a culturally congruent, community-based intervention that uses non-confrontational, non-judgmental motivational interviewing (MI) strategies in one-on-one sessions to address ART adherence challenges among Black people with HIV [111, 112]. To address mistrust, *Rise* is conducted in a trusted community setting, outside of a healthcare facility, by peer counselors from clients' communities and cultures – and, thus, counselors are not viewed as part of the medical system or as medical authority figures. *Rise* counselors acknowledge up-front historical challenges, mistreatment, and discrimination in healthcare that have led to medical mistrust in communities of color, and discuss how discrimination and mistrust can be barriers to adherence. *Rise* counselors then ask for permission (using a motivational interviewing style) to provide accurate information about treatment and HIV to counteract incorrect beliefs. A main goal of *Rise* is to break the link between mistrust and nonadherence to treatment by recognizing the justifiable and rational reasons for mistrust, as well as by raising awareness about how mistrust can lead to poor health, and offering guidance and accurate information about treatment. An initial randomized controlled trial (NCT01350544) demonstrated large effects of *Rise* on adherence; a large randomized controlled trial (NCT03331978) is currently being conducted that will have greater statistical power to assess the mechanisms through which the intervention affects adherence, including via reduced medical mistrust.

A second intervention uses cognitive behavioral therapy (CBT) and dialectical behavioral therapy (DBT) principles to address coping with discrimination among Black and Latinx sexual minority men in group sessions led by peer facilitators [113, 114]. The intervention was named by community stakeholders *Still Climbin'* for Black men (after *Mother to Son*, a Langston Hughes poem about resilience), and *Siempre Seguiré* for Latinx men ("I will always continue," after *¿A Quién le Importa? ("Who Cares?")*, a popular song that has become a message of gay empowerment). The intervention aims to raise awareness about coping responses to discrimination and how ineffective coping responses may negatively affect one's health behaviors and outcomes. Specific to mistrust, facilitators provide information about how discrimination has led to health disparities and discuss medical mistrust as a coping and survival mechanism that has arisen as a response to discrimination. Clients learn how to recognize when mistrust may impede their desire to be healthy, by leading to lack of healthcare engagement (e.g., because they mistrust healthcare providers and expect to experience discrimination) and nonadherence (e.g., because they do not believe that healthcare providers are acting in patients' best interest). Clients also discuss how to channel their mistrust into activism for community change. Two in-progress randomized controlled trials are testing the effects of the intervention on HIV testing and PrEP use among Latinx sexual minority men (NCT04225832), and healthcare and receipt of evidence-based healthcare among Black sexual minority men, as well as how mistrust mediates intervention effects on these outcomes.

LINK LA (Linking Inmates to Care in LA), a peer navigation intervention for HIV-positive cisgender men and transgender women released from a large municipal jail system, showed effects on maintenance of viral load suppression from baseline to 12 months; effects on general medical mistrust were not measured [115]. The intervention's peer navigator component builds on patient navigation, helping low-income, vulnerable patients find their way through complex healthcare systems to obtain timely diagnosis and treatment [116, 117]. Rather than include professionals such as case managers, as is commonly done [118], to promote trust among clients living with HIV, LINK LA's model of peer navigation utilizes strictly lay staff who could be considered peers – specifically Black or Latinx navigators with similar experiences as post-incarcerated people living with HIV (e.g., incarceration, being a patient retained in HIV care, and prior substance abuse recovery). Peer navigators aim to problem solve and build knowledge, skills, and self-efficacy regarding HIV care engagement and treatment adherence, accompany patients to healthcare appointments, assist with subsistence needs, and promote social support and trusting relationships with healthcare providers. The intervention addresses discrimination from and mistrust toward any healthcare provider, including nurses, pharmacists, and doctors. To further increase trust, sessions are conducted while clients are incarcerated and in transition to the community, rather than primarily in healthcare venues.

Other non-HIV-related work has aimed to increase patients' trust in their personal healthcare provider through patient education, such as describing treatment-related advantages and disadvantages that are tailored to the patient's subgroup, or disclosing information about the patient's physician (e.g., around conflict of interest) to address concerns about physicians' ulterior motives and transparency [119–122]. However, such interventions have had small or non-significant effects on trust [5], have not been tailored for HIV, and, importantly, focus on increasing trust in one's own provider, rather than increasing trust and reducing mistrust regarding the medical system, treatment, and healthcare providers in general. Interventions that focus on patients' overall mistrust-related beliefs, generalizing beyond their own provider, have been scarce in the research literature.

Social Network–Level Interventions At the *social network level*, we could find only one intervention study that addressed medical mistrust around HIV. Derose and colleagues [123] conducted a pilot intervention study to decrease HIV stigma and HIV conspiracy beliefs, and to increase HIV testing among congregants and their social network members in Black and Latinx churches. To encourage change at the individual level, pastors delivered a sermon that incorporated theological reflection and an imagined contact scenario with a person living with HIV, using principles from the contact hypothesis (i.e., congregants were asked to imagine a positive interaction with someone with HIV), to increase empathy and decrease HIV stigma [124]. To encourage change at the church level, congregants participated in educational workshops on HIV, testing, and stigma, in which they discussed HIV-related misconceptions and conspiracy beliefs present in their communities, were offered accurate information, and watched video testimonials about HIV meant to increase empathy and decrease stigma through indirect "contact" [125]. To encourage change at the social network and community levels, peer leaders were invited to workshops that used role-plays on how to deliver accurate HIV-related information and encourage HIV testing to social network members in the congregation and community, and congregants and community members were offered HIV testing through congregation-based HIV testing events. Results indicated greater HIV testing in intervention vs. control churches, and reductions in stigma and medical mistrust (measured as HIV conspiracy beliefs) in some but not all churches, with larger effects on mistrust in intervention than control churches. However, this study was a pilot and insufficiently powered to examine reasons for reductions in mistrust in some churches and not others, and effects at the community and social network levels were not measured. Nevertheless, we believe that this intervention serves as a good model for future research on reducing mistrust in communities, using faith-based organizations as a vehicle.

Structural-Level Interventions *Healthcare Provider Interventions to Reduce Mistrust*: Interventions have been conducted at the healthcare provider level to reduce mistrust and increase trust in healthcare, doctors, and treatment. Similar to the patient interventions discussed above, a handful of *healthcare provider interventions* aiming to increase providers' cultural competency and empathy for patients, in order to increase patients' trust in their own provider, have generally not shown effects on increasing trust [5, 126, 127]. Moreover, such studies have not aimed to address general medical mistrust and have not been developed for HIV care specifically [5]. One study found small effects for trust in patients' own provider and providers' increased empathetic responses for an intensive intervention in which hospital oncologists were instructed on how to improve empathetic responses, based on personalized feedback about their own consultations [127]. However, because the intervention requires intensive efforts to tailor feedback after observing physicians' consultations with patients, it may be challenging to implement on a large scale; also, the study did not assess, and the intervention did not target, general medical mistrust in healthcare systems, providers, and treatments.

Other research suggests that increasing patient-centered communication, in which providers incorporate patients' needs, preferences, and personal circumstances into the medical visit interaction, could help to decrease the association between medical mistrust and health decisions (e.g., around cardiovascular disease) by increasing satisfaction with the provider-patient interaction [128]. Under the Necessity-Concerns Framework [129], such patient-centered communication may help to increase patients' perceptions that treatment is necessary ("necessity beliefs," e.g., that it is effective) and decrease concerns and mistrust around the treatment (including conspiracy beliefs), both of which have been associated with treatment nonadherence in HIV and non-HIV research [35–37, 130]. However, it is unknown the extent to which existing healthcare provider interventions, which focus on increasing trust in a patient's own provider, generalize to decreased medical mistrust overall, and whether such interventions would be effective for HIV care specifically.

One untested strategy suggested by prior formative work [131] would be to educate healthcare providers about how to respond to mistrust in a sensitive manner while conveying accurate information in a way that is understandable and accessible to non-clinicians. For example, a qualitative study on how peer educators in South Africa address mistrust found that peer educators, as trusted and credible community members, attempt to address mistrust by offering accurate information about HIV and treatment using creative strategies such as metaphors from everyday life, to make complex scientific information more accessible. In the study, peer educators were well-versed in (and came from) the same community context, and had familiar, relevant experiences (and sources of mistrust) from which metaphors could be drawn, thus creating better understanding as well as credible stories about HIV treatment. Nevertheless, peer educators expressed that metaphors were not always well understood or well received [131] – suggesting that interventions are needed to train peer educators to harness their skills to be more effective. Given prior research, we recommend that future work could test the effects on mistrust of training non-clinical and clinical healthcare providers in motivational interviewing strategies that acknowledge and respond to mistrust in non-judgmental, non-confrontational ways using relevant community language, stories, and experiences.

Interventions to Reduce Discrimination in Healthcare: Given our conceptual model that perceived discrimination in healthcare is directly related to mistrust, another strategy could be to reduce interpersonal discrimination in healthcare, and thereby reduce levels of mistrust among patients. Importantly, healthcare providers' behaviors toward patients may be influenced by cultural and societal stereotypes about patients' groups (including HIV and related intersecting stigmas, e.g., minority race/ethnicity and sexual minority orientation), both consciously and unconsciously (i.e., outside of their awareness and control, through implicit bias) [132]. In addition to making differential treatment decisions, providers may treat patients of some groups differently than others in subtle ways that are reflected in vocal tones or non-verbal behaviors that make patients feel uncomfortable asking questions, for example. An early vignette study on HIV and antiretroviral treatment decisions found that physicians were less likely to believe that people of certain groups (e.g., Black men) would be adherent, and perceptions of adherence affected treatment decisions [133, 134]. A more recent study found similar results for PrEP prescription decisions [135]. Moreover, a systematic review concluded that implicit bias among healthcare providers is as common as it is in the general population, and implicit bias among healthcare professionals has been correlated with diagnosis and treatment decisions and quality of care, mostly using simulated patient interaction and vignette methods (although a small amount of research has shown effects through direct observations of patient-provider interactions) [136–138]. Thus, intervening on healthcare providers' biases and differential treatment could help to improve patients' experiences in healthcare, which in turn can help to change patients' beliefs about physicians and treatment, and reduce medical mistrust among patients and in their social networks and communities.

Several studies have tested healthcare provider interventions around stigma and discrimination [130, 139–141]. A meta-analysis found moderate-quality evidence that a social-networks-based popular opinion leader intervention, in which healthcare providers who were perceived to be more influential were trained to deliver HIV stigma reduction messages, showed significant effects on reducing HIV stigma among healthcare providers in their networks, with sustained effects after 12 months in a randomized controlled trial [139–141]. The quality of evidence was deemed low for other types of healthcare provider interventions (e.g., information-based), given poor study designs including measurement bias (e.g., no control group, confounding factors) [139]. Moreover, the popular opinion leader intervention trial, while promising, did not assess effects on providers' behaviors with patients, patients' attitudes and mistrust about healthcare, or patients' health outcomes. Thus, further research is needed to examine whether such healthcare provider network interventions can successfully address patient mistrust and improve patient outcomes. Moreover, additional research is needed to tailor such interventions for subgroups of patients at risk for HIV, who are likely to have multiple intersecting stigmatized identities.

Summary of Intervention Research The literature on intervention research that directly addresses medical mistrust and healthcare discrimination is meager and rarely addresses HIV-related medical mistrust specifically; moreover, few studies have been conducted in the context of HIV care. Research that has aimed to reduce mistrust as related to HIV is still in the pilot stages, and studies of provider interventions are especially lacking.

Recommendations for Next Steps on Medical Mistrust and HIV Research

Based on our synthesis of the literature and model of discrimination, mistrust, and HIV outcomes in Fig. 12.1, we propose a number of next steps for the field of medical mistrust and HIV.

Intervene on structural and interpersonal discrimination (both in healthcare and in general) to address mistrust Of course, it is essential to change federal and state policies and actions that are discriminatory or that lead to discrimination around HIV and intersectional stigmas around, for example, race/ethnicity, sexual and gender minority status, and immigration status (e.g., ban on transgender people in the US military; law enforcement policies that promote mistreatment, excessive force, and racial profiling, such as stop-and-frisk and immigration raids). Moreover, community leaders and policymakers at the local and federal level should host discussions of the implications of such policies for HIV prevention and treatment, as well as honest dialogue around HIV, race/ethnicity, and sexual and gender identity. However, policy change can be slow, especially given unwillingness of some lawmakers to address such issues constructively. Thus, we also recommend developing, evaluating, and implementing multilevel interventions to address stigma among healthcare providers, and to engage peer counselors from HIV-affected communities to address mistrust. For example, community members can be trained to discuss HIV openly, accurately, and without stigma within social networks, outside of healthcare (e.g., in faith-based organizations; places of recreation and business, such as parks and barbershops), in order to serve as peer educators and navigators as a bridge to healthcare. In addition, community stakeholders should be engaged formally in healthcare systems, in positions of leadership, as providers, and on community advisory boards, to inform how treatment-related decisions could affect communities of color. For example, a community advisory board associated with a healthcare organization could be helpful in disseminating information about new treatments that have been shown to be effective and safe for people of color, as well as community input to inform healthcare providers about how to present new treatments to patients in a culturally informed way. Moreover, healthcare providers who are from patients' communities are more likely to be perceived to be trustworthy and to be perceived to work in the patients' interests than healthcare providers who are not from patients' communities (who may be perceived as having ulterior motives) – which requires a commitment of educational institutions at all levels to increase the pipeline of medical providers of color.

As discussed above, one promising avenue may be to engage community members such as peer counselors, navigators, and educators, who may be perceived to be more trustworthy and credible than healthcare providers about the roots of mistrust and history of oppression, as well as more knowledgeable about current negative experiences and conditions in communities [142]. Peers can be trained in evidence-based communication skills (such as motivational interviewing and non-confrontational ways to initiate conversations) to be change agents for reducing stigma and mistrust in their communities and social networks. Peer-based interventions could be developed based on established social network approaches, including identifying change agents within the network for HIV-related activism and education, who could direct their efforts toward those most at risk for HIV and most mistrustful of HIV-related information and healthcare [143, 144, 145]. In this way, peers and credible community members can serve as a bridge to healthcare, increasing patients' willingness to engage with prevention and care.

Intervene on mechanisms of sustained mistrust in order to break the link between mistrust and health outcomes As noted above, mistrust can be conceptualized as a coping mechanism, and coping mechanisms can be effective or ineffective, depending on the context. Thus, mistrust is not necessarily harmful. Lack of trust can be advantageous in some situations, such as when new medications have not been fully tested on racial/ethnic subgroups or when a local healthcare organization or provider has received complaints or is not rated highly on quality of care measures. Thus, rather than reducing mistrust, which can be a healthy coping mechanism when channeled effectively, interventions can be developed to break the association between mistrust and less healthful behaviors and outcomes, and to harness mistrust for positive effects. Research could be done to investigate potential positive effects of mistrust, such as catalyzing individuals to educate themselves about quality of care of local organizations to be informed consumers, as well as for sociopolitical change – i.e., to empower communities for collective action to challenge existing power structures, and to vote and elect local leaders who have concrete policies on addressing healthcare disparities. Indeed, some research suggests that those who are marginalized may be more likely to engage with the political process. For example, the 2016 National Survey on HIV in the Black community found that Black individuals who reported same-sex sexual behavior were more likely to intend to vote in the 2016 presidential election [146] – which may reflect a heightened sense of civic duty when communities believe that their rights are in jeopardy. Studies are needed to determine ways that mistrust can be channeled for action within the healthcare realm as well.

Conclusion

A great deal of research suggests that medical mistrust is rooted in awareness of and experiences with discrimination, and that medical mistrust contributes substantially to HIV disparities. Moreover, at its core, mistrust is a survival mechanism that can be healthy or unhealthy, depending on the context. However, research is in its infancy regarding interventions to address mistrust at the individual and structural levels. Our review suggests that research is needed on multilevel approaches to address mistrust, including interventions that engage healthcare providers, such as clinicians and peer counselors, to communicate in a non-judgmental and accepting fashion; that engage community members as change agents in their social networks; and that empower individuals to channel mistrust into taking control of their health and engaging in activism to benefit themselves and their communities.

Acknowledgments The writing of this chapter was supported by National Institute of Nursing Research (NINR) R01NR017334, National Institute of Mental Health (NIMH) and National Institute on Minority Health and Health Disparities (NIMHD) R01MH121256, by Office of the Director, National Institutes of Health and National Institute on Minority Health and Health Disparities R01MD014722, and by NIMH R34MH113413 and P30MH058107 (Bogart); by NIMH P30MH58107 and R01MH103076, National Institute of Drug Abuse (NIDA) R01DA039934, National Institute of Aging (NIA) P30AG021684, NINR R01NR4014789, and the UCLA Clinical and Translational Science Institute (CTSI) NIH/NCATS UL1-TR001881 (This chapter is dedicated to the memory of Dr. William E. Cunningham, who devoted his career to addressing health disparities affecting people of color); and by the VA Office of Academic Affiliations through the National Clinician Scholars Program (Takada). The contents do not represent the views of the United States Department of Veterans Affairs or the United States Government.

References

1. Institute of Medicine Committee on Understanding Eliminating Racial Ethnic Disparities in Health Care. In: Smedley BD, Stith AY, Nelson AR, editors. Unequal treatment: confronting racial and ethnic disparities in health care. Washington, D.C.: National Academies Press (US); 2003.
2. Hall MA, Dugan E, Zheng B, Mishra AK. Trust in physicians and medical institutions: what is it, can it be measured, and does it matter? Milbank Q. 2001;79(4):613–39.
3. Pearson SD, Raeke LH. Patients' trust in physicians: many theories, few measures, and little data. J Gen Intern Med. 2000;15(7):509–13.
4. Williamson LD, Bigman CA. A systematic review of medical mistrust measures. Patient Educ Couns. 2018;101(10):1786–94.
5. Rolfe A, Cash-Gibson L, Car J, Sheikh A, McKinstry B. Interventions for improving patients' trust in doctors and groups of doctors. Cochrane Database Syst Rev. 2014;3:CD004134.
6. LaVeist TA, Nickerson KJ, Bowie JV. Attitudes about racism, medical mistrust, and satisfaction with care among African American and White cardiac patients. Med Care Res Rev. 2000;57(1_suppl):146–61.
7. Graham JL, Giordano TP, Grimes RM, Slomka J, Ross M, Hwang L-Y. Influence of trust on HIV diagnosis and care practices: a literature review. J Int Assoc Physicians AIDS Care (Chic). 2010;9(6):346–52.
8. Bogart LM, Wagner G, Galvan FH, Banks D. Conspiracy beliefs about HIV are related to antiretroviral treatment nonadherence among African American men with HIV. J Acquir Immune Defic Syndr. 2010;53(5):648–55.
9. Earnshaw VA, Bogart LM, Dovidio JF, Williams DR. Stigma and racial/ethnic HIV disparities: moving toward resilience. Am Psychol. 2015;68(4):225–36.
10. Jaiswal J. Whose responsibility is it to dismantle medical mistrust? Future directions for researchers and health care providers. Behav Med. 2019;45(2):188–96.
11. Arnett M, Thorpe RJ, Gaskin D, Bowie J, LaVeist T. Race, medical mistrust, and segregation in primary care as usual source of care: findings from the exploring health disparities in integrated communities study. J Urban Health. 2016;93(3):456–67.
12. Armstrong K, McMurphy S, Dean LT, Micco E, Putt M, Halbert CH, et al. Differences in the patterns of health care system distrust between Blacks and Whites. J Gen Intern Med. 2008;23(6):827–33.

13. Kinlock BL, Parker LJ, Bowie JV, Howard DL, LaVeist TA, Thorpe RJ Jr. High levels of medical mistrust are associated with low quality of life among Black and White men with prostate cancer. Cancer Control. 2017;24(1):72–7.
14. Boulware LE, Cooper LA, Ratner LE, LaVeist TA, Powe NR. Race and trust in the health care system. Public Health Rep. 2016;118:358–65.
15. Halbert CH, Armstrong K, Gandy OH, Shaker L. Racial differences in trust in health care providers. Arch Intern Med. 2006;166(8):896–901.
16. Musa D, Schulz R, Harris R, Silverman M, Thomas SB. Trust in the health care system and the use of preventive health services by older Black and White adults. Am J Public Health. 2009;99(7):1293–9.
17. Brandon DT, Isaac LA, LaVeist TA. The legacy of Tuskegee and trust in medical care: is Tuskegee responsible for race differences in mistrust of medical care? J Natl Med Assoc. 2005;97(7):951–6.
18. O'Malley AS, Sheppard VB, Schwartz M, Mandelblatt J. The role of trust in use of preventive services among low-income African-American women. Prev Med. 2004;38(6):777–85.
19. LaVeist TA, Isaac LA, Williams KP. Mistrust of health care organizations is associated with underutilization of health services. Health Serv Res. 2009;44(6):2093–105.
20. Thompson HS, Valdimarsdottir HB, Winkel G, Jandorf L, Redd W. The Group-Based Medical Mistrust Scale: psychometric properties and association with breast cancer screening. Prev Med. 2004;38(2):209–18.
21. Hammond WP. Psychosocial correlates of medical mistrust among African American men. Am J Community Psychol. 2010;45(1–2):87–106.
22. Powell W, Richmond J, Mohottige D, Yen I, Joslyn A, Corbie-Smith G. Medical mistrust, racism, and delays in preventive health screening among African-American men. Behav Med. 2019;45(2):102–17.
23. Brenick A, Romano K, Kegler C, Eaton LA. Understanding the influence of stigma and medical mistrust on engagement in routine healthcare among Black women who have sex with women. LGBT Health. 2017;4(1):4–10.
24. Hammond WP, Matthews D, Mohottige D, Agyemang A, Corbie-Smith G. Masculinity, medical mistrust, and preventive health services delays among community-dwelling African-American men. J Gen Intern Med. 2010;25(12):1300–8.
25. Benkert R, Cuevas A, Thompson HS, Dove-Meadows E, Knuckles D. Ubiquitous yet unclear: a systematic review of medical mistrust. Behav Med. 2019;45(2):86–101.
26. Scharff DP, Mathews KJ, Jackson P, Hoffsuemmer J, Martin E, Edwards D. More than Tuskegee: understanding mistrust about research participation. J Health Care Poor Underserved. 2010;21(3):879–97.
27. Corbie-Smith G, Thomas SB, George DM. Distrust, race, and research. Arch Intern Med. 2002;162(21):2458–63.
28. Drake BF, Boyd D, Carter K, Gehlert S, Thompson VS. Barriers and strategies to participation in tissue research among African-American men. J Cancer Educ. 2017;32(1):51–8.
29. Khanna AS, Schneider JA, Collier N, Ozik J, Issema R, di Paola A, et al. A modeling framework to inform PrEP initiation and retention scale-up in the context of Getting to Zero Initiatives. AIDS. 2019;33(12):1911–22.
30. Underhill K, Morrow KM, Colleran C, Holcomb R, Calabrese SK, Operario D, et al. A qualitative study of medical mistrust, perceived discrimination, and risk behavior disclosure to clinicians by US male sex workers and other men who have sex with men: implications for biomedical HIV prevention. J Urban Health. 2015;92(4):667–86.
31. Tekeste M, Hull S, Dovidio JF, Safon CB, Blackstock O, Taggart T, et al. Differences in medical mistrust between Black and White women: implications for patient-provider communication about PrEP. AIDS Behav. 2018;23(7):1737–48.
32. Dale SK, Bogart LM, Wagner GJ, Galvan FH, Klein DJ. Medical mistrust is related to lower longitudinal medication adherence among African-American males with HIV. J Health Psychol. 2016;21(7):1311–21.

33. Thrasher AD, Earp JAL, Golin CE, Zimmer CR. Discrimination, distrust, and racial/ethnic disparities in antiretroviral therapy adherence among a national sample of HIV-infected patients. J Acquir Immune Defic Syndr. 2008;49(1):84–93.
34. Kutnick AH, Leonard NR, Gwadz MV. "Like I have no choice": a qualitative exploration of HIV diagnosis and medical care experiences while incarcerated and their effects. Behav Med. 2019;45(2):153–65.
35. Kalichman SC, Eaton L, Kalichman MO, Cherry C. Medication beliefs mediate the association between medical mistrust and antiretroviral adherence among African Americans living with HIV/AIDS. J Health Psychol. 2017;22(3):269–79.
36. Kalichman SC, Eaton L, Kalichman MO, Grebler T, Merely C, Welles B. Race-based medical mistrust, medication beliefs and HIV treatment adherence: test of a mediation model in people living with HIV/AIDS. J Behav Med. 2016;39(6):1056–64.
37. Pellowski JA, Price DM, Allen AM, Eaton LA, Kalichman SC. The differences between medical trust and mistrust and their respective influences on medication beliefs and ART adherence among African-Americans living with HIV. Psychol Health. 2017;32(9):1127–39.
38. Quinn KG, Kelly JA, DiFranceisco WJ, Tarima SS, Petroll AE, Sanders C, et al. The health and sociocultural correlates of AIDS genocidal beliefs and medical mistrust among African American MSM. AIDS Behav. 2018;22(6):1814–25.
39. Sunstein CR, Vermeule A. Conspiracy theories: causes and cures. J Polit Philos. 2009;17(2):202–27.
40. Douglas KM, Uscinski JE, Sutton RM, Cichocka A, Nefes T, Ang CS, et al. Understanding conspiracy theories. Polit Psychol. 2019;40(S1):3–35.
41. Heller J. Rumors and realities: making sense of HIV/AIDS conspiracy narratives and contemporary legends. Am J Public Health. 2015;105(1):e43–50.
42. Bogart LM, Thorburn S. Are HIV/AIDS conspiracy beliefs a barrier to HIV prevention among African Americans? J Acquir Immune Defic Syndr. 2005;38(2):213–8.
43. Parsons S, Simmons W, Shinhoster F, Kilburn J. A test of the grapevine: an empirical examination of conspiracy theories among African Americans. Sociol Spectr. 1999;19(2):201–22.
44. Eaton LA, Kalichman SC, Price D, Finneran S, Allen A, Maksut J. Stigma and conspiracy beliefs related to pre-exposure prophylaxis (PrEP) and interest in using PrEP among Black and White men and transgender women who have sex with men. AIDS Behav. 2017;21(5):1236–46.
45. Hoyt MA, Rubin LR, Nemeroff CJ, Lee J, Huebner DM, Proeschold-Bell RJ. HIV/AIDS-related institutional mistrust among multiethnic men who have sex with men: effects on HIV testing and risk behaviors. Health Psychol. 2012;31(3):269–77.
46. Westergaard RP, Beach MC, Saha S, Jacobs EA. Racial/ethnic differences in trust in health care: HIV conspiracy beliefs and vaccine research participation. J Gen Intern Med. 2014;29(1):140–6.
47. Hutchinson AB, Begley EB, Sullivan P, Clark HA, Boyett BC, Kellerman SE. Conspiracy beliefs and trust in information about HIV/AIDS among minority men who have sex with men. J Acquir Immune Defic Syndr. 2007;45(5):603–5.
48. Olansky E, Mansergh G, Pitts N, Mimiaga MJ, Denson DJ, Landers S, et al. PrEP awareness in the context of HIV/AIDS conspiracy beliefs among Black/African American and Hispanic/Latino MSM in three urban US cities. J Homosex. 2019;67:1–11.
49. Ross MW, Essien EJ, Torres I. Conspiracy beliefs about the origin of HIV/AIDS in four racial/ethnic groups. J Acquir Immune Defic Syndr. 2006;41(3):342–4.
50. Bogart LM, Ransome Y, Allen W, Higgins-Biddle MBO. HIV-related medical mistrust, HIV testing, and HIV risk in the National Survey on HIV in the Black community. Behav Med. 2019;45(2):134–42.
51. Bogart LM, Thorburn S. Relationship of African Americans' sociodemographic characteristics to belief in conspiracies about HIV/AIDS and birth control. J Natl Med Assoc. 2006;98(7):1144–50.
52. Simmons WP, Parsons S. Beliefs in conspiracy theories among African Americans: a comparison of elites and masses. Soc Sci Q. 2005;86(3):582–98.

53. Gillman J, Davila J, Sansgiry S, Parkinson-Windross D, Miertschin N, Mitts B, et al. The effect of conspiracy beliefs and trust on HIV diagnosis, linkage, and retention in young MSM with HIV. J Health Care Poor Underserved. 2013;24(1):36–45.
54. Bogart LM, Galvan FH, Wagner GJ, Klein DJ. Longitudinal association of HIV conspiracy beliefs with sexual risk among Black males living with HIV. AIDS Behav. 2011;15(6):1180–6.
55. Bohnert AS, Latkin CA. HIV testing and conspiracy beliefs regarding the origins of HIV among African Americans. AIDS Patient Care STDs. 2009;23(9):759–63.
56. Brooks RA, Allen VC Jr, Regan R, Mutchler MG, Cervantes-Tadeo R, Lee S-J. HIV/AIDS conspiracy beliefs and intention to adopt preexposure prophylaxis among Black men who have sex with men in Los Angeles. Int J STD AIDS. 2018;29(4):375–81.
57. Bogart LM, Wagner GJ, Green HD Jr, Mutchler MG, Klein DJ, McDavitt B, et al. Medical mistrust among social network members may contribute to antiretroviral treatment nonadherence in African Americans living with HIV. Soc Sci Med. 2016;164:133–40.
58. Jaiswal J, Singer SN, Siegel K, Lekas H-M. HIV-related 'conspiracy beliefs': lived experiences of racism and socio-economic exclusion among people living with HIV in New York City. Cult Health Sex. 2019;21(4):373–86.
59. Mattocks KM, Gibert C, Fiellin D, Fiellin LE, Jamison A, Brown A, et al. Mistrust and endorsement of human immunodeficiency virus conspiracy theories among human immunodeficiency virus–infected African American veterans. Mil Med. 2017;182(11):e2073–e9.
60. Ford CL, Wallace SP, Newman PA, Lee S-J, Cunningham E. Belief in AIDS-related conspiracy theories and mistrust in the government: relationship with HIV testing among at-risk older adults. Gerontologist. 2013;53(6):973–84.
61. Ball K, Lawson W, Alim T. Medical mistrust, conspiracy beliefs & HIV related behavior among African Americans. J Psychol Behav Sci. 2013;1(1):1–7.
62. Brincks AM, Shiu-Yee K, Metsch LR, del Rio C, Schwartz RP, Jacobs P, et al. Physician mistrust, medical system mistrust, and perceived discrimination: associations with HIV care engagement and viral load. AIDS Behav. 2019;23(10):2859–69.
63. Gaston GB, Alleyne-Green B. The impact of African Americans' beliefs about HIV medical care on treatment adherence: a systematic review and recommendations for interventions. AIDS Behav. 2013;17(1):31–40.
64. Clark A, Mayben JK, Hartman C, Kallen MA, Giordano TP. Conspiracy beliefs about HIV infection are common but not associated with delayed diagnosis or adherence to care. AIDS Patient Care STDs. 2008;22(9):753–9.
65. Jaiswal J, Singer SN, Griffin Tomas M, Lekas HM. Conspiracy beliefs are not necessarily a barrier to engagement in HIV care among urban, low-income people of color living with HIV. J Racial Ethn Health Disparities. 2018;5(6):1192–201.
66. Bartholomew K, Horowitz LM. Attachment styles among young adults: a test of a four-category model. J Pers Soc Psychol. 1991;61(2):226–44.
67. Smith SS. Race and trust. Ann Rev Sociol. 2010;36(1):453–75.
68. Rotter JB. Generalized expectancies for interpersonal trust. Am Psychol. 1971;26(5):443–52.
69. Brotherton R, French CC, Pickering AD. Measuring belief in conspiracy theories: the generic conspiracist beliefs scale. Front Psychol. 2013;4(279):1–15.
70. Goreis A, Voracek M. A systematic review and meta-analysis of psychological research on conspiracy beliefs: field characteristics, measurement instruments, and associations with personality traits. Front Psychol. 2019;10(205):1–13.
71. Goertzel T. Belief in conspiracy theories. Polit Psychol. 1994;15(4):731–42.
72. Abalakina-Paap M, Stephan WG, Craig T, Gregory WL. Beliefs in conspiracies. Polit Psychol. 1999;20(3):637–47.
73. Darwin H, Neave N, Holmes J. Belief in conspiracy theories. The role of paranormal belief, paranoid ideation and schizotypy. Pers Individ Differ. 2011;50(8):1289–93.
74. Oliver JE, Wood TJ. Conspiracy theories and the paranoid style(s) of mass opinion. Am J Polit Sci. 2014;58(4):952–66.
75. Cichocka A, Marchlewska M, de Zavala AG. Does self-love or self-hate predict conspiracy beliefs? Narcissism, self-esteem, and the endorsement of conspiracy theories. Soc Psychol Personal Sci. 2016;7(2):157–66.

76. Rotter JB. A new scale for the measurement of interpersonal trust. J Pers. 1967;35(4):651–65.
77. Yeager DS, Purdie-Vaughns V, Garcia J, Apfel N, Brzustoski P, Master A, et al. Breaking the cycle of mistrust: wise interventions to provide critical feedback across the racial divide. J Exp Psychol. 2014;143(2):804–24.
78. Noguera PA. The trouble with Black boys: the role and influence of environmental and cultural factors on the academic performance of African American males. Urban Educ. 2003;38(4):431–59.
79. Ross CE, Mirowsky J, Pribesh S. Powerlessness and the amplification of threat: neighborhood disadvantage, disorder, and mistrust. Am Sociol Rev. 2001;66(4):568–91.
80. Hughes D. Correlates of African American and Latino parents' messages to children about ethnicity and race: a comparative study of racial socialization. Am J Community Psychol. 2003;31(1):15–33.
81. Hughes D, Chen L. When and what parents tell children about race: an examination of race-related socialization among African American families. Appl Dev Sci. 1997;1(4):200–14.
82. Jaiswal J, Halkitis PN. Towards a more inclusive and dynamic understanding of medical mistrust informed by science. Behav Med. 2019;45(2):79–85.
83. Gamble VN. Under the shadow of Tuskegee: African Americans and health care. Am J Public Health. 1997;87(11):1773–8.
84. Washington HA. Medical apartheid: the dark history of medical experimentation on Black Americans from colonial times to the present. New York: Doubleday Books; 2006.
85. King WD. Examining African Americans' mistrust of the health care system: expanding the research question. Commentary on "Race and trust in the health care system". Public Health Rep. 2003;118(4):366–7.
86. Alsan M, Wanamaker M. Tuskegee and the health of black men. Q J Econ. 2017;133(1):407–55.
87. Brandt AM. Racism and research: the case of the Tuskegee Syphilis Study. Hast Cent Rep. 1978;8(6):21–9.
88. Jones JH. Bad blood. London: Simon and Schuster; 1993.
89. Thomas SB, Quinn SC. The Tuskegee Syphilis Study, 1932 to 1972: implications for HIV education and AIDS risk education programs in the Black community. Am J Public Health. 1991;81(11):1498–505.
90. Nelson JC, Adams G, Branscombe NR, Schmitt MT. The role of historical knowledge in perception of race-based conspiracies. Race Soc Probl. 2010;2(2):69–80.
91. Cuevas AG, O'Brien K. Racial centrality may be linked to mistrust in healthcare institutions for African Americans. J Health Psychol. 2017;24(14):2022–30.
92. Hausmann LR, Kwoh CK, Hannon MJ, Ibrahim SA. Perceived racial discrimination in health care and race differences in physician trust. Race Soc Probl. 2013;5(2):113–20.
93. Kalichman S, Katner H, Banas E, Kalichman M. Population density and AIDS-related stigma in large-urban, small-urban, and rural communities of the southeastern USA. Prev Sci. 2017;18(5):517–25.
94. Galvan FH, Bogart LM, Klein DJ, Wagner GJ, Chen Y-T. Medical mistrust as a key mediator in the association between perceived discrimination and adherence to antiretroviral therapy among HIV-positive Latino men. J Behav Med. 2017;40(5):784–93.
95. Oakley LP, López-Cevallos DF, Harvey SM. The association of cultural and structural factors with perceived medical mistrust among young adult Latinos in rural Oregon. Behav Med. 2019;45(2):118–27.
96. Eaton LA, Driffin DD, Kegler C, Smith H, Conway-Washington C, White D, et al. The role of stigma and medical mistrust in the routine health care engagement of Black men who have sex with men. Am J Public Health. 2015;105(2):e75–82.
97. Newheiser A-K, Farias M, Tausch N. The functional nature of conspiracy beliefs: examining the underpinnings of belief in the Da Vinci Code conspiracy. Pers Indiv Differ. 2011;51(8):1007–11.
98. van Prooijen JW, Acker M. The influence of control on belief in conspiracy theories: conceptual and applied extensions. Appl Cogn Psychol. 2015;29(5):753–61.

99. Schul Y, Mayo R, Burnstein E. The value of distrust. J Exp Soc Psychol. 2008;44(5):1293–302.
100. Wyatt GE. Enhancing cultural and contextual intervention strategies to reduce HIV/AIDS among African Americans. Am J Public Health. 2009;99(11):1941–5.
101. Douglas KM, Sutton RM, Cichocka A. The psychology of conspiracy theories. Curr Dir Psychol Sci. 2017;26(6):538–42.
102. Rae J, Ball PhD K, Jeffers M, Sharlene L, Lawson M, DLFAPA P, et al. Medical mistrust, HIV-related conspiracy beliefs, and the need for cognitive closure among urban-residing African American women: an exploratory study. J Health Dispar Res Pract. 2018;11(4):138–48.
103. Whitson JA, Galinsky AD. Lacking control increases illusory pattern perception. Science. 2008;322(5898):115–7.
104. Crocker J, Luhtanen R, Broadnax S, Blaine BE. Belief in US government conspiracies against Blacks among Black and White college students: powerlessness or system blame? Personal Soc Psychol Bull. 1999;25(8):941–53.
105. Adams LM, Simoni JM. The need for multi-level mitigation of medical mistrust among social network members contributing to antiretroviral treatment nonadherence in African Americans living with HIV: comment on Bogart et al.(2016). Soc Sci Med. 2016;159:58–60.
106. Portes A. Social capital: its origins and applications in modern sociology. Ann Rev Sociol. 1998;24(1):1–24.
107. Bogart LM, Dale SK, Christian J, Patel K, Daffin GK, Mayer KH, et al. Coping with discrimination among HIV-positive Black men who have sex with men. Cult Health Sex. 2017;19(7):723–37.
108. Nattrass N. Understanding the origins and prevalence of AIDS conspiracy beliefs in the United States and South Africa. Sociol Health Illn. 2013;35(1):113–29.
109. Chigwedere P, Seage GR III, Gruskin S, Lee T-H, Essex M. Estimating the lost benefits of antiretroviral drug use in South Africa. J Acquir Immune Defic Syndr. 2008;49(4):410–5.
110. Rattani A, Syed RH, Sugarman J. HIV prevention and hip hop: what's the spin? Music Med. 2015;7(1):32–45.
111. Wagner GJ, Bogart LM, Mutchler MG, McDavitt B, Mutepfa KD, Risley B. Increasing antiretroviral adherence for HIV-positive African Americans (Project Rise): a treatment education intervention protocol. JMIR Res Protoc. 2016;5(1):e45.
112. Bogart LM, Mutchler MG, McDavitt B, Klein DJ, Cunningham WE, Goggin KJ, et al. A randomized controlled trial of Rise, a community-based culturally congruent adherence intervention for Black Americans living with HIV. Ann Behav Med. 2017;51(6):868–78.
113. Bogart LM, Dale SK, Daffin GK, Patel KN, Klein DJ, Mayer KH, et al. Pilot intervention for discrimination-related coping among HIV-positive Black sexual minority men. Cultur Divers Ethnic Minor Psychol. 2018;24(4):541–51.
114. Bogart LM, Galvan FH, Leija J, MacCarthy S, Klein DJ, Pantalone D. A pilot intervention addressing coping with discrimination among HIV-positive Latino sexual minority men. In Press. Annals of LGBTQ Public and Population Health.
115. Cunningham WE, Weiss RE, Nakazono T, Malek MA, Shoptaw SJ, Ettner SL, et al. Effectiveness of a peer navigation intervention to sustain viral suppression among HIV-positive men and transgender women released from jail: the LINK LA randomized clinical trial. JAMA Intern Med. 2018;178(4):542–53.
116. Bradford JB, Coleman S, Cunningham W. HIV System Navigation: an emerging model to improve HIV care access. AIDS Patient Care STDs. 2007;21(S1):S-49–58.
117. Higa DH, Marks G, Crepaz N, Liau A, Lyles CM. Interventions to improve retention in HIV primary care: a systematic review of US studies. Curr HIV/AIDS Rep. 2012;9(4):313–25.
118. Metsch LR, Feaster DJ, Gooden L, Matheson T, Stitzer M, Das M, et al. Effect of patient navigation with or without financial incentives on viral suppression among hospitalized patients with HIV infection and substance use: a randomized clinical trial. JAMA. 2016;316(2):156–70.
119. Pearson SD, Kleinman K, Rusinak D, Levinson W. A trial of disclosing physicians' financial incentives to patients. Arch Intern Med. 2006;166(6):623–8.

120. Nannenga MR, Montori VM, Weymiller AJ, Smith SA, Christianson TJ, Bryant SC, et al. A treatment decision aid may increase patient trust in the diabetes specialist. The Statin Choice randomized trial. Health Expect. 2009;12(1):38–44.
121. Clancy DE, Cope DW, Magruder KM, Huang P, Salter KH, Fields AW. Evaluating group visits in an uninsured or inadequately insured patient population with uncontrolled type 2 diabetes. Diabetes Educ. 2003;29(2):292–302.
122. Hall MA, Dugan E, Balkrishnan R, Bradley D. How disclosing HMO physician incentives affects trust. Health Aff. 2002;21(2):197–206.
123. Derose KP, Griffin BA, Kanouse DE, Bogart LM, Williams MV, Haas AC, et al. Effects of a pilot church-based intervention to reduce HIV stigma and promote HIV testing among African Americans and Latinos. AIDS Behav. 2016;20(8):1692–705.
124. Crisp RJ, Turner RN. Can imagined interactions produce positive perceptions?: reducing prejudice through simulated social contact. Am Pychol. 2009;64(4):231–40.
125. Pettigrew TF, Tropp LR. A meta-analytic test of intergroup contact theory. J Pers Soc Psychol. 2006;90(5):751–83.
126. Thom DH, Tirado MD, Woon TL, McBride MR. Development and evaluation of a cultural competency training curriculum. BMC Med Educ. 2006;6:38.
127. Tulsky JA, Arnold RM, Alexander SC, Olsen MK, Jeffreys AS, Rodriguez KL, et al. Enhancing communication between oncologists and patients with a computer-based training program: a randomized trial. Ann Intern Med. 2011;155(9):593–601.
128. Cuevas AG, O'Brien K, Saha S. Can patient-centered communication reduce the effects of medical mistrust on patients' decision making? Health Psychol. 2019;38(4):325–33.
129. Clifford S, Barber N, Horne R. Understanding different beliefs held by adherers, unintentional nonadherers, and intentional nonadherers: application of the necessity–concerns framework. J Psychosom Res. 2008;64(1):41–6.
130. Linn AJ, van Weert JC, van Dijk L, Horne R, Smit EG. The value of nurses' tailored communication when discussing medicines: exploring the relationship between satisfaction, beliefs and adherence. J Health Psychol. 2016;21(5):798–807.
131. Rubincam C. Peer educators' responses to mistrust and confusion about HIV and AIDS science in Khayelitsha. Cape Town: University of Cape Town; 2014. Available from: https://open.uct.ac.za/handle/11427/7879.
132. Dovidio JF, Penner LA, Albrecht TL, Norton WE, Gaertner SL, Shelton JN. Disparities and distrust: the implications of psychological processes for understanding racial disparities in health and health care. Soc Sci Med. 2008;67(3):478–86.
133. Bogart LM, Catz SL, Kelly JA, Benotsch EG. Factors influencing physicians' judgments of adherence and treatment decisions for patients with HIV disease. Med Decis Mak. 2001;21(1):28–36.
134. Bogart LM, Kelly JA, Catz SL, Sosman JM. Impact of medical and nonmedical factors on physician decision making for HIV/AIDS antiretroviral treatment. J Acquir Immune Defic Syndr. 2000;23(5):396–404.
135. Calabrese SK, Earnshaw VA, Underhill K, Hansen NB, Dovidio JF. The impact of patient race on clinical decisions related to prescribing HIV pre-exposure prophylaxis (PrEP): assumptions about sexual risk compensation and implications for access. AIDS Behav. 2014;18(2):226–40.
136. FitzGerald C, Hurst S. Implicit bias in healthcare professionals: a systematic review. BMC Med Ethics. 2017;18(1):1–18.
137. Hall WJ, Chapman MV, Lee KM, Merino YM, Thomas TW, Payne BK, et al. Implicit racial/ethnic bias among health care professionals and its influence on health care outcomes: a systematic review. Am J Public Health. 2015;105(12):e60–76.
138. Cooper LA, Roter DL, Carson KA, Beach MC, Sabin JA, Greenwald AG, et al. The associations of clinicians' implicit attitudes about race with medical visit communication and patient ratings of interpersonal care. Am J Public Health. 2012;102(5):979–87.

139. Feyissa GT, Lockwood C, Woldie M, Munn Z. Reducing HIV-related stigma and discrimination in healthcare settings: a systematic review of quantitative evidence. PLoS One. 2019;14(1):e0211298.
140. Wu S, Li L, Wu Z, Liang L-J, Cao H, Yan Z, et al. A brief HIV stigma reduction intervention for service providers in China. AIDS Patient Care STDs. 2008;22(6):513–20.
141. Li L, Wu Z, Liang L-J, Lin C, Guan J, Jia M, et al. Reducing HIV-related stigma in health care settings: a randomized controlled trial in China. Am J Public Health. 2013;103(2):286–92.
142. Natale-Pereira A, Enard KR, Nevarez L, Jones LA. The role of patient navigators in eliminating health disparities. Cancer. 2011;117(S15):3541–50.
143. Valente TW. Network interventions. Science. 2012;337(6090):49–53.
144. Valente TW, Palinkas LA, Czaja S, Chu K-H, Brown CH. Social network analysis for program implementation. PLoS One. 2015;10(6):e0131712.
145. Bogart LM, Matovu JK, Wagner GJ, Green HD, Storholm ED, Klein DJ, Marsh T, MacCarthy S, Kambugu A. A Pilot Test of Game Changers, a Social Network Intervention to Empower People with HIV to be Prevention Advocates in Uganda. AIDS and Behavior. 2020;6:1–9.
146. McGregor AJ, Bogart LM, Higgins-Biddle M, Strolovitch DZ, Ojikutu B. Marginalized yet mobilized: exploring the association between LGBT status, LGBT support, and voting intentions among African Americans in the 2016 election. Du Bois Rev. 2019;16:1–26.

Chapter 13
Incarceration and the HIV Epidemic

Ank Nijhawan, Nicholas Campalans, and Emily Hoff

Introduction

In this chapter, we provide an overview of the overlapping epidemics of incarceration and HIV and how they impact communities of color. First, we provide a brief overview of the epidemiology of incarceration itself – the epidemiology of HIV within the criminal justice (CJ) system – and review some of the interpersonal-, community-, and system-level factors that contribute to high rates of HIV among CJ-involved individuals. Second, we review HIV prevention in jails and prisons, including the evidence for behavioral and biomedical HIV prevention interventions. Third, we examine the HIV care cascade, extending from diagnosis to linkage to care, retention in care, antiretroviral therapy (ART), and virologic suppression in CJ-involved individuals, including key gaps in the cascade and differences in outcomes by race and ethnicity. Fourth, we examine the issue of re-entry, including the multiple barriers people living with HIV (PLWH) face after incarceration which impact continuity of HIV care and treatment. Lastly, we discuss the issue of stigma for CJ-involved PLWH, which may occur during and after incarceration, including the intersectional stigma and discrimination associated with being a racial or ethnic minority, sexual minority, and someone who has been incarcerated. Finally, we conclude with future directions, including national policies which aim to decrease

A. Nijhawan (✉)
Division of Infectious Diseases, University of Texas Southwestern Medical Center,
Dallas, TX, USA
e-mail: Ank.Nijhawan@Utsouthwestren.edu

N. Campalans
University of Texas Southwestern Medical Center, Dallas, TX, USA

E. Hoff
University of Texas Southwestern Medical Center/Parkland Health and Hospital Systems,
Dallas, TX, USA

© Springer Nature Switzerland AG 2021   233
B. O. Ojikutu, V. E. Stone (eds.), *HIV in US Communities of Color*,
https://doi.org/10.1007/978-3-030-48744-7_13

overall incarceration in the USA and promising partnerships and interventions to address health disparities in this vulnerable population.

Epidemiology of Incarceration and HIV and the Impact on Communities of Color

Epidemic of Incarceration in the USA

The USA incarcerates a larger proportion of its population than any other country in the world. Approximately 707/100,000 individuals are incarcerated in the USA, whereas other countries like Russia, the UK, and Finland incarcerate 474, 148, and 58 per 100,000, respectively [1]. Currently, about 2.1 million people are in US jails and prisons and another 4.5 million are on probation or parole [2]. People are detained in jails for relatively short periods of time (typically weeks to months), and the majority will return to the community from jail. Individuals in prison are incarcerated for longer periods, usually for years, though the majority will also return to the community. These data highlight not only the overall magnitude of the impact of incarceration on the US population as a whole, but also the potential impact on communities (family structure, economic, workforce, public health, public safety) as large numbers of individuals are removed from and later return to their local communities.

Epidemiology of Incarceration by Geography, Race/Ethnicity

Incarceration does not impact communities across the USA equally. For example, southern US states have the highest incarceration rates (157,000 behind bars in Texas, a rate of 553/100,000; Louisiana has 33,000 in prison, a rate of 719/100,000). The ratio of black:white prisoners in both of these states are 4:1 and Hispanic:whites in Texas is 1.2:1. Other parts of the country have much lower rates of incarceration, but more pronounced racial and ethnic disparities. For example, Minnesota has a state imprisonment rate of 151/100,000, though the ratio of black:white is 11:1 and Hispanic:white is 2.6:1 [3]. It is estimated that on average 1 in 100 adults are incarcerated in the USA at any given time [4], though this varies widely by demographic groups. For women, 1 in 265 is incarcerated at any given time, whereas for men, 1 in 54 is incarcerated. Race and ethnicity also play a role, with white men (1 in 106) incarcerated less often than Hispanic men (1 in 36) and black men (1 in 15). When examining lifetime likelihood of imprisonment, 1 in 3 black men (versus 1 in 6 Latino men, 1 in 17 white men). Will be incarcerated during theirs [5, 6] understanding the differential impact of mass incarceration on communities of color is key to understanding and addressing health disparities in these groups.

Prevalence of HIV in Jails and Prisons

One in seven PLWH pass through jail or prison each year [5]. As a result, the prevalence of HIV in the CJ system is three to five times higher than in the general population. Based on data from the Bureau of prisons, HIV prevalence is 1.3% in prison [7], and certain incarcerated groups have higher HIV prevalence, including those in jail rather than prison, women, and black individuals [8]. Though limited data exist on men who have sex with men who are incarcerated, per a study of over 1500 black men who have sex with men (MSM) enrolled in an HIV prevention trial, 60% had been incarcerated in their lifetime [9]. Similarly, a history of recent arrest was more common among black MSM compared to white MSM (OR 1.6). MSM who reported an arrest history were less likely to identify as homosexual and reported more substance use and HIV sexual risk than those were not arrested in the past 12 months [10]. Therefore, within the already elevated HIV risk group of incarcerated individuals, subgroups such as black MSM may be at even higher risk of acquiring HIV.

Factors Contributing to Overlap of HIV and Incarceration

The reason for the high prevalence of HIV in US jails and prisons are multifold. Many of the risk factors associated with incarceration may directly or indirectly place individuals at risk for HIV. With the "war on drugs" and mandatory minimum sentencing laws beginning in the 1970s, many individuals with substance use disorder were incarcerated. Whether through injection drug use or high-risk sexual encounters while using drugs or alcohol, substance use is also associated with increased risk of HIV acquisition [11]. In addition, trading sex for drugs or money increases the risk for both incarceration and HIV. Communities highly impacted by incarceration often have high rates of poverty, violence, and low male:female gender ratios [12]. When a large proportion of eligible men in a community are incarcerated, there are higher rates of concurrent partnerships, which can increase the risk of sexually transmitted infections (STIs) as well as HIV, especially in limited social and sexual networks [13, 14]. Barriers to medical treatment such as medical mistrust among communities of color and limited access to medical care in underserved areas can lead to high rates of undiagnosed STIs and HIV (which are often asymptomatic), facilitating the spread of disease [15]. For these reasons, there is substantial overlap in the communities most heavily impacted by incarceration and HIV.

Incarceration, HIV, and Health Disparities

With high rates of incarceration in communities of color, where HIV and other health outcomes are already suboptimal compared to white populations [16], health disparities are perpetuated by the disruptive nature of incarceration. For PLWH, there are often interruptions in HIV treatment at the time of arrest. Though the time spent in jail or prison may be a period of relative stability from a healthcare perspective, with regular access to medical care and medications, the gains made during incarceration are usually lost after release. In fact, rates of engagement in HIV care, treatment with ART, and virologic suppression after incarceration are lower than they were before incarceration, indicating a net negative effect [17]. In addition to the individual health impact of incarceration on PLWH, incarceration increases the risk of HIV acquisition in communities with high rates of incarceration. In a study of 9 southern US cities, a 10 person increase in the prison release rate in a given zip code was associated with a 4% increase in HIV diagnoses [18]. Therefore, in order to decrease disparities in the HIV outcomes between communities of color and their white counterparts, dedicated efforts to addressing HIV prevention, testing, care, and treatment in justice-involved individuals and communities are needed [19].

HIV Prevention in CJ Settings

Approaches to HIV Prevention in CJ System

CJ settings represent a key venue for implementing HIV prevention strategies. Multiple studies demonstrate that upon return to the community, released individuals engage in high-risk sexual and injection risk behaviors, often in the context of significant psychosocial and environmental stressors [20–22]. Therefore, the time period immediately following incarceration is characterized by increased HIV acquisition and transmission. Incarceration represents a reachable moment where people are temporarily removed from community stressors and are able to engage in HIV prevention education and intervention. HIV prevention interventions aim to identify those at risk of HIV infection and use a multimodal approach including behavioral education, risk reduction, and biomedical methods that can indirectly and directly prevent HIV infection.

HIV Prevention: Behavioral Interventions

Different psychosocial interventions focused on HIV prevention have been tested in individuals at risk for HIV either within the CJ system or with justice-involved individuals in the community.

These interventions are based on various theories, including motivational interviewing, health belief model, transtheoretical model, and social cognitive models. A systematic review of randomized controlled trials (RCTs) and quasi-RCTs published in 2014 identified 37 different prevention studies with CJ-involved populations, including 26 of psychosocial interventions conducted in the USA [23].

Strategies included HIV education, negotiation skills, peer education, HIV testing and counseling, case management, training on condom use, needle cleaning, and intimate partner violence intervention. These interventions were mainly delivered one-on-one to individuals, though some were in group sessions.

Behavioral Outcomes and Changes in HIV Knowledge and Attitudes

Most psychosocial interventions examined changes in sexual risk behavior—condomless sexual intercourse, condom use, transactional sex, sex under the influence of drugs or alcohol—and some studies also measured self-reported frequency of injection drug use. Several studies reported a decrease in condomless sex [23–26] and increases in condom use [27, 28] with other studies finding a decrease in transactional sex [29]. With regards to injection drug use, one study showed a decrease in the frequency of injection through methadone maintenance [30] treatment or case management. None of the published behavioral intervention studies for HIV prevention were designed with long-term follow-up to detect biological endpoints (STIs, HIV), though in studies which did measure these outcomes, there was no significant impact of behavioral interventions on STI or HIV incidence. Other HIV prevention studies in incarcerated populations have focused on education as a means of achieving intermediate endpoints such as increasing HIV/AIDS knowledge, reducing misconceptions about HIV, improving understanding of risk reduction strategies, and increasing HIV testing. Many of these educational interventions were peer-led and interactive [31]. Most educational interventions showed a significant increase in HIV knowledge [32–34], while others also noted changes in attitudes toward condom use and increases in condom self-efficacy [32, 35]. One intervention also showed a doubling of requests for HIV testing among those completing a peer-led educational intervention [36].

Gaps in HIV Prevention Behavioral Interventions in CJ-Involved

Overall, psychosocial and educational interventions focused on HIV prevention were feasible and demonstrated changes in risk behavior, knowledge, and attitudes around HIV, both in the incarcerated setting and through programs which included CJ-involved populations after release. However, important gaps in the literature remain. There are limited data in the USA on the implementation of prevention tools within jails and prisons, since very few programs offer condoms and access to clean needles or sterilization supplies [37, 38]. Also, few studies focused on sexual or gender minorities or described interventions tailored to race or ethnic group, though up to 50% of participants in prevention studies are African American. One prevention study focused solely on black MSM [39]. A separate ongoing trial is studying the implementation of a group-based computerized HIV/STI and intimate partner violence prevention intervention focused on African-American women who use drugs and are in the CJ system [40]. These data will help inform the acceptability, feasibility, and efficacy of an intervention tailored to specific racial or ethnic groups.

Biomedical HIV Prevention – Substance Use Treatment

The majority of the published literature focused on HIV prevention in CJ populations using biomedical methods involves treatment for opiate use disorder, such as methadone [41–43] or buprenorphine [44, 45]. Through treatment of substance use disorder, individuals can decrease their HIV risk by reducing substance use and specifically injection drug use (including sharing needles, reusing needles) as well as by decreasing sexual risk such as condomless sex while under the influence of drugs or exchange of sex for drugs or money [44]. In addition, through treatment of opiate use disorder for those who are living with HIV, improved HIV virological outcomes have implications for secondary HIV prevention and extended-release naltrexone, an opioid antagonist that has been shown to improve or maintain virologic suppression in PLWH with opioid use disorder and alcohol use disorder released from prison [46, 47].

Biomedical HIV Prevention – Pre-exposure Prophylaxis

Pre-exposure prophylaxis, or PrEP, an effective biomedical tool for HIV prevention and a key pillar to ending the HIV epidemic, has been understudied in CJ-involved populations. Interest in PrEP is high among incarcerated women [48]; however, despite HIV risk factors among this group, awareness and use of PrEP are low. Incarcerated MSM also report a high level of risk for HIV acquisition, low level of PrEP knowledge, but the majority are interested in PrEP. A pilot study that is examining linkage to community-based PrEP for women who have been incarcerated is ongoing [49]. Additional studies are needed to evaluate the implementation of this evidence-based strategy in the CJ system, including identifying best practices for the timing of HIV and PrEP screening and linkage to PrEP care; developing standards of care for PrEP care tailored to different CJ settings [50]; and educating CJ medical staff about PrEP and evaluating which PrEP methods (injections, pills, vaginal rings) are most feasible and acceptable in this setting. The focus of current research has been on PrEP provided in the community setting, given elevated risk of HIV acquisition in the community and limited data on HIV transmission during incarceration [51, 52]. Given the geographic and racial/ethnic disparities in the uptake of PrEP [53], with low rates of PrEP use among African American and Latinx MSM in the South, implementation of PrEP care with CJ-involved populations has the potential to have a large impact on these disparities.

HIV Care Cascade Prior to, During, and After Incarceration

Impact of Incarceration on HIV Care Cascade

The HIV care cascade extends from HIV testing to linkage to HIV care, retention in care, receipt of ART, and finally viral suppression [54]. A systematic review of the literature found that overall, PLWH entering jails and prisons have lower rates of being aware of HIV infection, being engaged in care, receiving treatment, and being virologically suppressed at the time of incarceration than the general population. Though each step of the care cascade improved substantially during incarceration, often exceeding community rates for each care cascade milestone, these same measures decreased to levels below where they were prior to incarceration, i.e., lower engagement in care, ART receipt, and virologic suppression, after release, indicating a net negative effect of incarceration on HIV outcomes [17]. These data highlight not only the elevated need for HIV care and treatment that newly incarcerated individuals have but also the disruptive nature of incarceration on an individual's health. The decline in HIV care, treatment, and virologic suppression after incarceration perpetuates existing racial/ethnic disparities, as communities of color are more affected by incarceration, resulting in increased HIV transmission in these vulnerable communities [14, 18, 55].

HIV Testing in Jails and Prisons

Testing individuals for HIV who are entering the CJ system has a high potential impact given the elevated prevalence of HIV and generally low rates of routine health care engagement in this patient population. HIV testing in jails and prisons has been demonstrated to be acceptable and feasible [56], including rapid point-of-care tests. The Centers for Disease Control and Prevention recommends offering HIV testing to all CJ-involved individuals using a routine, opt-out method. A study conducted in the Washington state Department of Corrections showed that offering HIV testing using an opt-out testing approach resulted in higher uptake of testing (70–100%) than either opt-in (60–90%) or voluntary testing (under 20%) [57]. However, per a recent survey, only 35% of jails and 19% of prisons offer opt-out HIV testing [58]. These gaps in testing represent an important missed opportunity, particularly for sexual and racial minorities. A study examining reasons for low rates of HIV testing among black MSM identified deficiencies in HIV testing services in correctional facilities, along with stigma and discrimination, as an important structural barrier to accessing HIV testing [59].

HIV Care, Treatment, and Viral Suppression in CJ System

Though HIV testing in the CJ system is important for identifying previously undiagnosed infections, many testing studies identify PLWH who had a previously known HIV infection but were not engaged in care [60, 61]. Incarceration therefore represents a key opportunity to re-engage PLWH in HIV treatment. Many PLWH entering jails and prisons have either never linked to HIV care (44%) or have not been retained in care (60%), with the majority not actively taking ART prior to incarceration and 79% have a detectable viral load [17]. Individuals who are incarcerated are legally entitled to the same level of medical care as is available in the community, including HIV treatment and care. A survey of correctional facilities indicated that the majority (92%) do offer HIV treatment [62] to inmates, though some gaps remain. During incarceration, a large proportion of PLWH will achieve an undetectable viral load, and the likelihood of this outcome increases with the duration of incarceration [63].

Disparities in HIV Care Cascade Within Incarcerated Population

However, certain subgroups are less likely to achieve these outcomes than others. For example, among HIV-positive jail entrants, black individuals had more advanced HIV disease than other HIV-positive inmates [64]. In a large multicenter demonstration grant of incarcated PLWH, young (under age 30) black MSM, were less likely to have health insurance, access to a care provider before incarceration, receive disease management interventions during incarceration or link to HIV care after jail release in a large multicenter demonstration project of incarcerated PLWH [65]. Given the disruptive nature of incarceration and the over-representation of minorities, the criminal justice system can worsen existing health disparities in PLWH.

Re-entry

Transition from Incarceration to Community

The transition from incarceration back to the community, or re-entry, is a particularly challenging and vulnerable time period which involves balancing personal needs and obligations imposed by community supervision. For many, securing necessities, such as housing, transportation, and employment, represent challenges which precede medical care in Maslow's hierarchy of needs [66]. Obtaining access to medical care after discharge from a correctional facility is hindered by suspension of Medicaid benefits for incarcerated individuals, disproportionately impacting states which did not expand Medicaid under the Affordable Care Act [67, 68]. Furthermore, relapse to substance use is common and during the 2 weeks following incarceration, mortality is over 12-fold higher than in the general population, a statistic that is mostly driven by overdose deaths [69].

Re-entry Barriers and HIV

PLWH often experience addition barriers while transitioning back into their communities. Homelessness, substance use disorders, mental illness, stigma, and loss of social or medical benefits are common barriers to continuing HIV care after release [70–73]. In addition, the first several weeks to months after incarceration is characterized by risk behaviors which may increase HIV transmission including unprotected sex, exchanging sex for drugs or money, and sharing needles [12, 15, 55]. Given the key strategy of treatment as prevention, where undetectable HIV viral load translates into untransmittable HIV to others, these findings highlight the public health implications of uninterrupted HIV treatment across the continuum from corrections to community-based HIV care.

Linkage to HIV Care Post-incarceration

Systematic measurement of linkage to HIV care after incarceration is limited by electronic medical records and health systems in jails and prisons which are not connected to the community systems. However, when linkage to care has been evaluated through various research programs and demonstration projects, estimates of linkage to HIV care in the community vary widely by setting. For example, only 34% of incarcerations among PLWH which resulted in release from the Dallas County Jail were followed by a clinic visit within 90 days [74]. Data from Rhode Island and North Carolina show that 43% and 49%, respectively, linked to HIV care within 90 days after prison release [75]. The control arm in research study may also provide an indication of baseline linkage to HIV care, with 70% of PLWH linked to care within 90 days in a Maryland study of intensive case management for probationers/parolees [76], and 78% linked to care within 3 months in a randomized controlled trial of case management after release from prison in North Carolina [77]. However, given the varying resources for discharge planning and care coordination in different settings and enhanced retention efforts in the context of a research trial, it is difficult to make meaningful comparisons between these groups.

Linkage to Post-incarceration HIV Care Interventions

Several interventions focused on improving linkage to post-incarceration HIV care have been evaluated, though with mixed results. Intensive case management has been proposed as a potential intervention to improve linkage to care and achieve viral suppression for PLWH transitioning out of correctional facilities [70], and several non-randomized studies have shown a positive impact on linkage to care [78]. A multicenter demonstration project involving various site-specific interventions (e.g., needs assessment, counseling, discharge planning) found that 79% of released inmates linked to HIV care within 1 month [79]. Also, a study of patient navigation with enhanced case management after jail release found significant increases in linkage to HIV care and sustained retention in the intervention arm [80]. However, a randomized controlled trial of intensive case management was no more successful than standard discharge planning in healthcare utilization post-release [77]. Similarly, a different study of intensive case management showed no difference in linkage to HIV care among probationers/parolees [76], though both of these studies had very high linkage to care rates in the treatment as usual arm.

Post-incarceration Viral Suppression Interventions

Subsequent studies have included viral load as an outcome. Intensive case management with motivational interviewing and mobile phone support produced no difference in viral load suppression over the treatment as usual group among individuals released from prison [81]. However, a different randomized trial found that peer navigation resulted in higher rates of sustained viral load suppression in PLWH released from jail [82]. Improving our understanding of which interventions will be successful in a given setting may inform future adaptations of these interventions. For example, high recidivism rates which limit interpretation of community outcomes may argue for a combined medical-legal intervention. Also, patients released from jails (which have rapid turnover, small time window for intervention but local release) may benefit from caretain interventions, such as in person navigation efforts, whereas those released from prisons (longer stays, more opportunity for medical stabilization and discharge planning, but release to a wide geographical area) may need the flexibility of virtiual care coordination. Despite generally suboptimal rates of re-engagement in HIV care after jail release outside of the context of a research study, there are certain racial/ethnic groups which may experience differences in outcomes. In Dallas, whites and African Americans living with HIV were less likely to link to care within 90 days of release than Latinx PLWH [74]. However, an intervention study in California found that Latinx individuals were less likely to link to post-release HIV care [80].

HIV-Related Stigma and Relationship with Clinical Outcomes

According to the CDC, HIV-related stigma refers to "negative beliefs, feelings and attitudes towards people living with HIV, their families, people who work with them and members of groups that have been heavily impacted by HIV, such as gay and bisexual men, homeless people, street youth, and mentally ill people" [83]. Though experiences with stigma have decreased since the beginning of the HIV epidemic [84], many PLWH continue to experience stigma, significantly impacting quality of life, social relationships, and clinical outcomes. Data from the medical monitoring project, with a nationally representative group of PLWH, found that 79% endorsed ≥1 HIV-related stigma statement and stigma was especially prevalent among PLWH under age 50 and Latinx [85]. Stigma is associated with social isolation [86] and depression and negatively impacts physical health [87, 88]. Among African-American women living with HIV, both perceived and internalized stigma correlated with depression [89]. HIV-related stigma also has implications for HIV prevention and care, as stigma has been associated with lower likelihood of disclosing HIV status to a partner [87, 90], less engagement in medical care [91], poorer medication adherence [88, 92], and increased viral load [93].

Stigma and Discrimination During Incarceration

PLWH who are incarcerated may be additionally stigmatized. A survey among prison inmates being offered HIV testing revealed high levels of HIV-related fear, stigma, homophobia, and incomplete understanding of HIV transmission [94]. In addition to other inmates, stigmatizing attitudes against PLWHA may come from correctional staff [95, 96]. During incarceration, PLWH may be assigned segregated housing or be treated differently from the general population in terms of diet, job opportunities, and medication access, leading to increased stigma [97]. Stigma during incarceration can impact willingness to be tested for HIV and/or for PLWH to disclose their HIV status [95], thereby interfering with HIV care, treatment, and treatment outcomes [98]. In one study of incarcerated men and transgender women, interpersonal violence and a lack of safety and perceived threats to privacy were cited as barriers to care and adherence to ART while incarcerated [99]. A qualitative study described incarcerated PLWH avoiding care since particular doctors were associated with HIV. They feared seeking treatment would indicate their status to other inmates and correctional staff and compromise their safety [100].

Intersectional Stigma During Re-entry

Upon release from incarceration, PLWH may face additional, intersectional stigma including discrimination or fear of discrimination related to being a minority, having a history of incarceration, and having HIV. HIV-positive African-American men with a history of incarceration described feeling inadequate, isolated, and dangerous due to their HV status. They also reported traveling long distances to access medical and social services to avoid being seen by people they may know, or not using services altogether [101]. Mental health issues such as depression and anxiety, which carry their own stigma, may compound this issue, increasing internalized stigma and avoidance of care [102]. Sexual orientation can also contribute to feeling stigmatized, and black MSM specifically report inadequate access to culturally competent services, stigma, and discrimination that impede access to services, deficiency of services in correctional institutions, and limited services in areas where black MSM live [59]. Lastly, given the overlap between substance use and CJ involvement, stigma associated with substance use can have a substantial impact on PLWH released from incarceration, and anticipated substance use stigma is associated with decreased adherence to HIV medications. Overall, the potential for stigma in various forms and related to different issues to affect and serve as a barrier to HIV care for PLWH released from incarceration is very high.

Summary

In sum, the overlapping epidemics of incarceration and HIV have created a public health crisis, perpetuating and worsening HIV health disparities for people of color. We have reviewed the epidemiology of both of these epidemics as well as some of the contributing factors, such as sentencing policies around drug use, poverty, violence, imbalance in gender ratios, concurrent partnerships, discrimination, and medical mistrust, which contribute to the overlap of HIV and criminal justice involvement. We review HIV prevention interventions, both behavioral and biomedical (including substance use treatment and PrEP) in this setting, including the pressing need to expand these efforts. We also examine the HIV care cascade – including testing; engagement in care; and virologic suppression before, during, and after incarceration – to identify persistent gaps and the impact on racial and ethnic minorities. We specifically focus on re-entry, and the need for new, culturally competent, patient-centered interventions to improve very low rates of re-engagement in care after incarceration. Lastly, we briefly discuss the overlapping stigma, as both overt discrimination and internalized stigma, related to HIV, incarceration, being a racial and/or sexual minority, mental health, and substance use.

Future Directions

The current rate of incarceration in the USA is not only destructive to highly impacted communities but it is also financially unsustainable. There is bipartisan governmental support for criminal justice reform, and in the context of the current opioid epidemic with rising numbers of overdose deaths, policymakers are exploring alternatives to incarceration such as intensive substance use treatment. In addition, partnerships between departments of public health and corrections are important cornerstones for improving HIV prevention, treatment, retention in care, and virologic outcomes, and these partnerships will be critical to achieve the goals established in the *Ending the HIV Epidemic* National Plan [103]. Additional focus on the transition from incarceration to community is needed, including universal discharge planning and care coordination with involvement of peer navigators as well as medical-legal partnerships which provide integrated services focused on improving clinical outcomes while also reducing recidivism. With regards to stigma, the CDC has outlined efforts to combat HIV-related stigma which include building capacity nationwide for a HIV prevention workforce that is aware of and actively combatting stigma, increasing monitoring of stigma and research on stigma, and disseminating stigma reduction communication campaigns [104]. Include "ban the box", an initiative in which employers remove the requirement for job applicants to disclose prior criminal justice involvement, as well as expungement of criminal records [105]. Lastly, public health providers and academic researchers are needed to implement innovative approaches to HIV care in this setting, including expansion of integrated HIV and substance use disorder treatment services and evaluation of long-acting injectable antiretroviral therapies in the CJ system and shared electronic health records between the CJ system and the community.

References

1. Council NR. Jeremy Travis BW, Redburn S, editors. The growth of incarceration in the United States: exploring causes and consequences (2014). Washington, D.C.: The National Academies Press. p. 2014.
2. Kaeble D, Cowhig M. Correctional populations in the United States, 2016. Washington, D.C.: Department of Justice, Office of Justice Programs; 2018.
3. Project TS. State by state data Washington DC 2019 [Source: US Bureau of Justice Statistics data for 2017]. Available from: https://www.sentencingproject.org/the-facts/#map.
4. Trusts PC. One in 100: behind bars in America 2008. Available from: https://www.pewtrusts.org/-/media/legacy/uploadedfiles/pcs_assets/2008/one20in20100pdf.pdf.
5. Spaulding AC, Seals RM, Page MJ, Brzozowski AK, Rhodes W, Hammett TM. HIV/AIDS among inmates of and releases from US correctional facilities, 2006: declining share of epidemic but persistent public health opportunity. PLoS One. 2009;4(11):e7558.
6. Bonczar TP. Prevalence of Imprisonment in the US Population, 1974-2001. Washington, D.C.: US Department of Justice; 2003.
7. Laura M Maruschak. HIV in prisons, 2001-2010. Washington, D.C.: US Department of Justice; 2015.
8. Beckwith CG, Zaller ND, Fu JJ, Montague BT, Rich JD. Opportunities to diagnose, treat, and prevent HIV in the criminal justice system. J Acquir Immune Defic Syndr. 2010;55(Suppl 1):S49–55.
9. Brewer RA, Magnus M, Kuo I, Wang L, Liu TY, Mayer KH. The high prevalence of incarceration history among Black men who have sex with men in the United States: associations and implications. Am J Public Health. 2014;104(3):448–54.
10. Lim JR, Sullivan PS, Salazar L, Spaulding AC, Dinenno EA. History of arrest and associated factors among men who have sex with men. J Urban Health. 2011;88(4):677–89.

11. Altice FL, Kamarulzaman A, Soriano VV, Schechter M, Friedland GH. Treatment of medical, psychiatric, and substance-use comorbidities in people infected with HIV who use drugs. Lancet. 2010;376(9738):367–87.
12. Khan MR, Golin CE, Friedman SR, Scheidell JD, Adimora AA, Judon-Monk S, et al. STI/HIV sexual risk behavior and prevalent STI among incarcerated African American men in committed partnerships: the significance of poverty, mood disorders, and substance use. AIDS Behav. 2015;19(8):1478–90.
13. Adimora AA, Schoenbach VJ, Doherty IA. Concurrent sexual partnerships among men in the United States. Am J Public Health. 2007;97(12):2230–7.
14. Khan MR, Behrend L, Adimora AA, Weir SS, Tisdale C, Wohl DA. Dissolution of primary intimate relationships during incarceration and associations with post-release STI/HIV risk behavior in a Southeastern city. Sex Transm Dis. 2011;38(1):43–7.
15. Adams JW, Lurie MN, King MRF, Brady KA, Galea S, Friedman SR, et al. Potential drivers of HIV acquisition in African-American women related to mass incarceration: an agent-based modelling study. BMC Public Health. 2018;18(1):1387.
16. Crepaz N, Dong X, Wang X, Hernandez AL, Hall HI. Racial and ethnic disparities in sustained viral suppression and transmission risk potential among persons receiving HIV care - United States, 2014. MMWR Morb Mortal Wkly Rep. 2018;67(4):113–8.
17. Iroh PA, Mayo H, Nijhawan AE. The HIV care Cascade before, during, and after incarceration: a systematic review and data synthesis. Am J Public Health. 2015;105(7):e5–16.
18. Ojikutu BO, Srinivasan S, Bogart LM, Subramanian SV, Mayer KH. Mass incarceration and the impact of prison release on HIV diagnoses in the US South. PLoS One. 2018;13(6):e0198258.
19. Rich JD, DiClemente R, Levy J, Lyda K, Ruiz MS, Rosen DL, et al. Correctional facilities as partners in reducing HIV disparities. J Acquir Immune Defic Syndr. 2013;63(Suppl 1):S49–53.
20. Belenko S, Langley S, Crimmins S, Chaple M. HIV risk behaviors, knowledge, and prevention education among offenders under community supervision: a hidden risk group. AIDS Educ Prev. 2004;16(4):367–85.
21. Green TC, Pouget ER, Harrington M, Taxman FS, Rhodes AG, O'Connell D, et al. Limiting options: sex ratios, incarceration rates, and sexual risk behavior among people on probation and parole. Sex Transm Dis. 2012;39(6):424–30.
22. Adams LM, Kendall S, Smith A, Quigley E, Stuewig JB, Tangney JP. HIV risk behaviors of male and female jail inmates prior to incarceration and one year post-release. AIDS Behav. 2013;17(8):2685–94.
23. Underhill K, Dumont D, Operario D. HIV prevention for adults with criminal justice involvement: a systematic review of HIV risk-reduction interventions in incarceration and community settings. Am J Public Health. 2014;104(11):e27–53.
24. Martin SS, O'Connell DJ, Inciardi JA, Surratt HL, Maiden KM. Integrating an HIV/HCV brief intervention in prisoner reentry: results of a multisite prospective study. J Psychoactive Drugs. 2008;40(4):427–36.
25. Weir BW, O'Brien K, Bard RS, Casciato CJ, Maher JE, Dent CW, et al. Reducing HIV and partner violence risk among women with criminal justice system involvement: a randomized controlled trial of two motivational interviewing-based interventions. AIDS Behav. 2009;13(3):509–22.
26. Wolitski RJ, Group PSW. Relative efficacy of a multisession sexual risk–reduction intervention for young men released from prisons in 4 states. Am J Public Health. 2006;96(10):1854–61.
27. Eldridge GD, St Lawrence JS, Little CE, Shelby MC, Brasfield TL, Service JW, et al. Evaluation of the HIV risk reduction intervention for women entering inpatient substance abuse treatment. AIDS Educ Prev. 1997;9(1 Suppl):62–76.
28. Lurigio AJ, Petraitis J, Johnson BR. Joining the front line against HIV: an education program for adult probationers. AIDS Educ Prev. 1992;4(3):205–18.

29. Sacks JY, McKendrick K, Hamilton Z. A randomized clinical trial of a therapeutic community treatment for female inmates: outcomes at 6 and 12 months after prison release. J Addict Dis. 2012;31(3):258–69.

30. Dolan KA, Shearer J, White B, Zhou J, Kaldor J, Wodak AD. Four-year follow-up of imprisoned male heroin users and methadone treatment: mortality, re-incarceration and hepatitis C infection. Addiction. 2005;100(6):820–8.

31. Valera P, Chang Y, Lian Z. HIV risk inside U.S. prisons: a systematic review of risk reduction interventions conducted in U.S. prisons. AIDS Care. 2017;29(8):943–52.

32. Bryan A, Robbins RN, Ruiz MS, O'Neill D. Effectiveness of an HIV prevention intervention in prison among African Americans, Hispanics, and Caucasians. Health Educ Behav. 2006;33(2):154–77.

33. Fasula AM, Fogel CI, Gelaude D, Carry M, Gaiter J, Parker S. Project power: adapting an evidence-based HIV/STI prevention intervention for incarcerated women. AIDS Educ Prev. 2013;25(3):203–15.

34. Fogel CI, Crandell JL, Neevel AM, Parker SD, Carry M, White BL, et al. Efficacy of an adapted HIV and sexually transmitted infection prevention intervention for incarcerated women: a randomized controlled trial. Am J Public Health. 2015;105(4):802–9.

35. Bauserman RL, Richardson D, Ward M, Shea M, Bowlin C, Tomoyasu N, et al. HIV prevention with jail and prison inmates: Maryland's prevention case management program. AIDS Educ Prev. 2003;15(5):465–80.

36. Ross MW, Harzke AJ, Scott DP, McCann K, Kelley M. Outcomes of project wall talk: an HIV/AIDS peer education program implemented within the Texas State Prison System. AIDS Educ Prev. 2006;18(6):504–17.

37. Hammett TM, Harmon P, Maruschak LM. 1996-1997 update: HIV/AIDS, STDs, and TB in correctional facilities. Washington, D.C.: US Department of Justice; 1999.

38. Tucker JD, Chang SW, Tulsky JP. The catch 22 of condoms in US correctional facilities. BMC Public Health. 2007;7:296.

39. Harawa NT, Brewer R, Buckman V, Ramani S, Khanna A, Fujimoto K, et al. HIV, sexually transmitted infection, and substance use continuum of care interventions among criminal justice-involved Black men who have sex with men: a systematic review. Am J Public Health. 2018;108(S4):e1–9.

40. Welle D, Falkin GP, Jainchill N. Current approaches to drug treatment for women offenders. Project WORTH. Women's options for recovery, treatment, and health. J Subst Abus Treat. 1998;15(2):151–63.

41. Kinlock TW, Gordon MS, Schwartz RP, O'Grady K, Fitzgerald TT, Wilson M. A randomized clinical trial of methadone maintenance for prisoners: results at 1-month post-release. Drug Alcohol Depend. 2007;91(2-3):220–7.

42. Magura S, Lee JD, Hershberger J, Joseph H, Marsch L, Shropshire C, et al. Buprenorphine and methadone maintenance in jail and post-release: a randomized clinical trial. Drug Alcohol Depend. 2009;99(1–3):222–30.

43. McKenzie M, Zaller N, Dickman SL, Green TC, Parihk A, Friedmann PD, et al. A randomized trial of methadone initiation prior to release from incarceration. Subst Abus. 2012;33(1):19–29.

44. Brown R, Gassman M, Hetzel S, Berger L. Community-based treatment for opioid dependent offenders: a pilot study. Am J Addict. 2013;22(5):500–2.

45. Cropsey KL, Lane PS, Hale GJ, Jackson DO, Clark CB, Ingersoll KS, et al. Results of a pilot randomized controlled trial of buprenorphine for opioid dependent women in the criminal justice system. Drug Alcohol Depend. 2011;119(3):172–8.

46. Springer SA, Di Paola A, Barbour R, Azar MM, Altice FL. Extended-release naltrexone improves viral suppression among incarcerated persons living with HIV and alcohol use disorders transitioning to the community: results from a double-blind, placebo-controlled trial. J Acquir Immune Defic Syndr. 2018;79(1):92–100.

47. Springer SA, Di Paola A, Azar MM, Barbour R, Biondi BE, Desabrais M, et al. Extended-release naltrexone improves viral suppression among incarcerated persons living with HIV with opioid use disorders transitioning to the community: results of a double-blind, placebo-controlled randomized trial. J Acquir Immune Defic Syndr. 2018;78(1):43–53.
48. Rutledge R, Madden L, Ogbuagu O, Meyer JP. HIV risk perception and eligibility for pre-exposure prophylaxis in women involved in the criminal justice system. AIDS Care. 2018;30(10):1282–9.
49. Ramsey SE, Ames EG, Brinkley-Rubinstein L, Teitelman AM, Clarke J, Kaplan C. Linking women experiencing incarceration to community-based HIV pre-exposure prophylaxis care: protocol of a pilot trial. Addict Sci Clin Pract. 2019;14(1):8.
50. Brinkley-Rubinstein L, Dauria E, Tolou-Shams M, Christopoulos K, Chan PA, Beckwith CG, et al. The path to implementation of HIV pre-exposure prophylaxis for people involved in criminal justice systems. Curr HIV/AIDS Rep. 2018;15(2):93–5.
51. Jafa K, McElroy P, Fitzpatrick L, Borkowf CB, MacGowan R, Margolis A, et al. HIV transmission in a state prison system, 1988–2005. PLoS One. 2009;4(5):e5416.
52. Macalino GE, Vlahov D, Sanford-Colby S, Patel S, Sabin K, Salas C, et al. Prevalence and incidence of HIV, hepatitis B virus, and hepatitis C virus infections among males in Rhode Island prisons. Am J Public Health. 2004;94(7):1218–23.
53. Huang YA, Zhu W, Smith DK, Harris N, Hoover KW. HIV preexposure prophylaxis, by race and ethnicity - United States, 2014-2016. MMWR Morb Mortal Wkly Rep. 2018;67(41):1147–50.
54. Gardner EM, McLees MP, Steiner JF, Del Rio C, Burman WJ. The spectrum of engagement in HIV care and its relevance to test-and-treat strategies for prevention of HIV infection. Clin Infect Dis. 2011;52(6):793–800.
55. Khan MR, McGinnis KA, Grov C, Scheidell JD, Hawks L, Edelman EJ, et al. Past year and prior incarceration and HIV transmission risk among HIV-positive men who have sex with men in the US(.). AIDS Care. 2019;31(3):349–56.
56. Beckwith CG, Atunah-Jay S, Cohen J, Macalino G, Poshkus M, Rich JD, et al. Feasibility and acceptability of rapid HIV testing in jail. AIDS Patient Care STDs. 2007;21(1):41–7.
57. Centers for Disease Control and Prevention (CDC). HIV screening of male inmates during prison intake medical evaluation--Washington, 2006-2010. MMWR Morb Mortal Wkly Rep. 2011;60(24):811–3.
58. Solomon L, Montague BT, Beckwith CG, Baillargeon J, Costa M, Dumont D, et al. Survey finds that many prisons and jails have room to improve HIV testing and coordination of postrelease treatment. Health Aff (Millwood). 2014;33(3):434–42.
59. Levy ME, Wilton L, Phillips G 2nd, Glick SN, Kuo I, Brewer RA, et al. Understanding structural barriers to accessing HIV testing and prevention services among black men who have sex with men (BMSM) in the United States. AIDS Behav. 2014;18(5):972–96.
60. Spaulding AC, Kim MJ, Corpening KT, Carpenter T, Watlington P, Bowden CJ. Establishing an HIV screening program led by staff nurses in a county jail. J Public Health Manag Pract. 2015;21(6):538–45.
61. de la Flor C, Porsa E, Nijhawan AE. Opt-out HIV and hepatitis C testing at the Dallas County jail: uptake, prevalence, and demographic characteristics of testers. Public Health Rep. 2017;132(6):617–21.
62. Belenko S, Hiller M, Visher C, Copenhaver M, O'Connell D, Burdon W, et al. Policies and practices in the delivery of HIV services in correctional agencies and facilities: results from a multisite survey. J Correct Health Care. 2013;19(4):293–310.
63. Westergaard RP, Hess T, Astemborski J, Mehta SH, Kirk GD. Longitudinal changes in engagement in care and viral suppression for HIV-infected injection drug users. AIDS. 2013;27(16):2559–66.
64. Stein MS, Spaulding AC, Cunningham M, Messina LC, Kim BI, Chung KW, et al. HIV-positive and in jail: race, risk factors, and prior access to care. AIDS Behav. 2013;17(Suppl 2):S108–17.

65. Vagenas P, Zelenev A, Altice FL, Di Paola A, Jordan AO, Teixeira PA, et al. HIV-infected men who have sex with men, before and after release from jail: the impact of age and race, results from a multi-site study. AIDS Care. 2016;28(1):22–31.
66. Springer SA, Spaulding AC, Meyer JP, Altice FL. Public health implications for adequate transitional care for HIV-infected prisoners: five essential components. Clin Infect Dis. 2011;53(5):469–79.
67. Wakeman SE, McKinney ME, Rich JD. Filling the gap: the importance of Medicaid continuity for former inmates. J Gen Intern Med. 2009;24(7):860–2.
68. Zaller ND, Cloud DH, Brinkley-Rubinstein L, Martino S, Bouvier B, Brockmann B. Commentary: the importance of Medicaid expansion for criminal justice populations in the south. Health Justice. 2017;5(1):2.
69. Binswanger IA, Stern MF, Deyo RA, Heagerty PJ, Cheadle A, Elmore JG, et al. Release from prison--a high risk of death for former inmates. N Engl J Med. 2007;356(2):157–65.
70. Nunn A, Cornwall A, Fu J, Bazerman L, Loewenthal H, Beckwith C. Linking HIV-positive jail inmates to treatment, care, and social services after release: results from a qualitative assessment of the COMPASS program. J Urban Health. 2010;87(6):954–68.
71. Meyer JP, Chen NE, Springer SA. HIV Treatment in the Criminal Justice System: Critical Knowledge and Intervention Gaps. AIDS Res Treat. 2011;2011:680617.
72. Aidala AA, Wilson MG, Shubert V, Gogolishvili D, Globerman J, Rueda S, et al. Housing status, medical care, and health outcomes among people living with HIV/AIDS: a systematic review. Am J Public Health. 2016;106(1):e1–e23.
73. Chen NE, Meyer JP, Avery AK, Draine J, Flanigan TP, Lincoln T, et al. Adherence to HIV treatment and care among previously homeless jail detainees. AIDS Behav. 2013;17(8):2654–66.
74. Ammon B, Iroh P, Tiruneh Y, Li X, Montague BT, Rich JD, et al. HIV care after jail: low rates of engagement in a vulnerable population. J Urban Health. 2018;95(4):488–98.
75. Montague BT, Rosen DL, Sammartino C, Costa M, Gutman R, Solomon L, et al. Systematic assessment of linkage to care for persons with HIV released from corrections facilities using existing datasets. AIDS Patient Care STDs. 2016;30(2):84–91.
76. Gordon MS, Crable EL, Carswell SB, Leopold J, Hodo-Powell J, McKenzie M, et al. A randomized controlled trial of intensive case management (project bridge) for HIV-infected probationers and parolees. AIDS Behav. 2018;22(3):1030–8.
77. Wohl DA, Scheyett A, Golin CE, White B, Matuszewski J, Bowling M, et al. Intensive case management before and after prison release is no more effective than comprehensive pre-release discharge planning in linking HIV-infected prisoners to care: a randomized trial. AIDS Behav. 2011;15(2):356–64.
78. Rich JD, Holmes L, Salas C, Macalino G, Davis D, Ryczek J, et al. Successful linkage of medical care and community services for HIV-positive offenders being released from prison. J Urban Health. 2001;78(2):279–89.
79. Booker CA, Flygare CT, Solomon L, Ball SW, Pustell MR, Bazerman LB, et al. Linkage to HIV care for jail detainees: findings from detention to the first 30 days after release. AIDS Behav. 2013;17(2):128–36.
80. Myers JJ, Kang Dufour MS, Koester KA, Morewitz M, Packard R, Monico Klein K, et al. The effect of patient navigation on the likelihood of engagement in clinical care for HIV-infected individuals leaving jail. Am J Public Health. 2018;108(3):385–92.
81. Wohl DA, Golin CE, Knight K, Gould M, Carda-Auten J, Groves JS, et al. Randomized controlled trial of an intervention to maintain suppression of HIV Viremia after prison release: the imPACT trial. J Acquir Immune Defic Syndr. 2017;75(1):81–90.
82. Cunningham WE, Weiss RE, Nakazono T, Malek MA, Shoptaw SJ, Ettner SL, et al. Effectiveness of a peer navigation intervention to sustain viral suppression among HIV-positive men and transgender women released from jail: the LINK LA randomized clinical trial. JAMA Intern Med. 2018;178(4):542–53.
83. Centers for Disease C. Dealing with stigma and discrimination 2019. Available from: https://www.cdc.gov/hiv/basics/livingwithhiv/stigma-discrimination.html.

84. Herek GM, Capitanio JP, Widaman KF. HIV-related stigma and knowledge in the United States: prevalence and trends, 1991-1999. Am J Public Health. 2002;92(3):371–7.
85. Baugher AR, Beer L, Fagan JL, Mattson CL, Freedman M, Skarbinski J, et al. Prevalence of internalized HIV-related stigma among HIV-infected adults in care, United States, 2011-2013. AIDS Behav. 2017;21(9):2600–8.
86. Courtenay-Quirk C, Wolitski RJ, Parsons JT, Gomez CA. Is HIV/AIDS stigma dividing the gay community? Perceptions of HIV-positive men who have sex with men. AIDS Educ Prev. 2006;18(1):56–67.
87. Overstreet NM, Earnshaw VA, Kalichman SC, Quinn DM. Internalized stigma and HIV status disclosure among HIV-positive black men who have sex with men. AIDS Care. 2013;25(4):466–71.
88. Sweeney SM, Vanable PA. The association of HIV-related stigma to HIV medication adherence: a systematic review and synthesis of the literature. AIDS Behav. 2016;20(1):29–50.
89. Vyavaharkar M, Moneyham L, Corwin S, Saunders R, Annang L, Tavakoli A. Relationships between stigma, social support, and depression in HIV-infected African American women living in the rural Southeastern United States. J Assoc Nurses AIDS Care. 2010;21(2):144–52.
90. Wolitski RJ, Pals SL, Kidder DP, Courtenay-Quirk C, Holtgrave DR. The effects of HIV stigma on health, disclosure of HIV status, and risk behavior of homeless and unstably housed persons living with HIV. AIDS Behav. 2009;13(6):1222–32.
91. Yehia BR, Stewart L, Momplaisir F, Mody A, Holtzman CW, Jacobs LM, et al. Barriers and facilitators to patient retention in HIV care. BMC Infect Dis. 2015;15:246.
92. Sayles JN, Wong MD, Kinsler JJ, Martins D, Cunningham WE. The association of stigma with self-reported access to medical care and antiretroviral therapy adherence in persons living with HIV/AIDS. J Gen Intern Med. 2009;24(10):1101–8.
93. Golub SA, Gamarel KE. The impact of anticipated HIV stigma on delays in HIV testing behaviors: findings from a community-based sample of men who have sex with men and transgender women in New York City. AIDS Patient Care STDs. 2013;27(11):621–7.
94. Muessig KE, Rosen DL, Farel CE, White BL, Filene EJ, Wohl DA. "Inside these fences is our own Little world": prison-based HIV testing and HIV-related stigma among incarcerated men and women. AIDS Educ Prev. 2016;28(2):103–16.
95. Derlega VJ, Winstead BA, Brockington JE Jr. AIDS stigma among inmates and staff in a USA state prison. Int J STD AIDS. 2008;19(4):259–63.
96. Belenko S, Dembo R, Copenhaver M, Hiller M, Swan H, Albizu Garcia C, et al. HIV stigma in prisons and jails: results from a staff survey. AIDS Behav. 2016;20(1):71–84.
97. Sprague C, Scanlon ML, Radhakrishnan B, Pantalone DW. The HIV prison paradox: agency and HIV-positive Women's experiences in jail and prison in Alabama. Qual Health Res. 2017;27(10):1427–44.
98. Meyer CL, Tangney JP, Stuewig J, Moore KE. Why do some jail inmates not engage in treatment and services? Int J Offender Ther Comp Criminol. 2014;58(8):914–30.
99. Culbert GJ. Violence and the perceived risks of taking antiretroviral therapy in US jails and prisons. Int J Prison Health. 2014;10(2):94–110.
100. Remien RH, Bauman LJ, Mantell JE, Tsoi B, Lopez-Rios J, Chhabra R, et al. Barriers and facilitators to engagement of vulnerable populations in HIV primary care in New York City. J Acquir Immune Defic Syndr. 2015;69(Suppl 1):S16–24.
101. Brinkley-Rubinstein L. Understanding the effects of multiple stigmas among formerly incarcerated HIV-positive African American men. AIDS Educ Prev. 2015;27(2):167–79.
102. Kemnitz R, Kuehl TC, Hochstatter KR, Barker E, Corey A, Jacobs EA, et al. Manifestations of HIV stigma and their impact on retention in care for people transitioning from prisons to communities. Health Justice. 2017;5(1):7.
103. Fauci AS, Redfield RR, Sigounas G, Weahkee MD, Giroir BP. Ending the HIV epidemic: a plan for the United States. JAMA. 2019;321(9):844–5.

104. Beer L, McCree DH, Jeffries WL, Lemons A, Sionean C. Recent US centers for disease control and prevention activities to reduce HIV stigma. J Int Assoc Provid AIDS Care. 2019;18:2325958218823541.
105. Agan A, Starr S. Ban the box, criminal records, and racial discrimination: a field experiment*. Q J Econ. 2017;133(1):191–235.

Index